NEW TRENDS IN HEPATOLOGY

NEW TRENDS IN HEPATOLOGY

The Proceedings of the Annual Meeting of the Italian National Programme on Liver Cirrhosis and Viral Hepatitis, San Miniato (Pisa), Italy, 7–9 January, 1996

edited by

Paolo Gentilini

Institute of Internal Medicine, School of Medicine, University of Florence, Florence, Italy

and

Mario Umberto Dianzani

Department of Experimental Medicine and Oncology, Section of General Pathology, University of Turin, Turin, Italy

KLUWER ACADEMIC PUBLISHERS
DORDRECHT / BOSTON / LONDON

Distributors

for the United States and Canada: Kluwer Academic Publishers, PO Box 358, Accord Station, Hingham, MA 02018-0358, USA

for all other countries: Kluwer Academic Publishers Group, Distribution Center, PO Box 322, 3300 AH Dordrecht, The Netherlands

A catalogue record for this book is available from the British Library.
ISBN-13:978-94-010-6646-4 e-ISBN-13:978-94-009-0357-9
DOI:10.1007/978-94-009-0357-9

Kluwer Academic Publishers BV incorporates the publishing programmes of
D. Reidel, Martinus Nijhoff, Dr W. Junk and MTP Press.

CONTENTS

Section 5. CLINICAL ASPECTS OF CHRONIC LIVER DISEASE

FOREWORD

The Italian Group for the Study of Liver Cirrhosis began its activity in 1980 on the basis of recognition and financial support from the Italian Ministry of the University, Scientific Research and Technology, having been chosen from several other scientific programs. The group is now called the National Group for the Study of Liver Cirrhosis and Viral Hepatitis and includes more than 40 centers throughout the nation under the auspices of the universities.

The primary initiative of the group, to combine experimental and clinical approaches in the study of liver pathophysiology, remains unchanged. Annual meetings in January provide the possibility of comparing experimental and clinical results in the spirit of mutual comprehension and criticism. After 15 years and 6 volumes (published biannually), the actual improvement of Italian research in liver pathophysiology is evident. In fact, in order to let other researchers know what has been achieved we chose to publish the 7th volume, in spite of the economic difficulties at hand.

We have gathered specific experiences of all the centers included in the national program. Each group was required to present an update in its own field of research, rather than specific or recently obtained results, which could have been reported only in relationship with other data already published by others. Like the 6th edition in our series, this volume affirms the specific competence of all the participants and summarizes the most important updates in liver pathophysiology.

The volume is divided into 5 sections dealing with different aspects of liver pathophisiology. Many contributions are focused on the pathophysiology of liver injury and on clinical and pathogenetical aspects of hepatitis C virus infection, which today are representative of emergent fields. Other important aspects include the pathophysiology of liver cancer and clinical and therapeutical approaches in liver cirrhosis.

All Italian centers, whether participants in the National program or not, are invited to consider the level of the results obtained, the possibility of establishing new relationships or collaboration in Italy and abroad and the

P. Gentilini and M. U. Dianzani. New Trends in Hepatology, ix-x

perspective of the latest scientific program of research. This is what we aim to achieve in proposing this edition of the National Group for the Study of Liver Cirrhosis and Viral Hepatitis in addition to being open to collaborating with any Italian or foreign researcher who may be interested in this program.

Paolo Gentilini
Mario Umberto Dianzani

Editors

Scientific Secretariat

V. Casini Raggi
G. La Villa
R. Mazzanti
R.G. Romanelli

Institute of Internal Medicine
University of Florence
Florence, Italy

Acknowledgment
We are grateful to Mary Diamond of the Fondazione Italiana per lo Studio del Fegato - Italian Liver Foundation, for English revision.

Section I

PATHOGENETIC MECHANISMS OF LIVER INJURY

CHAPTER 1

4-HYDROXY-ALKENALS, PRODUCTS OF LIPID PEROXIDATION, AS SIGNALS FOR BIOCHEMICAL FUNCTIONS OF NORMAL CELLS

M.U. DIANZANI

Department of Experimental Medicine and Oncology, Section of General Pathology, University of Torino, Corso Raffaello 30, 10125 Torino, Italy

Summary

Several aldehydic compounds which originate from the oxidative breakdown of membrane lipids exert biochemical effects of interest in physiopathology. The actual result of their interaction with a variety of molecular targets depends on the aldehyde steady-state concentration reached in a defined tissue damage. However, aldehydic concentrations below 10^{-6} M, i.e. those detectable under basal conditions, exert positive effects on cell migration, activation and function. A physiological role of defined classes of biogenic aldehydes is thus proposed.

Lipid peroxidation has for a long time been considered a mechanism in cell damage. It acts first of all by provoking anatomical damage to cellular membranes; moreover, it gives origin to many toxic compounds that can move from the production site to reach distant targets (protein, enzymes, nucleotides) (1-4). Among these toxic substances, a relevant importance has been attributed to aldehydes which represent the major end products of lipid peroxidation inside the cells. The collaborative work of three laboratories, the Department of Biochemistry of the University of Graz, the Department of Biochemistry of the Brunel University of West-London and this Section of Turin, led to the isolation and identification of several of these aldehydes (5, 6). They belong to three types: 1. saturated aldehydes, such as hexanal, butanal, octanal, nonanal, decanal and others; 2. 2.3-trans-unsaturated aldehydes, such as hexenal, octenal, nonenal decenal, undecenal and others; 3. 4-hydroxy-2,3-trans-unsaturated aldehydes, such as 4-hydroxy-hexenal, 4-hydroxy-octenal, 4-hydroxy-nonenal, 4-hydroxy-undecenal, 4,5-di-hydroxy-decenal, 4-hydroxy-nonenal, first identified by Benedetti et al. (7) among the toxic products of peroxidizing microsomes, being most abundat in the third type. Aldehyde toxicity largely depends upon the

P. Gentilini and M. U. Dianzani. New Trends in Hepatology, 3-16

reaction of their -CHO group with either -SH or -NH2 groups of reactant molecules, but the 4-hydroxy group and the double bond must be considered important in the selection of the targets. In fact, the reactivity of the carbonyl group with sulphidryl or amino groups is a general property of aldehydes, but not all the aldehydes display the same degree of toxicity. The most abundant final carbonyl compound of lipid peroxidation, malonildialdehyde, contains two -CHO groups, but it is practically non toxic. The list of damaging effects on cellular biochemical functions is shown in Tab.1.

TABLE 1. Damaging effects of 4-hydroxynonenal on cellular biochemical functions

Active concentrations range from 10 μM to 1 mM

Block in protein synthesis
Block in the secretion of lipoproteins and proteins
Block in tubulin polymerization
Inhibition of ornithine decarboxylase
Inhibition of mithocondrial respiratory chain
Partial inhibition of the cytochrome P450-depending microsomal chain
Inhibition of microsomal glucose-6-phosphatase
Inhibition of Golgi galactosyltransferase

The common characteristics of such actions is that they are displayed at relatively high concentrations of the aldehyde, ranging from 10 μM to 1 mM. 10 μM have been reported to be present in liver tissue during the late phases of CCl4 poisoning (6). It is, however, of note that inside the cell the concentration of the aldehyde is not homogenous, due to its lipophilic nature. So, membranes, which are rich in lipids, are expected to contain more HNE than the cytosol. Moreover, what is possible to measure at a given time in damaged tissues does not represent the whole amount of aldehyde produced during the lipoperoxidative process. In fact, several enzymes present which are present in the tissues are able to continuously remove the formed aldehydes, thus their actual concentration is only the result of a balance between production and removal. In principle, stechiometrically only one molecule of the aldehyde is needed to react with a single -SH or NH2 group. So, it is possible to predict, therefore, that the continuous flux of aldehydes from the production sites to the targets will produce the inactivation of more and more molecules of the target, until a detectable inhibition of the function takes place.

When studying the effects of 4-hydroxynonenal (HNE) on single cellular fractions, we discovered, however, that some of these effects are displayed at concentrations of 1 μM or less, that is to say at concentrations most authors report as "normal" content of HNE in "normal" cells. Of course, the so called "normal" isolated cells or cell subfractions may not exactly correspond to their real normal state inside the tissues since the isolation techniques themselves may produce some damage. For instance, some lipid peroxidation might have been provoked by the changes in membrane geography, producing spacial derangements between natural antioxidants and peroxidizable substrates contained in the membranes. Some evidence, however, suggests that lipid peroxidation can occur even in normal tissues, and especially in those whose cells belong to the post-mitotic type (2, 7-9). In such cells, the life span of subcellular organelles is much shorter than that of the cells themselves. The presence of autophagic vacuoles, containing peroxidizing lipid remnants of such structures is frequently detectable in such cells, both by electron microscopy and by chemiluminescence methods. It is also noteworthy that the P450-depending drug metabolizing system can afford lipid peroxidation in normal conditions by diversion of an electron at the level of FADH2 to oxygen, thereby forming the superoxide anion O_2^-. Moreover, the plasma of normal subjects always contains measurable amounts of aldehydes produced during lipid peroxidation, especially malonildialdehyde (very poorly toxic) and HNE (much more toxic). The aldehydes are usually bound to plasma albumin, with which they form adducts (10).

Such adducts, at least in the case of HNE, are not entirely stable since they can release small amounts of free aldehyde in the medium, depending upon its external concentration. This seems to be a possible way for aldehydes to reach distant targets, since the aldehydes bound to proteins are not substrates for the enzymes, which are able to destroy them when in the free state. Even lipoproteins contain aldehydes, including HNE and MDA. In fact, lipids contained in lipoproteins can undergo peroxidation at a rate possibly depending upon the balance between antioxidants and prooxidants or pro-oxidant stimuli (11-13). This phenomenon is now considered with great attention to be possibly important in the pathogenesis of atherosclerosis. It has been shown that acetylated lipoproteins (14), as well as HNE-modified lipoproteins (15-17) form more stable

bonds with surface receptors on endothelial cells. This may be cause of increased endocytosis of lipoproteins themselves.
To my knowledge, the first demonstration of a physiological role of 4-hydroxy-alkenals was by M. Curzio et al. (18-21), confirmed by Schaur et al. (22, 23). Curzio and collaborators found that aldehydes display chemotactic activity on rat polymorphonucleates leukocytes (PMNL), as well as chemokinetic activity on human PMNL. Such activities are maximally afforded at concentrations of 1 μM in the case of HNE, and even lower concentrations in the case of 4-hydroxy-octenal (HOE), but remain detectable even at concentrations less than nanomolar. The most effective aldehyde of the series is HOE (19), which is present in microsomal extracts submitted to stimulation of lipid peroxidation at a concentration of about 100 times lower than HNE. Great stimulating activity on both oriented migration (chemotaxis) and random migration (chemokinesis) is displayed even by 4-hydroxy-hexenal,4-hydroxy-undecenal and by the long-chained non natural aldehydes 4-hydroxy-tetradecenal, 4-hydroxypentadecenal and 4-hydroxy-heptadecenal (18-21). Hexanal, hexenal, nonanal and nonenal are unable to attract leukocytes. So, it seems that this property is related to the presence of the 4-hydroxy-group in unsaturated aldehydes. At higher concentrations (10 μM or more) HNE, as well as other aldehydes, independently from their chemical structure, decrease leukocyte mobility. This may be due to the block that aldehydes produce at the level of tubulin polymerization. Tubulin is the major protein of microtubules which are involved in cell movements (1, 2).
The comparison between HNE action on chemotaxis and chemokinesis and that afforded by other known chemoattractants shows that HNE behaves in a very peculiar way. Formylmethionylleucylphenylalanine (fmlp), a tripeptide from bacterial origin, is one of the most powerful chemoattractants known. HNE is less powerful than fmlp and seems to be able to stimulate only a portion of the tested leukocyte population. Cells submitted to fmlp, do not respond a second time to the same substance, but retain their responsiveness to HNE. The exact same reaction occurs with cells submitted to HNE action. After having been attracted a first time, they do not respond a second time to the aldehyde, but retain their responsiveness to fmlp. This phenomenon is known as deactivation. The lack of cross deactivation may be interpreted to be related to a difference between the specific receptors of fmlp and aldehydes. Fmlp receptors have been identified on the leukocyte surface. In the case of HNE, experiments have been done by Curzio et al. (24) using tritiated HNE. This substance binds to proteins contained in the cytosol, whereas apparently there is no binding to the plasma membranes. Of course, this might have been due to a displacement towards the

cytosol of substances previously sited inside the membrane, but there is no evidence for this. Moreover, HNE, which is lipophillic, does not need to bind to a receptor on the membrane. In fact, it may be simply dissolved in the lipid phase of the membrane, like other liposoluble substances do, including some hormones. Quite recently, Parola et al. (unpublished experiments) noted by confocal microscopy that added HNE can be recognized by specific fluorescent antibodies at the level of the surface of certain types of cells. The distribution, however, is not homogenous. The bond of tritiated HNE to cytosolic receptors is not stable. In fact, tritiated HNE can be displaced by excess unlabeled HNE, as well as by excess 4-hydroxyoctenal or 4-hydroxyhexenal. No displacement, however, occurs with nonenal or nonanal. It seems, therefore, that the bond involves the 4-hydroxy group in some way. The use of Scatchard plats made it possible to conclude that the bond obeys the laws of agonist-receptor interactions. Thus, the cytosolic target behaves like a medium affinity receptor. Further work is needed on this point, but the existence in normal cells of a receptor for a product of lipid peroxidation would be strongly suggestive for a physiological role of this process. Most chemoattractants, such as fmlp, provoke an increase in the activity of NADPH oxidase, which results in increased production and release in the medium of superoxide anion (25-29). This phenomenon is usually referred to as "respiratory burst". This is not the case, however, with HNE, which attracts PMNL without producing respiratory burst (30, 31). Moreover, chemoattractants very frequently provoke an increased synthesis of another free radical, i.e. $NO^{\cdot}$. This can react with O_2^-, providing peroxynitrate, which is another damaging substance. In the case of HNE, however, $NO^{\cdot}$ synthesis from L-arginine is blocked (30). So, it is clear that the mechanism of chemotaxis stimulation by HNE is different from those displayed by other chemoattractants. Nevertheless, the production of HNE in the inflammatory sites is consistently increased (22, 23), and its concentration in the exudates is rather high (20). This may represent another mechanism for recruitment of PMNL and for the propagation of inflammation.

Other actions displayed by HNE at low concentration are the effects on membrane G-proteins, and especially on those involved in the functioning of adenylate cyclase (7-9, 32) and of phosphatidylinositol-4,5-diphosphate hydrolase, also usually called phospholipase C (9, 30, 33-35). Both enzymes are strongly stimulated by concentrations of HNE ranging from 0.1 to 1μM, the stimulation starting immediately after HNE addition of the aldehyde to hepatocyte isolated plasmamembranes and lasting for about 10 minutes. Maximal stimulation of adenylate cyclase occurs with 1μM HNE, whereas in the case of phospholipase C maximal stimulation occurs with 0.1 μM. The enzymatic system is better known in the case of adenylate cyclase. It consist of a catalytic unit sited across the leaflet of the plasmamembrane facing the cytosol, of a stimulatory G-protein system and of an inhibitory G-protein system, each of them connected to a surface receptor binding the agonists. The involved G proteins (respectively referred to as G-stimulatory, or Gs and G-inhibitory, Gi) consists of three different chains or subunits, respectively referred to as α, ß and V. When bound together, the subunits display a high GTPase activity that disappears after binding of the agonist to the competent receptor. The disappearance of GTPase activity is due to the separation of α from ß-V. This event results either in activation (in the case of Gs) or in inhibition (in the case of Gi) of the catalytic unit. Forskolin is a strong activator of adenylate cyclase, probably acting on the catalytic unit. Cholera toxin also activates adenylate cyclase by acting on Gs system. Pertussis toxin also activates by inhibiting the Gi system. HNE, as well as HOE and HHE, activates adenylate cyclase apparently by inhibiting the Gi system, like pertussis toxin, whereas it does not influence the response to cholera toxin, forskolin or glucagon, an agonist binding the stimulatory receptor (Rs). The potentiation regards not only the enzymatic activity, but also the adenosylribosylation of Gi proteins (30), whereas that of Gs proteins is less influenced. As a result of adenylate cyclase stimulation, an increase in the production of cAMP is expected. This might influence the activity of the cAMP-dependent kinases (protein kinases A).

A similar activation is produced by HNE on phospholipase C. The structure of this system not as deeply investigated, but it is certain that G-proteins are also involved in this case. It is noteworthy that both in the case of adenylate cyclase and of phospholipase C, stimulation is afforded by all tested 4-hydroxy-2,3-trans-alkenals, whereas the corresponding non 4-hydroxylated saturated or unsaturated aldehydes are devoid of any effect at low concentrations, and are inhibitory at high concentration. As a result of the increase in phospholipase C activity, an increased production of inositol-triphosphate (IP_3) and of diacylglycerol (DAG) are expected. IP_3 is known to increase the cytosolic Ca^{2+} from either mitochondria or from microsomal vesicles into the cytosol. DAG is known to act as a stimulator of protein kinases C, that are involved in chemotaxis, as well as in other important cytoplasmic and nuclear functions. With isolated hepatocytes, low concentrations of HNE have been reported to produce a slight but significant increase on protein kinase C activity (36, 37). A sudden increase has been seen, even shortly, after CCl_4 treatment, in conditions of stimulated lipid peroxidation. As far as Ca^{2+} content of hepatocytes is concerned, 1 μM HNE provokes a biphasic increase. During a first phase, only a moderate increase in cytosolic Ca^{2+} can be observed, occuring even with hepatocytes incubated in a medium not containing external Ca^{2+} and containing Ca^{2+} chelators. A second phase is characterized by a much more intense increase in cytosolic Ca^{2+}, surely corresponding to an increased influx of this cation from the incubation medium. In fact, this phase does not occur when the incubation medium is devoid of Ca^{2+} and contains chelators (38). So, it seems that HNE influences Ca^{2+} influx, and it is possible that this effect is the consequence of HNE action on a Ca^{2+} channel. As far as the nature of the chemical interaction of HNE with the G-proteins is concerned, it is noteworthy that its effect on Gi proteins in the adenylate cyclase system is mimiced by the sulphidryl reagent N-ethyl-maleimide, acting however at much higher concentration. So, it seems possible that a specific -SH group in Gi is involved. The 4-hydroxy-2,3-trans-alkenal structure might act as an adapter, allowing an effect of the aldehyde at lower concentration. It is in any case important to state that adenylate cyclase and phospholipase C are specifically inhibited. In fact, other enzymes contained in plasma membrane, such as 5'-nucleotidase or cytochrome P450-depending enzymes, which is poorly represented in this structure, but in any case present, are not influenced by 1 μM HNE, and are inhibited at high concentration. Guanylate cyclase, another plasmamembrane enzyme, is stimulated by 1 μM HNE, but only to a small extent (7-9). Another important function of HNE and related aldehydes is displayed on the genetic program of several types of cells, including tumor cells. In working on two types of human leukemias, K562 erythroleukemia and HL-60 myeloblastic-promyelocytic leukemia, Barrera et al., (39-41) and Fazio et al. (42) found that the addition of 1 μM HNE or related aldehydes to the coltures, decreases the multiplication rate, promotes differentiation and at the same time cancels the high expression of the oncogene c-myc, which is characteristic of these tumor cells. In the case of HL-60 cells, even the high expression of the oncogene c-myb is blocked, but with different kinetics. It is difficult at present to decide if all these phenomena are sequential, and represent the consequence of the impact of HNE on unique target. Concerning K562 cells, it is noteworthy that the effect on c-myc expression, which starts within 1 hour after the addition of the aldehydes to the cells, and lasts for 2-4 hours, is displayed when added HNE has practically disappeared from the cells, due to its quick removal by the specific enzymes. The effect can be prolonged if HNE treatments are repeated several times on the same sample of cells. Apparently there is an effect requiring a continous supplementation of the aldehyde. Fazio et al. (42) have shown that this effect is due to the impact of HNE on the third hexon of the promoter gene for c-myc. It is still unclear, however, if this effect is related to a direct reaction of HNE with an amino group in a nucleotide, or if it is mediated through the interaction with some inhibiting protein. When added to isolated hepatocytes, 1 μM of HNE is able to provoke the expression of a subset of heat shock proteins; in this case, it seems that HNE acts on the cytoplasmic heat shock promoter factor (HSF) (43-45).

Other interesting effects of HNE and related alkenals have been shown to occur on human cultivated fat storing cells (FSC), also called "Ito cells". These cells are thought to play an important role in liver fibrogenesis, especially during the development of cirrhosis. In fact they are able to express the gene for the procollagen α 2 (I), as well as the related protein product. Such cells develop lipid peroxidation when incubated in vitro in the presence of these conditions. The expression of the mRNA for the procollagen α 2 (I) is strongly stimulated, and even the synthesis of its protein product increases. These effects are prevented in the presence of vitamin E or of other antioxidants, so it is clear that the genic effects are lipid peroxidation-dependent. An increased expression of the same gene, as well as of its protein product, occurs when FSC are incubated in the presence of 1 μM of HNE, or of related 4-hydroxy-alkenals, but not in the presence of the corresponding saturated or unsaturated non-4-hydroxylated aldehydes. In this case, the addition to the medium of antioxidants has no effect.

It seems therefore that the effect of lipid peroxidation on the genetic expression of the gene for procollagen α 2 (I) is exerted through its products (46-48). It is noteworthy that the HNE effect is specific, since the procollagen α 1 (III) gene is not influenced. It is important to remember that CCl_4^- mediated fibrosis is largely prevented in rats by loading with vitamin E during the experimental period (49-51), and that even in the case of fibrosis following bile duct ligation there is increased lipid peroxidation. Therefore, it is possible that the mechanism for fibrosis is similar to that occuring in CCl_4^--treated rats. For the moment it is difficult to say whether these phenomena are the consequence of the direct impact of HNE with genomic structures, or its action is an indirect one.

HNE provokes, in FSC, the expression of the transcription factor AP 1, as well as of the c-phos oncogene, whereas no effect has been observed on the transcription factor NF-kB (48).

All such effects are transient, probably due to the continuous removal of HNE from the medium by the existing enzymes. In fact, several enzymes (alcohol dehydrogenase, aldehyde oxidases, NAD- and NADP-dependent aldehyde dehydrogenases, glutathione transferase) which present in all tissues are able to remove the aldehydes. Their activity can therefore modulate aldehyde action on genomic targets. In any case, it has been shown in cultivated cells that the genomic effects last for several hours, when most of the added aldehyde has been removed from the medium. A summary of the effects displayed by low concentration of HNE is given in Tab.2.

TABLE 2. Effects of HNE and related aldehydes at concentrations of 1 μM or lower

1.	Stimulation of chemotaxis in rat PMN leukocytes
2.	Stimulation of random movements (chemokinesis) in human leukocytes
3.	Strong activation of membranes adenylate cyclase in hepatocytes
4.	Strong stimulation of phopholipase C in hepatocyte and PMN leukocyte plasmamembranes
5.	Slight stimulation of hepatocyte protein kinase C
6.	Discharge of Ca^{2+} from intracellular stores to the cytosol; increase in the Ca^{2+} influx from the suspension medium into the hepatocyte.
7.	Block in the expression of the oncogene c-myc in K562 erythroleukemic and in HL-60 myeloblastic-pro-myelocitic leukemic cells
8.	Block in the expression of the oncogene c-myb in HL-60 cells. No effects on the Ras oncogene series.
9.	Reexpression of gamma globin gene and protein product in K562 cells
10.	Maturation of chemiluminescent granules in HL-60 cells; differentiation towards the granulocyte line
11.	Stimulation of the expression of heat shock proteins (HSP70) in hepatocytes
12.	Stimulation of the expression of mRNA for procollagen α 2 (I) and of its protein product in FSC.
13.	Stimulation of the expression of the transcription factor AP 1 in FSC.

At the end of this short survey on the effects of 4-hydroxy-alkenals at physiological doses, are we allowed to conclude that lipid peroxidation displays a physiological role, regulating cell functions through the production of aldehydes acting as signals for biochemical functions? I think it is too early to draw this conclusion, but that a mass of data now exist to support it. Thus, there is sufficient emphasis to make deeper analysis.

References

1) Dianzani, M.U. (1982) Biochemical effects of saturated and unsaturated aldehydes, in D.C.H. McBrien, and T.F. Slater (eds), Free Radicals, Lipid Peroxidation and Cancer, Academic Press, London, 129-158.

2) Dianzani, M.U. (1991) Biochemical aspects of fatty liver, in R.G. Meeks, S.D. Harrison and R.J. Bull (eds), Hepatotoxicology, CRC Press; Boca Raton, 327-399.

3) Comporti, M. (1985) Biology of the disease. Lipid peroxidation and liver damage in toxic liver injury, Lab. Invest. 53,599-623.

4) Poli, G., Albano, E. and Dianzani, M.U. (1987) The role of lipid peroxidation in liver damage. Chem.-Phys. Lipids, 45,117-142.

5) Esterbauer, H., Cheeseman, K.H., Dianzani, M.U., Poli, G. e Slater, T.F. (1982) Separation and characterization in the aldehydic products of lipid peroxidation stimulated by ADP-Fe2+ in rat liver microsomes, Biochem. J., 208,129-140

6) Poli, G., Dianzani, M.U., Cheeseman, K.H., Slater, T.F., Lang, J. and Esterbauer H., (1985) Separation and characterization of the aldehydic products of lipid peroxidation stimulated by carbon tetrachloride or ADP-iron in isolated rat hepatocytes and rat liver microsomal suspensions, Biochem. J., 227,629-638.

7) Benedetti, A., Comporti, M. and Esterbauer, H. (1980) Identification of 4-hydroxynonenal as a cytotoxic product originating from the peroxidation of liver microsomal lipids, Biochim. Biophys. Acta, 620,281-296,

8) Dianzani, M.U., Paradisi, L., Barrera, G., Rossi, M.A. and Parola, M. (1990) The action of 4-hydroxynonenal on the plasma membrane enzymes from rat hepatocytes, in P.C.Beaumont, D.C. Parson and C. Rice-Evans (eds.), Free radicals, metal ions and biopolymers, Richelieu Press, London, 329-346.

9) Dianzani, M.U., Paradisi, L., Di Mauro, C., Cervo, A., Barrera, G. and Rossi, M.A. (1991) Evidence of the effects of 4-hydroxynonenal an adenylate cyclase activity of plasma membranes via the guanine regulatory g-proteins., in K.A. Davies (eds.), Oxidative damage and repair, Pergamon Press, Oxford, 487-493.

10) Curzio, M., Di Mauro, C., Esterbauer, H. and Dianzani, M.U. (1987) Chemotactic activity of aldehydes. Structural requirements. role in inflammatory process, Biomed. Pharmacother. 41, 304-314.

11) Jürgens, G., Lang, J. and Esterbauer, H. (1986) Modification of human low-density lipoprotein by the lipid peroxidation product 4-hydroxynonenal, Biochem. Biophys. Acta, 875,103-112.

12) Heinicke, J.W. (1987) Free radical modification of low density lipoproteins, mechanisms and biological consequences, Free Rad. Biol. Med.,3,65-75.

13) Esterbauer, H., Jürgens, J.C. e Quehenberger, O. (1988) Modification of human low-density lipoprotein by lipid peroxidation, in G. Simic, K.A. Taylor, J.F. Ward and von Sonntag (eds.), *Oxygen free radicals in biology and medicine*, Basic Life Sciences, Plenum Press, New York, vol. 49, 369-375.

14) Goldstein, J.L., Ho, Y.K., Basu, S.K. and Brown, M. (1979) Binding site in macrophages that mediates uptake and degradation of acetylated low density lipoprotein producing massive cholesterol deposition, Proc. Natl. Acad. Sci. U.S.A., 76,33-336.

15) Haberland, M.E., Fogelman, A.M. and Edwards, P.A. (1982). Specificity of receptor-mediated recognition of malonaldehyde modified low density lipoproteins, Proc. Natl. Acad. Sci U.S.A.,79,1712-1713.

16) Steinbrecher, U.P., Parthasarathy, S., leake, D.S., Witztum, J.L., and Steinberg, D., (1984) Modification of low density lipoprotein by endothelial cells involves lipid peroxidation and degradation of low density lipoprotein phospholipids. Proc. Natl. Acad. Sci. U.S.A., 81,3883-3885.

17) Kurth, H.S., Skarlatos, S.I., Lilly, K., Chang, J. and Ifrim, I. (1995) Sequestration of acetylated LDL and cholesterol cristals by human monocyte-derived macrophages, J. Cell Biol., 129,133-145.

18) Curzio, M., Torrielli, M.V., Giroud, J.P., Esterbauer, H. and Dianzani, M.U. (1982) Neutrophil chemotactic responses to aldehydes, Res. Comm. Chem. Pathol. Pharmacol. 36,463-476.

19) Curzio, M., Esterbauer, H. and Dianzani, M.U. (1983) Chemotactic power of 4-hydroxyoctenal. IRCS Med. Sci. 11,521.

20) Curzio, M., Esterbauer, H., Di Mauro, C., Cecchini, G. and Dianzani, M.U. (1986) Chemotactic activity of the lipid peroxidation product 4-hydroxy-nonenal and homologous aldehydes, Biol.Chem. Hoppe Seyler's 367,321-329.

21) Curzio, M., Poli, G., Esterbauer, H. and Dianzani M.U. (1986) Detection of carbonyl products of lipid peroxidation in rat pleural exsudates, IRCS Med. Sci.,14,984-985.

22) Schaur, J.R. and Curzio, M. (1995) On the role of hydroxyalkenals in inflammation. Recent Topics in Biophysics, 18,238-244.

23) Schaur, J.R., Dussing, G., Kink, E., Schauenstein, E., Posh, K., Kukovetz, E. and Egger, G. (1994) The lipid peroxidation product 4-hydroxy-nonenal is formed and is able to attract rat neutrophils in vivo. Free Rad. Res.,20,365-373.

24) Curzio, M., Ferretti, C, Stephens, R.J., Esterbauer, H. and Dianzani, M.U. (1994) Binding of the lipid peroxidation product 4-hydroxynonenal to human polymorphonuclear leukocytes, Cell Biochem. Funct. 12,57-62.

25) Babior, B.M., Kipnes, R.S. and Curnutte, G.T. (1973). Biological defense mechanisms. The production by leukocytes of superoxide, a potential bactericidal agent, J.Clin. Invest., 52, 741-755.

26) Babior, B.M. (1977) Recent studies on oxygen metabolism in human neutrophils, superoxide and chemiluminescence, in A.M. Michelson, J.M. McCord and Fridovich (eds.), Superoxide and Superoxide Dismutase, Acad. Press, London, pp.271-281.

27) Babior, B.M. and Peters, W.A. (1981) The 0_2^- producing enzyme of human neutrophils: Further Properties, J.Biol. Chem, 256,2321-2323.

28) Babior, B.M. (1988) The respiratory burst oxidase, in Oxygen Radicals in Biology and Medicine, in M.G. Simic, K.A. Taylor, J.F. Ward, C. von Sonntag (eds.), Basic Life Sciences, Plenum Press, New York, vol 49, pp. 815-821.

29) Rossi, F. and Zatti, M. (1964) Biochemical aspects of phagocytosis in polymorphonuclear leococytes: NADPH oxidation by the granules of the resting and phagocytizing cells, Experientia, 20,21-26.

30) Di Mauro, C., Cavalli, G., Curzio, M., Ferretti, C., Mengozzi, G., Rossi, M.A., Paradisi, L. and Dianzani, M.U. (1995) Evidences of 4-hydroxynonenal involvement in modulation of phagocyte activities, Inter. J. Tissue Reactions, 17, 61-72.

31) Rossi, M.A. (1991) Experimental studies on the mechanism of action of 4-hydroxy-2,3-trans-nonenal, a lipid peroxidation product displaying chemotactic activity toward rat neutrophils. Cell Biochem. Funct., 9,163-170.

32) Paradisi, L., Panagini, C., Parola, M., Barrera, G. and Dianzani, M.U. (1985) Effects of 4-hydroxynonenal on adenylate cyclase and 5'-nucleotidase activities in rat liver plasma membranes, Chem.-Biol.Interact., 53, 209-217.

33) Rossi, M.A., Garramone, A. and Dianzani, M.U. (1988) Stimulation of 4-hydroxy-2,3-trans-nonenal, a lippid peroxidation product, on hepatic phospholipase C., J. Tissue React.,10,321-325.

34) Rossi, M.A., Fidale, F., Garramone, A., Esterbauer, H. and Dianzani, M.U. (1990) effectof 4-hydroxyalkenals on hepatic phosphatidylinositol-4,5-diphosphate phospholipase C. Biochem. Pharmacol.,39,1715-1719.

35) Rossi, M.A., Di Mauro, C., Esterbauer, H., Fidale, F. and Dianzani, M.U. (1994) Activation of phosphoinositide-specific phospholipase C of rat neutrophils by the chemotactic aldehyde 4-hydroxy-2,3-trans-nonenal and 4-hydroxy-2,3-trans-octenal, Cell Biochem.Funct., 12,275-280.Rossi, M.A., Fidale,

36) Pronzato, M.A., Domenicotti, C., Biasi, F., Chiarpotto, E., Cottalasso, D., Viotti, P., Melloni, E., Marinari, U.M. and Poli, G. (1991) Inactivation of hepatocyte protein kinase C by carbon tetrachloride: involvement of drug's metabolic activation and prooxidant effect. Biochem Biophys.Res. Comm., 171,1353-1360.

37) Pronzato, M.A., Domenicotti, C., Rosso, E., Bellocchio, A., Patrone, M., Marinari, U.M., Melloni, E. and Poli, G. (1993) Modulation of rat liver protein kinase C during "in vivo" CCl4-inducedoxidative stress, Biochem.Biophys. Res. Comm., 194,635-641.

38) Carini, R., Bellomo, G., Paradisi, L., Dianzani, M.U. and Albano, E. (1996) 4-hydroxynonenal triggers Ca2+-influx in isolated rat hepatocytes, Accepted for publication in Biochem. Biophys. Res. Comm..

39) Barrera, G., Martinotti, S., Fazio, V., Manzari, V., Paradisi, L., Parola, M., Frati, L. and Dianzani M.U. (1987) Effect of 4-hydroxynonenal on c- myc expression, Toxicol. Pathol., 15,238-240.

40) Barrera, G., Di Mauro, C., Muraca, R., Ferrero, D., Cavalli, G., Fazio, V.M., Paradisi, L. and Dianzani, M.U. (1991) Induction of Differentiation in Human HL-60 Cells by 4-Hydroxynonenal, a Product of Lipid Peroxidation, Exp. Cell Res., 197,148-152.

41) Barrera, G., Muraca, R., Pizzimenti, S.S., Serra, A., Rosso, C., Saglio, G., Farace, M.G., Fazio, V.M. and Dianzani, M.U. (1994) Inhibition on c-myc expression induced by 4-hydroxynonenal, a product of lipid peroxidation, in the HL-60 human leukemic cell line, Biochem. Biophys. Res. Comm., 203,553-561.

42) Fazio, V.M., Barrera, G., Martinotti, S., Farace, M.G., Giglioni, B., Fratti, L., Manzari, V. and Dianzani, M.U. (1992) 4-hydroxynonenal, a product of lipid peroxidation, which modulates c-myc and globin-gene expression in K562 erytroleukemic cells, Cancer Res., 52, 4866-4871.

43) Cajone, F. and Bernelli, Zazzera A. (1988) Oxidative stress induces a subset of heat shock proteins in rat hepatocytes and MH1C1 cells, Chem. Biol. Interact., 65,235-246.

44) Cajone F., Salina, M. and Bernelli Zazzera, A. (1989) 4-hydroxynonenal induces a DNA-binding protein similar to heat shock factor, Biochem. J., 262,977-979.

45) Cajone, F. and Crescente, M., (1992) In vitro activation of heat shock transcription factor by 4-hydroxy-nonenal Chem.-Biol. Interact., 84,97-112.

46) Parola, M., Albano, E., Leonarduzzi, G., Muraca, R., Dianzani, I., Poli, G. and Dianzani, M.U., (1993) Evidence for a possible role of lipid peroxidation in experimental liver fibrosis, in G.Poli, E. Albano and M.U.Dianzani (eds). Free Radicals: from Basic Science to Medicine, Birkhaüser Verlag, Basel, 274-286.

47) Parola, M., Pinzani, M., Casini, A., Albano, E., Poli G., Gentilini, A., Gentilini, P. and Dianzani, M.U. (1993) Stimulation of lipid peroxidation or 4-hydroxynonenal treatment increases procollagen 1 (1) gene expression in human liver fat-storing cells, Biochem. Biophys. Res. Comm., 194,1044-1050.

48) Parola, M., Leonarduzzi, G., Robino, G., Albano, E., Poli, G. and Dianzani, M.U. (1996) On the role of lipid peroxidation in the pathogenesis of liver damage induced by long-standing cholestasis, accepted for publication in Free Rad. Biol. Med., 20.

49) Parola, M., Leonarduzzi, G., Biasi, F., Albano, E., Biocca, M.E., Poli, G., e Dianzani, M.U. (1992) Vitamin E dietary supplementation protects against carbon tetrachloride-induced chronic liver damage and cirrhosis, Hepatology, 16,1014-1021.

50) Parola, M., Muraca, R., Dianzani, I., Barrera, G., Leonarduzzi, G., Bendinelli, R., Piccoletti, R. and Poli, G. (1992) Vitamin E dietary supplementation inhibits transforming growth factor ß1 gene expression in the rat liver, FEBS, 308,267-270.
51) Parola, M., Leonarduzzi, G., Albano, E., Poli, G. and Dianzani, M.U. (1994) Oxidative damage in the pathogenesis of liver cirrhosis, in M.U. Dianzani and P. Gentilini (eds.) Liver Pathophysiology, Elsevier Science, Amsterdam, 3-12.

CHAPTER 2

OXIDATIVE STRESS AND PROTEIN KINASE C ACTIVITY MODULATION

C. DOMENICOTTI, G. SANTORI, M.A. PRONZATO, D. COTTALASSO, R. RICCIARELLI, A. LAMEDICA, D. PAOLA, U.M. MARINARI
Institute of General Pathology, University of Genoa, Via L.B.Alberti 2, 16132 Genoa, Italy

Summary

The conventional protein kinase C (PKC) is a family of cytoplasmic calcium (Ca^{2+})- and phospholipid (PL)- dependent serine-threonine kinases. Recently, it has been proposed that oxidative stress plays a role in both the up-regulation and the down-regulation of PKC. Our experimental studies "in vitro" and "in vivo" have shown that rat intoxication with prooxidant concentrations of carbon tetrachloride (CCl_4) induced significant changes in the liver PKC activity.

Oxygen free radicals and subsequent lipid peroxidation may participate in the pathogenesis of tissue injury, including the brain injury induced by hypoxia and cardiac injury arising from ischemia and reperfusion [1, 2]. Mechanisms by which the initial oxidative insult leads to cellular and tissue damages are not well understood. Many reports have indicated that PKC may be activated following oxidative stress and that this enzyme may play an important role in the pathways leading to cellular injury. The thiol-rich regions in regulatory and catalytic domains of PKC are extremely sensitive to oxidative modifications. A selective oxidative alteration of the regulatory domain results in a Ca^{2+}/lipid independent activation of the kinase with a loss of phorbol ester binding [3]. Further oxidation leads to inactivation of the kinase, because of a presumable modification of the catalytic domain [4]. According to various "in vitro" investigations, oxidants may lead to either up- or down-regulation of PKC, depending on the intensity of the oxidative stimulus. The kinase has shown to be activated by fatty acid hydroperoxides [5], oxygenation products of arachidonic acid [6], redox-cycling quinones [7] and lipid peroxidation [8]. Our experimental studies have demonstrated that the exposure of isolated rat hepatocytes to prooxidant concentrations of CCl4 led to a marked decrease in the kinase activity [9] and that aldehydic products of lipid peroxidation inhibited the enzyme at micromolar

P. Gentilini and M. U. Dianzani. New Trends in Hepatology, 17-23

concentrations [10]. Recently, the "in vivo" acute intoxication with CCl_4 has revealed that low oxidative stress can stimulate liver PKC while a strong oxidative stress leads to a marked inactivation of the enzyme [11].

The main types of protein kinase (PK) present in isolated hepatocytes have been separated and examined [12, 13]. Both the particulate and cytosolic fractions obtained from isolated hepatocytes contained two major PK activities. One of them showed an absolute requirement of Ca^{2+}, PLs and diacylglycerol for the enzyme function and was ascribed to PKC; the other PK activity did not require Ca^{2+} and PLs and was recognized as Ca^{2+}-/PLs-independent PK [9, 14]. After 30 min exposure of rat hepatocytes to a prooxidant concentration of CCl_4 (0.129 mM) the PKC activity was decreased by 50 %, while that of Ca^{2+}-/PLs-independent PK remained unchanged.

In order to verify the involvement of CCl_4 metabolism in PKC inactivation, the early phases of CCl_4 exposure were analyzed in hepatocytes from PB untreated and PB pre-treated rats (*Figure 1*).

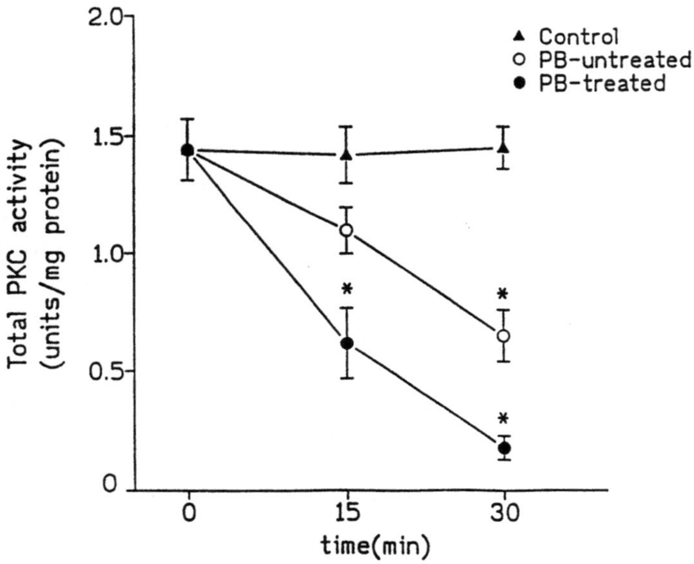

Figure 1. Enhancement of PKC inactivation due to CCl_4 by rat pre-treatment with a single dose of Na-phenobarbital (PB), 80 mg/kg i.p., followed by the administration of a 0.1% PB solution in drinking water for 7 days until sacrifice (*$p < 0.01$ vs control).

PB induces overexpression in cytochrome P-450 content, so enhancing CCl_4 metabolism to free radical species [10, 15]. In hepatocytes from PB untreated rats, 30 min CCl_4 exposure significantly impaired both the cytosolic and the particulate PKC activity. In hepatocytes from PB-treated rats a significant inactivation of the enzyme was monitored at 15 min CCl_4 exposure, and PKC activity was completely depressed after 30 min of the haloalkane treatment.
To investigate the role of two main mechanisms of CCl_4 toxicity, i.e. haloalkylation and lipid peroxidation, the experimental model was modulated by addition of a free radical scavenger, able to protect from lipid peroxidation without interfering with the other mechanism. The pre-incubation of isolated hepatocytes with Trolox, an hydrosoluble vitamin E analogue, allowed a complete protection against CCl_4-induced stimulation of lipid peroxidation measured in terms of malondialdehyde production [10]. Cell supplementation with Trolox did not affect the covalent binding of CCl_4 metabolites to hepatocyte total proteins. A marked but not complete protection of cytosolic and particulate PKC activity was observed both in PB untreated and PB pre-treated rats.
This "in vitro" evidence suggests that CCl_4 metabolism and in particular lipid peroxidation induced by CCl_4 radicals are partially involved in the loss of PKC activity. A similar degree of enzymatic inhibition was observed in both the particulate and cytosolic compartments, suggesting that the effects of the haloalkane on PKC may spread from the site of metabolic activation of CCl_4 to the cytosol. In a cell free system, partially purified liver cPKC containing a mixture of α and β isoforms was directly exposed to different concentrations of the alkanal hexanal or of the hydroxyalkenals (4-hydroxypentenal, 4-hydroxyexenal, 4-hydroxyoctenal and 4-hydroxynonenal), which are the main products of CCl_4-induced lipid peroxidation. A 50 % inhibition of PKC activity was observed at micromolar concentrations of these products [16].
In the "in vivo" experiments, rat intoxication carried out with different concentrations of CCl_4 (from 12.5 µl to 250 µl % g bwt/4 h) induced significant changes in hepatic cPKC activity [11]. The enzymatic activity was stimulated at low CCl_4 concentrations (12.5 - 25 µl % g bwt) while it showed a progressive inhibition at higher doses (150 - 250 µl % g bwt) of haloalkane (*Figure 2a*). Therefore, these data support the hypothesis that a shift in cellular redox equilibrium towards a moderate oxidative stress stimulates PKC function while a more intense oxidative stress decreases the enzymatic activity.
The CCl_4-induced oxidative inactivation of cPKC was further analyzed after a different time treatment with a standard prooxidant concentration of CCl_4 i.e. 250 µl % g bwt (*Figure 2b*).

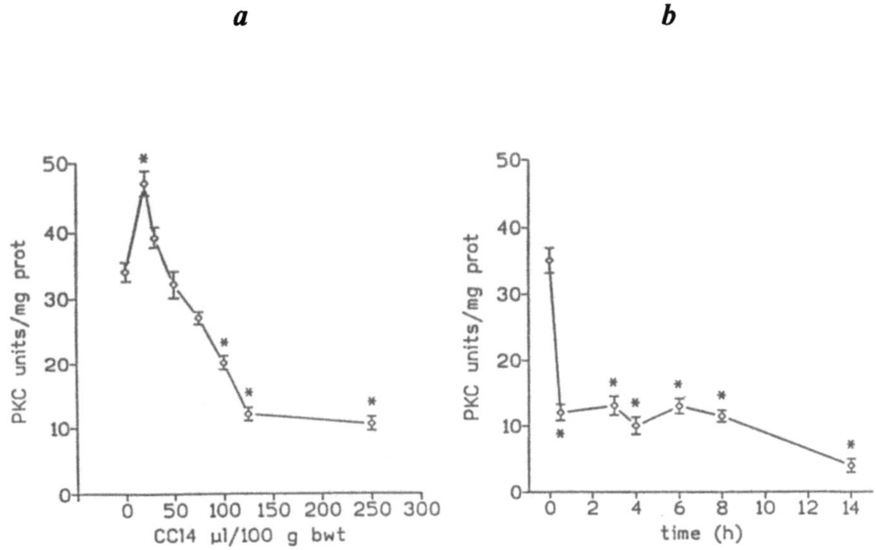

Figure 2. a) rat liver PKC activity after 4 h intoxication with increasing amounts of CCl_4 (* $p < 0.05$ vs control).
b) time course of rat liver PKC inactivation after 250 µl/% g bwt CCl_4 (* $p < 0.001$ vs control).

In this latter experimental model, PKC activity decreased showing a triphasic, time-dependent behaviour. Firstly, enzyme activity fell to 30 % of control levels after 30 min; secondly it stayed steady for 8 h of treatment and finally after 14 h only 10% of PKC was detectable. In the immunoblot analysis, the immunoreactive PKC was still present after 3 h of CCl_4 exposure, while a significant decrease of the protein was observed after 14 h of treatment (*Figure 3*).

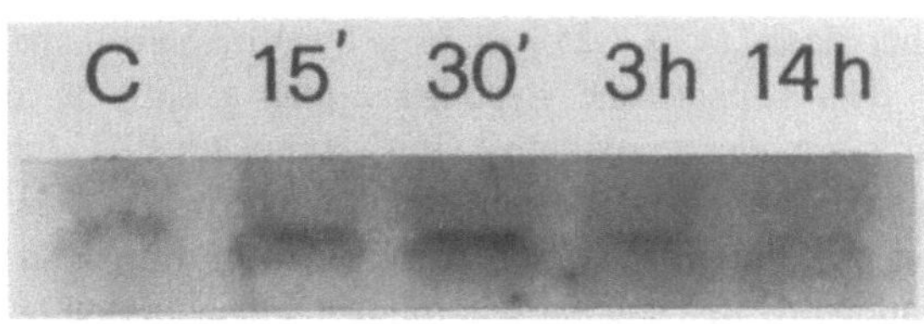

Figure 3. Immunoblot analysis of liver PKC following rat intoxication with a prooxidant dose of CCl_4 (250 µl/% g bwt).

Two different mechanisms are probably involved in this loss of PKC activity. CCl_4 radical metabolites may play an important role in the rapid enzyme inactivation and subsequently a proteolytic degradation of the enzyme might occur. The proteolytic degradation of PKC is probably the result of an extensive activation of calpain and calpastatin, the Ca^{2+}-dependent proteolytic system which regulates the PKC activity. In fact, a significant increase of intracellular Ca^{2+} occurred as early as 30 min after CCl_4 treatment [17]. Therefore, the activities of calpain I, II and their natural inhibitor calpastatin in the liver of CCl_4-treated rats were monitored up to 14 h of intoxication [11]. While calpain I activity was only slightly affected, calpain II and calpastatin showed a marked and progressive decrease. Inactivation of calpain-calpastatin system could be considered the result of its autoproteolytic activation [15]. This inactivation appeared statistically significant after 1 h treatment, when the first PKC damage had already started. The kinetics of inactivation of calpain-calpastatin system and of PKC are different, suggesting that the impairment of proteases is not dependent on reactive species produced during CCl_4-induced oxidative stress. These products, including aldehydes, are able to inactivate the PKC and also favour an early and excessive Ca^{2+} flow from the extracellular compartment into the hepatocyte. This latter event may trigger a pathological stimulation of calpain II, leading to the proteolytic degradation of PKC. Therefore, inactivation and also proteolytic degradation of the enzyme take place, because of the Ca^{2+}-dependent recruitment of calpain II (*Figure 4*).

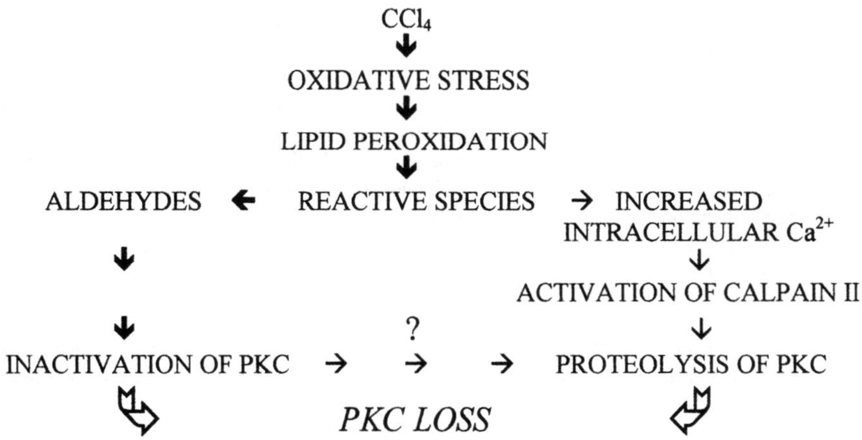

Figure 4. Putative processes involved in the loss of PKC activity by CCl_4-induced lipid peroxidation.

Both of these processes, inactivation and proteolysis, contribute to the PKC loss. As for other proteins, the inactive oxidatively modified form of PKC may be more susceptible to proteolysis. The early oxidant-induced activation of PKC is followed by enzyme inhibition and proteolytic degradation, with the final loss of enzymatic function.

Ackowledgments
This work was supported by grants from CNR (Project ACRO) and MURST 40% and 60%.

References

1. Halliwell, B.: Oxidants and human disease : some new concepts, *FASEB Journal* **1** (1987), 358-364.
2. Werns, S.W. and Lucchesi, B.R.: Free radicals and ischemic tissue injury, *Trends in Pharmacological Sciences* **11** (1990), 161-166.
3. Gopalakrishna, R. and Anderson, W.B.: Ca^{2+}- and phospholipid-independent activation of protein kinase C by selective oxidative modification of the regulatory domain, *Proc. Natl. Acad. Sci. USA* **86** (1989), 6758-6762.
4. Gopalakrishna, R. and Anderson, W.B.: Reversible oxidative activation and inactivation of protein kinase C by the mitogen/tumour promoter periodate, *Arch. Biochem. Biophys. Res. Commun.* **285** (1991), 382-387.
5. O'Brian, C.A., Ward, N.E., Weinstein, L.B., Bull, A.W. and Marnett, L.J.: Activation of rat brain protein kinase C by lipid oxidation products, *Biochem. Biophys. Res. Commun.* **155** (1988), 1374-1380.
6. Hansson, A., Serhan, C.N., Haeggstrom, J., Ingelman-Sundberg, M. and Samuelsson, B.: Activation of protein kinase C by lipoxin A and other eicosanoids. Intracellular action of oxygenation products of arachidonic acid, *Biochem. Biophys. Res. Commun.* **134** (1986), 1215-1222.
7. Kass, G.E.N., Duddy, S.K. and Orrenius, S.: Activation of hepatocyte protein kinase C by redox cycling quinones, *Biochem. J.* **266** (1989), 499-507.
8. Von Ruecker, A.A., Han-Jeon, B.G., Wild, M. and Bidlingmaier, F.: Protein kinase C involvement in lipid peroxidation and cell membrane damage induced by oxygen based radicals in hepatocytes, *Biochem Biophys. Res. Commun.* **163** (1989), 836-842.
9. Poli, G., Albano, E., Dianzani, M.U., Melloni, E., Pontremoli, S., Marinari, U.M., Pronzato, M.A. and Cottalasso, D.: Carbon tetrachloride-induced inhibition of protein kinase C in isolated rat hepatocytes, *Biochem. Biophys. Res. Commun.* **153** (1988), 591-597.
10. Pronzato, M.A., Domenicotti, C., Biasi, F., Chiarpotto, E., Cottalasso, D., Viotti, P., Melloni, E., Marinari, U.M. and Poli, G.: Inactivation of hepatocyte protein kinase C by carbon tetrachloride : involvement of drug's metabolic activation and prooxidant effect, *Biochem. Biophys. Res. Commun.* **171** (1990), 1353-1360.
11. Pronzato, M.A., Domenicotti, C., Rosso, E., Bellocchio, A., Patrone, M., Marinari, U.M., Melloni, E. and Poli, G.: Modulation of rat liver protein kinase C during "in vivo" CCl_4-induced oxidative stress, *Biochem. Biophys. Res. Commun.* **194** (1993), 635-641.

12.Poli, G., Gravela, E., Albano, E. and Dianzani, M.U.: Studies on fatty liver with isolated hepatocytes. II- The action of carbon tetrachloride on lipid peroxidation, protein and trygliceride synthesis and secretion, *Exp. Mol. Pathol.* **30** (1979), 116-127.

13.Tapley, P.M. and Murray, A.W.: Platelet Ca^{2+} activated, phospholipid dependent protein kinase evidence for proteolytic activation of the enzyme in cells treated with phospholipase C_1, *Biochem. Biophys. Res. Commun.* **118** (1984), 835-841.

14.Melloni, E. and Pontremoli, S.: The calpain-calpastatin system : structural and functional properties, *J. Nutr. Biochem.* **2** (1991), 467-476.

15.Pronzato, M.A., Marinari, U.M., Domenicotti, C., Rosso, E., Cottalasso, D., Nanni, G., Melloni, E., and Poli, G.:.Effects of carbon tetrachloride on the regulatory system of transmembrane signalling, *Oxigen Radicals*, Elsevier Science Publishers (1992), 501-504.

16.Marinari, U.M., Pronzato, M.A., Viotti, P., Domenicotti, C., Chiarpotto, E., Cottalasso, D., Melloni, E., Poli, G. and Dianzani, M.U.: Effect of lipid peroxidation carbonyl products on rat hepatocyte protein kinases, *Medical, Biochemical and Chemical aspects of Free Radicals*, Elsevier Science Publishers (1989), 1049-1052.

17.Biasi F., Albano E., Chiarpotto E., Corongiu F.P., Pronzato M.A., Marinari U.M., Parola M., Dianzani M.U. and Poli G.: In vivo and in vitro evidence concerning the role of lipid peroxidation in the mechanism of hepatocyte death due to carbon tetrachloride, *Cell Biochemistry and Function* **9** (1991), 111-118.

CHAPTER 3

OXIDATIVE DAMAGE IN CHRONIC AND ACUTE LIVER DISEASE.

ELISABETTA BALDI, PATRIZIA BURRA, ROMILDA CARDIN, MARIA CHIARAMONTE, STEFANO FAGIUOLI, FABIO FARINATI, ANNAROSA FLOREANI, CINZIA MESTRINER, GIACOMO CARLO STURNIOLO and REMO NACCARATO.

Liver Unit, Department of Gastroenterology, Padua University.
Cattedra Malattie Apparato Digerente, Istituto di Medicina Interna, Policlinico Universitario, Via Giustiniani 2, 35128, Padova, Italy.

Summary

This paper discusses the role and the biochemical and clinical effects of oxidative damage in liver diseases such as HCV-related chronic hepatitis, primary biliary cirrhosis, Wilson's disease and in liver transplantation. In particular, data are reported on lipid peroxidation, hepatocyte proliferation, DNA adducts formation in relation to free radical-mediated damage, and on glutathione metabolism, as a measure of antioxidant defense. The results presented demonstrate that oxidative damage is an important pathologic mediator in liver disease.

INTRODUCTION

The terms "free radicals" and "reactive oxygen species (ROS)" are used to characterize metabolites of low molecular weight, which are reactive enough to damage essential biological molecules. Injury is mediated by reaction of the ROS with essential cell and tissue components, such as proteins, lipids and DNA (1) as in the process of lipid peroxidation, which consists in a variety of reactions, creating cell damage by destroying membrane integrity and producing toxic compounds (2). Many observations indicate that oxygen free radical events may also have a causative role in carcinogenesis. During this process, ROS may damage specific genes that control cell growth and differentiation during the initiation/promotion phase (3), or that increase the activity of carcinogenic xenobiotics (4). They may also stimulate a more rapid growth of malignant cells (progression phase) (5), and may interact directly with genomic DNA (6). With this in mind, in the last few years we have attempted to evaluate the relevance of oxidative damage in several liver diseases, aiming to clarify the mechanisms of damage and carcinogenesis and the effect of drug administration.

P. Gentilini and M. U. Dianzani. New Trends in Hepatology, 24-32

OXIDATIVE DAMAGE AND HCV-RELATED CHRONIC HEPATITIS

While the mechanisms underlying hepatitis B virus (HBV) mediated liver damage have been clarified (7), it is still debatable whether HCV is directly cytopathic or the associated liver damage is immunologically mediated. Some histological features peculiar to the HCV-infected liver, such as the presence of steatosis (8), suggest a direct cytopathic effect. It has recently been shown (9) that some viruses may promote hepatocyte damage by activating lipid peroxidation via an iron-mediated mechanism. The above findings, in association with the anecdotal report of increased ferritin levels in HCV-related hepatitis, prompted us to ascertain whether a similar metabolic mechanism could be involved in HCV-mediated liver damage. Our study (10) involved 63 patients, subgrouped as HCV-positive [HCV+]), HBsAg-positive ([HBV+]), with chronic alcoholic liver disease [CALD], with both alcohol abuse and HCV-related liver damage [HCV+ETOH], and with genetic hemochromatosis [HEMO]: we determined serum iron, ferritin and also, in subfragments of the liver biopsy, tissue iron, glutathione and malondialdehyde (MDA). The pathologist indicated the score for disease staging according to Knodell (11).

Liver glutathione in its reduced (GSH) and oxidized (GSSG) forms was determined according to Reed's method (12). GSSG was also calculated as a percentage of total glutathione (GS) (GSSG/GSH+GSSG,%) to provide a measure of the actual consumption of GSH in relation to its production. Liver lipoperoxide determination was performed by the thiobarbituric acid reaction using a modified version of Masugi's method (13). Liver iron concentrations were measured by atomic absorption spectrophotometry (14) and the iron index was calculated (14).

The most relevant findings were as follows. Serum ferritin levels were significantly higher in HCV+ versus HBV+ patients. An uneven distribution of tissue iron was confirmed with significant differences between HCV+ and HBV+ patients and between HCV+ETOH and HBV+ patients. By stepwise multiple regression analysis only the iron index and serum ferritin correlated with tissue iron levels. Liver GSH levels were significantly higher in HCV+ than in HBV+ patients. Liver GSSG was also significantly higher in HCV+ and in HCV+ETOH than in HBV+ patients. MDA liver levels were significantly higher in HCV and CALD with respect to HBV+ patients and correlated with both tissue iron and serum ferritin.

The overall meaning of these data is, in our minds, that HCV- and HBV-related chronic liver damage, though caused by a virus in both cases, clearly follows two different pathways, and in HCV+ patients a pattern involving free radical production and lipid peroxidation is activated, which correlates with the presence of steatosis and the activation of glutathione metabolism. All these aspects are apparently linked to a local and systemic iron metabolism derangement with a clear-cut increase in liver iron storage, which reflects raised serum ferritin levels. Finally, since HCV-positive patients are at high risk for hepatocellular carcinoma (15), a potential effect of increased free radical production and liver iron storage could be hypothesized in liver carcinogenesis, as described in other models.

HCV, OXIDATIVE DAMAGE AND CARCINOGENESIS

With respect to the mechanisms underlying the development of hepatocellular carcinoma in HCV-positive patients, it is worth bearing in mind that HCV is a single-stranded RNA virus and such viruses have never been associated with oncogenesis. We therefore evaluated hepatocyte proliferation in patients with HCV-related liver damage in regards to disease activity and free-radical production, aiming to establish whether studying cytoproliferation in HCV-positive patients can improve our understanding of their risk of cancer.

The proliferative index was assessed using the Ki67 monoclonal antibody MIB1 (AMAC Inc., Westbrook, USA), one of three monoclonal antibodies reactive to parts of the Ki67 antigen (16). The proliferation rate, as a labeling index, was assessed in the periportal area (zone 1), and in the intermediate and perivenular zones (2 and 3) together (17).

HCV-positive patients had a median number of MIB1-positive cells significantly higher than the other groups. To be more precise, a statistically significant difference was documented between HCV-positive patients and HBV-positive, alcoholics and hemochromatosis patients. The percentage of patients with MIB1-positive cells in zones 2 and 3 was significantly higher in HCV-positive patients, and in those with HCV plus alcohol abuse, than in the other groups considered.

In a multiple regression analysis significant correlations of the MIB-1 score were found with ALT levels, etiology and Knodell index, but not with liver MDA levels.

Information on the proliferative activity of the liver in patients with chronic liver damage might be relevant because chronic hepatitis and cirrhosis might be viewed as precancerous steps in the lengthy progression of chronic liver damage towards hepatocellular carcinoma. Our data indicate that liver proliferative activity in chronic hepatitis is clearly modulated by both the etiology and the activity of the disease, and that oxidative damage has no role.

In conclusion, the use of monoclonal Ki67 MIB1 enabled us to document a direct effect of HCV on the extent and qualitative expression of hepatocyte proliferation in chronic hepatitis and cirrhosis. Whether the specific aspect of abnormal hepatocyte proliferation - that we documented mainly (though not exclusively) in

HCV-positive patients and that is generally found only after massive necrosis or carcinogen administration (18) - might be one of the factors involved in HCV-related liver carcinogenesis remains to be seen.

We then evaluated the extent of oxidative DNA damage in the circulating leukocytes of patients with various stages of HCV-related chronic hepatic disease in an attempt to further clarify the mechanisms and timing of events underlying the increased risk of hepatocellular carcinoma (HCC) in HCV-related liver cirrhosis.
The DNA was purified from circulating leukocytes according to Fraga et al. (19).
The separation of 8OHdG and normal deoxynucleosides was performed in HPLC-ECD according to Degan et al. (20).
The results indicated that patients with chronic active hepatitis had higher 8OHdG levels in DNA than controls, cirrhotics or patients with HCC. 8OHdG levels were correlated with the presence of relevant steatosis to confirm the relationship with peroxidation.
To date, the role of oxidative DNA adducts in human carcinogenesis is inadequately understood, but the presence and persistence of DNA adducts in human tissue can clearly have considerable relevance with respect to cancer risk (4). Although the effect of this damage *in vivo* remains unknown, this oxidatively-modified residue may accumulate, causing mispairing and thus becoming mutagenic and, as a consequence, potentially carcinogenic (21).
Our findings that DNA oxidative damage, as assessed by demonstrating the accumulation of 8OHdG in circulating leukocyte DNA, is increased in patients with chronic HCV-mediated liver damage and appears to specifically characterize the early phases of the disease therefore appear to be relevant.

OXIDATIVE DAMAGE AND SULFOXIDATION CAPACITY IN PRIMARY BILIARY CIRRHOSIS

Sulfoxidation is a hepatic function that is important in the oxidative metabolism of many compounds. An impaired sulfoxidation has been reported to be closely associated with primary biliary cirrhosis (PBC) (22), but the same Authors recently failed to confirm the primary defect in sulfoxidation (23). To assess the turnover of sulfhydryl groups and evaluate the tissue content of cysteine in PBC, we studied a group of 12 female pre-cirrhotic PBC patients. Cysteine (CYSH) and reduced and oxidized glutathione (GSH/GSSG) contents were evaluated as described above (12), together with the GSSG/GSH+GSSG ratio (as a measure of glutathione turnover), the CYSH/GSH ratio (as a measure of CYSH utilization), and liver MDA. Patients with chronic HCV-related liver damage or with HBV-related hepatitis were used for control purposes. Basically, the PBC patients presented the lowest liver CYSH levels and CYSH/GSH ratio, and the highest

GSSG levels and GSSG/GSH+GSSG ratio, though they had low MDA levels. Said results testify to an increased glutathione turnover, associated with CYSH consumption and an increased GSSG production in the liver.
There was an apparent contradiction between the high plasma CYSH levels reported in the above-mentioned papers and the very low liver CYSH levels we detected. A possible explanation could be that CYSH levels are reduced in the liver due to a high glutathione turnover. GSH is indeed quite low in the liver of PBC patients, possibly due to its use as a scavenger and its catabolism by liver gamma-glutamiltrans-peptidase, responsible for GSH splitting (24) and possibly also involved in causing the reported high plasma CYSH levels (25).

OXIDATIVE DAMAGE IN WILSON'S DISEASE

The hepatic accumulation of excess copper in Wilson's disease results in the onset of cirrhosis, liver failure and eventually death. There is still debate, however, as to the cellular and biochemical mechanisms whereby copper induces liver damage. Several different mechanisms have been suggested for the damaging effects of copper (26-29) and a role has recently been proposed for copper in triggering peroxidative damage, with free radical production and consequent oxidant hepatic injury (30). With this in mind, we wondered to what extent liver copper status and treatment modalities could modulate lipoperoxide production and glutathione turnover in Wilson's disease.
Patients with Wilson's disease were included in the study (31) at the time of a clinical and bioptic follow-up, when they were admitted for a control liver biopsy, after at least 12 months of penicillamine or zinc therapy. Patients with chronic HCV- or HBV-related liver disease were also included in the study for control purposes.
In essence, the results showed that GSH levels were significantly lower in Wilson's disease patients than in HBV- or HCV-positive patients. On the other hand, the % GSSG/GSH+GSSG was significantly higher and the CYSH levels were significantly lower. The comparison of patients under zinc or penicillamine treatment showed that the liver GSH levels were significantly lower and the % of GSSG/GSH+GSSG and MDA were significantly higher in the penicillamine-treated patients, whose copper tissue levels were lower than in the zinc-treated subjects (though not significantly so) but, as a mean, were still significantly higher than the normal range.
The role of zinc as an anti-oxidant in Wilson's disease may be important through: 1. its participation in superoxide dismutase (32); 2. interaction with cellular membranes (33); 3. the induction of sulfur-rich metallothionein in the liver (34); 4. the prevention of iron accumulation (35); and 5. the modulation of glutathione

status (36). The above data suggest that zinc treatment protects against free radical-induced liver damage and ameliorates GSH availability.

LIPID PEROXIDATION DURING LIVER TRANSPLANTATION

Orthotopic liver transplantation is the treatment of choice for patients with end-stage liver disease, no longer responsive to medical treatment. However, in spite of an overall improved survival, early postoperative graft dysfunction still remains a relevant event in liver transplant recipients (37). It is well recognized that ischemia-reperfusion injury represents a key event leading to primary graft malfunction after prolonged graft storage (38), but the underlying mechanisms have yet to be fully elucidated. Activation of the Kupffer cells with the release of superoxide anion and other mediators directly into the blood (39) may aggravate the liver injury or promote the development of oxygen species-related reactions (40,41). Oxygen free radicals may act as chemoattractants stimulating neutrophil margination: this could explain why superoxide dismutase reduces neutrophil infiltration in reperfused liver after both warm and cold ischemia (42,43). Irreversible endothelial cell injury after reperfusion of rat livers occurs at the time of activation of Kupffer cells (44), probably because of superoxide formation during reperfusion, leading to hydroxyl radical production, with subsequent tissue injury (45).

The aim of our study was to confirm whether lipid peroxidation is increased during liver transplantation and plays a role in hepatocellular damage. Twenty-nine transplanted patients were studied. All donor livers were procured using well-described techniques and preserved with the University of Wisconsin solution. Patients were studied at the time of transplant surgery and for 5 consecutive days. The indications for liver transplantation were HBV and/or HCV related cirrhosis in 12 cases (2 with hepatocellular carcinoma), alcoholic cirrhosis in 7, cholestatic liver disease in 6, miscellanea in 4. Venous blood samples were drawn from all patients at the baseline (before surgery), after anesthetic induction, at the anhepatic phase, at graft reperfusion, and then daily for 5 consecutive days. Malondialdehyde (MDA), AST, ALT, lactic acid (LA), and prothrombin time (PT) were measured. CO_2 production (VCO_2) and oxygen consumption (VO_2) were also assessed at the same time. MDA was assessed using the standard procedure (46). Oxygen consumption and carbon dioxide production were estimated by respiratory mode indirect calorimetry (Deltatrac Datex, Finland).

MDA levels remained stable during the surgical procedure, but were significantly higher at day 5 than at day 1 (mean ±SD, 3.05±0.5 nmol/ml vs 2.67±0.5 nmol/ml; $p<0.05$). No correlation was found with AST, ALT, LA, PT values. VO_2 and VCO_2 dropped rapidly during the anhepatic phase but increased after the operation. No significant correlations were found between MDA levels and VO2 and VCO2 values.

In conclusion, serum MDA increases after OLTx up to 5 days from transplantation, but does not correlate with markers of hepatocellular necrosis. The increased oxygen consumption and CO2 production, seen after reperfusion and during the days that follow and linked to glucose utilization and lipid oxidation, follows a trend similar to MDA production and may also be associated with metabolic changes in the hepatocytes.

CONCLUSIONS

In conclusion, all the above-reported data point to the importance of oxidative damage and its effects in liver pathologies in which free radical formation is not generally considered a pathogenic factor (with the sole exception of reperfusion injury). Our studies, and their clinical consequences, suggest stimulating possibilities for further investigations on the pathophysiologic and therapeutic aspects of liver damage.

REFERENCES

1. de Groot, H. (1994) Reactive oxygen species in tissue injury, Hepato-Gastroenterol. 41,328-332.
2. Comporti, M. (1985) Biology of disease. Lipid peroxidation and cellular damage in toxic liver injury, Lab. Invest. 53,599-623.
3. Crawford, D. and Cerutti, P. (1988) Expression of oxidant stress-related genes in tumor promotion of mouse epidermal cells JB6, in: Nygaard O. Simic M, Cerutti P (eds): "Anticarcinogenesis and Radiation Protection", New York: Plenum Press, pp 183-190.
4. Ames, B.N. (1989) Mutagenesis and Carcinogenesis: Endogenous and exogenous factors, Environmental and Molecular Mutagenesis, 14, 16, 66-77.
5. Troll, W. and Wiesner, R. (1985) The role of oxygen radicals as a possible mechanism of tumor promotion, Ann Re. Pharmacol. Toxical., 25, 509-528.
6. Adelman, R., Saul, R.L. and Ames, B.N. (1988) Oxidative damage to DNA: Relation to species metabolic rate and life span, Proc. Natl. Acad. Sci., 85, 2706-2708.
7. Chisari, F.V., Ferrari, C. and Mondelli, M.U. (1989) Hepatitis B virus structure and biology, Microbial. Pathogenesis, 6, 311-325.
8. Scheuer, P.J., Ashrafzadeh, P., Sherlock, S. et al. (1991) The pathology of hepatitis C, Hepatology, 15, 567-571.
9. Schwarz, K.B., Larroya, S., Vogler, C., et al. (1990) Role of influenza B virus in hepatic steatosis and mitochondrial abnormalities in a mouse model of Reye syndrome, Hepatology, 13, 96-103.
10. Farinati, F., Cardin, R., De Maria, N., et al. (1995) Iron storage, lipid peroxidation and glutathione turnover in chronic anti-HCV positive hepatitis, J. Hepatol., 22, 449-456.
11. Knodell, R.G., Ishak, K.G., Black, W.C. et al. (1981) Formulation and application of a numerical scoring system for assessing histological activity in asymptomatic chronic active hepatitis, Hepatology, 1, 431-435.
12. Reed, D.J., Babson, J.R., Beatty, P.W. et al. (1980) High-performance liquid chromatography analysis of nanomole levels of glutathione, glutathione disulphide, and related thiols and disulphides, Anal. Biochem., 106, 55-62.
13. Masugi, F., and Nakamura. T. (1977) Measurement of thiobarbituric acid value in liver homogenate solubilized with sodium dodecyl sulphate and variation of the values affected by vitamin E and drugs, Vitamins, 51, 21-29.

14. Bassett, M.L., Halliday, J.W., and Powell, L.W. (1986) Value of hepatic measurements in early hemochromatosis and determination of the critical iron level associated with fibrosis, Hepatology, 61, 24-29.
15. Farinati, F., Fagiuoli, S., De Maria, N. et al. (1992) Anti-HCV positive hepatocellular carcinoma in cirrhosis. Prevalence, risk factors and clinical features, J. Hepatol., 14, 183-186.
16. Sternberger, LA. (1979) Immunocytochemistry. 2nd edition.
17. Rappaport, A.M. (1973) The microcirculatory hepatic unit, Microvascular Research, 6, 212-228.
18. Paolucci, F., Mancini, R., Marucci, L., et al. (1990) Immunohistochemical identification of proliferating cells following dimethylnitrosamine-induced liver injury, Liver, 10, 278-281
19. Fraga, C.G., Shigenaga, M.K., Park, J.W., et al. (1990) Oxidative damage to DNA during aging: 8-hydroxy-2'-deoxyguanosine in rat organ DNA and urine, Proc. Natl. Acad. Sci., 87, 4533-4537.
20. Degan, P., Shigenaga, M.K., Park, E.M., et al. (1991) Immunoaffinity isolation of urinary 8-hydroxy-2'deoxyguanosine and 8-hydroxyguanine and quantitation of 8-hydroxyguanosine in DNA by polyclonal antibodies, Carcinogenesis, 12, 865-871.
21. Kuchino, Y., Mori, F., Kasai, H., et al. (1987) Misreading of DNA templates containing 8-hydroxydeoxyguanosine at the modified base and at adjacent residues, Nature, 327, 77-79.
22. Davies, M.H., Ngong, J.M., Pean, A., et al. (1995) Sulphoxidation and sulphation capacity in patients with primary biliary cirrhosis, J. Hepatol., 22, 551-560.
23. Olomu, A.B., Vickers, C.R., Waring, R.H., et al. (1988) High incidence of poor sulfoxidation in patients with primary biliary cirrhosis, N. Eng. J. Med., 318, 1089-1092.
24. Griffith, O.W., Meister, A. (1979) Glutathione: Interorgan translocation, turnover, and metabolism, Proc. Natl. Acad. Sci. USA, 76, 5606-5610.
25. Davies, M.H., Klovrza, L., Waring, R.H., et al. (1994) Plasma cysteine and sulphate levels in patients with cirrhosis of the liver, Clin. Sci. Colch., 87, 357-362
26. Roth, L.E., and Shigenaka, T. (1970) Microtubules in the heliozoan axopodium. II. Rapid degradation by cupric and nickelous, J. Ultrastruct. Res., 31, 356-374.
27. Wallin, M., Larsson, H., and Edstrom, A. (1970) Tubulin sulfhydryl groups and polymerization in vitro. Effects of di- and trivalent cations, Exp. Cell Res., 31, 356-374.
28. Eichhorn, G.L., and Clark, P. (1965) The unwinding and rewinding of DNA strands under the influence of copper (II) ions, Proc. Natl. Acad. Sci. USA, 53, 586-593.
29. Sternlieb, I., and Quintana, N. (1982) Abnormalities of human hepatocellular peroxisomes, Ann. Natl. Acad. Sci., 386, 530-533.
30. Sokol, R.J., Twedt, D., McKim, J.M. Jr., et al. (1994) Oxidant injury to hepatic mitochondria in patients with Wilson's disease and Bedlington Terriers with copper toxicosis, Gastroenterology, 107, 1788-1798
31. Farinati, F., Cardin, R., Mestriner, C., et al. (1995) Mechanisms of Pennicillamine and Zinc in the treatment of Wilson's disease, Am.J. Gastroenterol., 90, 2264-2265.
32. Taylor, O.G., Bettger, W.J., and Bray, T.M. (1988) Effect of dietary zinc or copper deficiency on the primary free radical defense system in rats, J.Nutr., 118, 613-621.
33. Chvapil, M., and Zukowski, C.F. (1974) New concept on the mechanism(s) of the biological effect of zinc, in: Clinical applications of zinc metabolism, WJ Pories, WH Strain, JM Hsu, RL Woosley (eds.), CT Thomas, Springfield, IL, 75-86.
34. Shiraishi, N., Aono, K., and Utsumi, K. (1983) Increased metallothionein content in rat liver induced by x irradiation and exposure to high oxygen tension, Radiat. Res., 95, 298-302.
35. Keen, C.L., and Graham, T.W. (1989) Trace elements, in: Kaneko, J.J. (ed.) , Clinical Biochemistry of Domestic Animals, 4th Ed., New York: Academic, 753-795.
36. Hsu, J.M., Anthony, W.L., and Buchanan, P.J. (1968) Incorporation of glycine-1-14C into liver glutathione in zinc deficient rats, Proc. Soc. Exp. Biol. Med., 127, 1048-1051
37. Shaw, S.E., Gordon, R.D., Iwatsuki, S., et al. (1985) Hepatic transplantation, Transplant Proc, 17, 264
38. Lemasters, J.J., Bunzendahl, H., and Thurman, R.G. (1955) Reperfusion injury to donor livers stored for transplantation, Liver Transplantation and Surgery, 1, 124-138
39. Wake, K., Decker, K., Kirn, A., et al. (1989) Cell biology and the kinetics of Kupffer cells in the liver, Int. Rev. Cytol., 118, 173-229
40. Granger, D.N., Hollwarth, M.E., and Parks, D.A. (1986) Ischemia-reperfusion injury: role of oxygen-derived free radicals, Acta Physiol. Scand., Suppl, 548, 47-63

41. Dawson, T.L., Gores, G.J., Nieminen, A-L., et al. (1993) Mitochondria as a source of reactive oxygen species during reductive stress in rat hepatocytes, Am. J. Physiol., 264, C961-C967
42. Koo, A., Komatsu, H., Tao, G., et al. (1992) Contribution of no-reflow phenomenon to hepatic injury after ischemia-reperfusion: evidence of a role for superoxide anion, Hepatology, 15, 507-514.
43. Marzi, I., Knee, J., Buhren, V., et al. (1992) Reduction by superoxide dismutase of leukocyte-endothelial adherence after liver transplantation, Surgery, 111, 90-97
44. Caldwell-Kenkel, J.C., Currin, R.T., Coote, A., et al. (1995) Reperfusion injury to endothelial cells after cold storage of rat livers: protection by mildly acidic pH and lack of protection by antioxidants, Transpl. Int., 8, 77-85.
45. Jaeschke, H. (1991) Reactive oxygen and ischemia/reperfusion injury of the liver, Chem. Biol. Interact., 79, 115-136.
46. Yagi, K. (1976) A simple fluorimetric assay for lipoperoxide in blood plasma, Biochem. Med., 15, 212-215.

CHAPTER 4

CHRONIC ETHANOL CONSUMPTION IMPAIRS DOLICHOL LEVELS AND GLYCOSYLATION PROCESSES IN RAT LIVER MICROSOMES AND GOLGI APPARATUS

D. COTTALASSO, C. DOMENICOTTI, M.A. PRONZATO,
N. TRAVERSO, A. BELLOCCHIO, D. DAPINO, P. GAZZO,
U.M. MARINARI, G. NANNI.
Institute of General Pathology, University of Genoa, Via L.B. Alberti 2, 16132 Genova, Italy

Summary

The purpose of this study was to investigate whether chronic ethanol intake may induce changes in the rat liver glycoprotein processing. Isolated hepatocytes prelabelled with [^{3}H]-Na-palmitate and [^{14}C]-glucosamine showed a significant storage of the lipid and carbohydrate radioactivity in Golgi apparatus and a significant impairment of labelled glycoprotein secretion. At the same time, changes of the glycosylation steps were observed: in endoplasmic reticulum Dolichyl-Posphate, which is rate limiting for the synthesis of glycoprotein, showed a significant reduction; in the Golgi apparatus the activity of the main enzyme responsible for the terminal glycosylation processes was significantly decreased.

Data obtained in our laboratory indicated that acute ethanol administration produces a precocious and selective impairment of protein glycosylation mechanisms both in liver endoplasmic reticulum (ER) at the level of glycosyl carriers, such as dolichol, and in the Golgi apparatus (GA) where terminal glycosylation occurs (1, 2, 3). Dolichols are a family of long-chain polyisoprenoid alcohols usually containing 14-24 isoprene units with the alfa-isoprene unit being saturated. They exist as free dolichol (free-Dol), fatty acyl dolichyl esters (Dol-FA) or dolichyl phosphate (Dol-P) (4). A function for Dol-P in the rough endoplasmic reticulum (RER) has been established as glycosyl carrier during the membrane-directed biosynthesis of the N-linked oligosaccharide chains of glycoproteins. In fact, it is known that the initial stages of asparagine-linked oligosaccharide synthesis start in the RER where involving Dol-P in the translocation of activated glycosyl units across these

P. Gentilini and M. U. Dianzani. New Trends in Hepatology, 33-41

membranes [5].Nearly all of the other steps concerning the glycosylation of proteins occur in GA but little is known about the functions of neutral dolichols in this area where these compounds might have a role either in the terminal glycoprotein processing or in their secretion in the blood stream [6]. The final steps in the synthesis of the oligosaccharide chains occur in GA where the distal sugar N-acetylglucosamine, galactose and sialyc acid are enzimatically added from their nucleotide precursors [7].

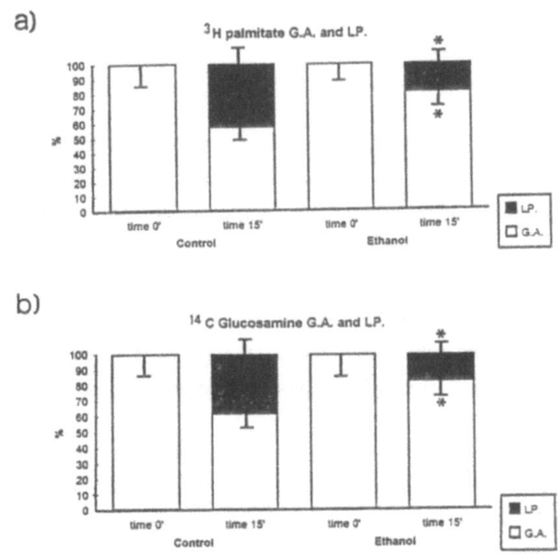

Figure 1. Per cent of (a) [^{3}H]-Na-palmitate and (b) [^{14}C]-glucosamine distribution in total Golgi apparatus and (2,3) lipoproteins secreted from rats hepatocyte chronically intoxicated with ethanol.
Isolated hepatocytes (5-7x10^6cells/ml) from Collagenase perfused rat liver were prelabelled with 1.5 μCi/ml of 5% bovine albumin-bound [9-10 ^{3}H]-Na-palmitate and with 0.16 μCi/ml of [^{14}C]-glucosamine for 45 and 15 mins, respectively [8]. After this time the cells were washed with saline medium, centrifuged and resuspended in the same saline medium. The intracellular distribution and the lipoprotein secretion of labelled precursors was measured after the washing (time 0') and after 15' incubation at 37°C.
Isolation of liver GA was carried out from total microsomal fraction of isolated hepatocytes, by discontinuous sucrose density gradient ultracentrifugation as previously described by Nanni et al. [2,3].
The values represent the mean ± SD of 6-8 preparations of hepatocytes isolated from different rats. Each group of rats, initially weighing 100 ± 12 g, was fed for 8 weeks Lieber De Carli liquid diet containing ethanol (36% caloric content) or isocalorically balanced with dextrin-maltose (pair-fed controls).

* Significant as 15' pair-fed control ($p<0.01$)

Nevertheless, different changes of the dolichols level were described in some pathological conditions, e.g. in aging (9) and in neurodegenerative disease (10). To our knowledge, at present there is no information about dolichol level changes in liver diseases, in addition to those described in our laboratory. An increase of dolichol level in urine of alcoholics has been described by Roine at al. (11), but this data are not confirmed by Stetter at al. (12).

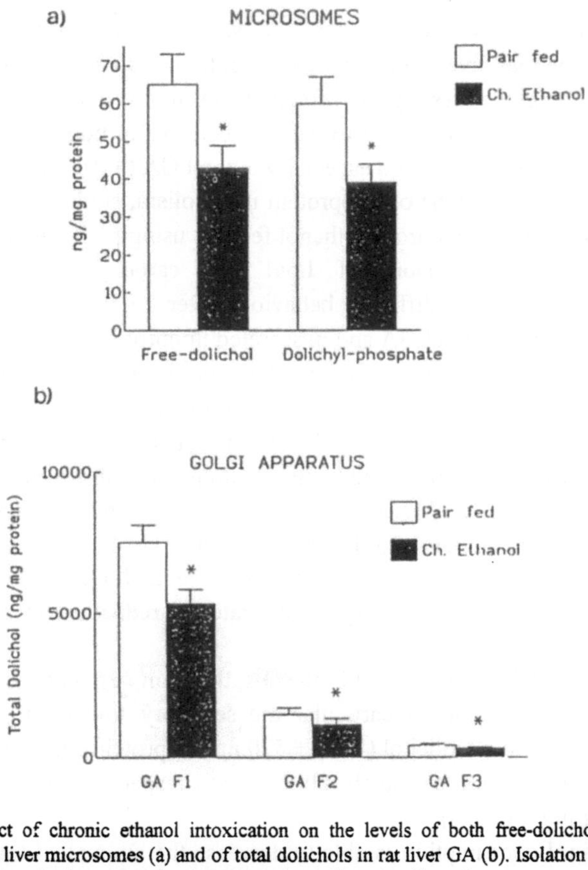

Figure 2. Effect of chronic ethanol intoxication on the levels of both free-dolichol and dolichyl-phosphate in rat liver microsomes (a) and of total dolichols in rat liver GA (b). Isolation of liver GA was carried out from total microsomal fraction of whole rat liver, by discontinuous sucrose density gradient ultracentrifugation as previously described by Nanni et al. [2,3].
The HPLC determination of dolichols (total, free+Dol-FA and phosphate) was carried out as previously described [3].
The values represent the means of 6-8 rats per groups. Other conditions as in Fig.1.

* Significant as to corresponding pair fed group ($p<0.01$)

After partial hepatectomy and after the treatment of rats with inducers of the ER, an increase in dolichol levels in liver was observed (13, 14).
The purpose of this study was to determine the effects of chronic ethanol feeding on protein glycosylation in rat liver ER and GA, using Female Sprague Dawley rats (initial body weight 100 ± 12 g (Morini, Italy) housed in wired bottomed cages in a thermostatically controlled room (22°) with a relative humidity of about 50% and 12h/12h dark/light cycle), fed a Lieber De Carli diet.
The chronic ethanol consumption increased weakly the liver weight (+8%) and significantly the total liver protein with respect to the pair fed control (+16%).
The ratio of triglycerides/mg of protein showed a significant increase in ethanol-treated rats, as compared to pair-fed controls in homogenate (+88%), in total microsomes (+66%) and especially in total GA (+101%).
The intracellular alterations of lipoprotein metabolism, studied in hepatocytes isolated from control and chronic ethanol fed rats using [^{3}H]-Na-palmitate and [^{14}C]-glucosamine precursors of lipid and carbohydrate moieties of lipoproteins, revealing a different behaviour after 15 min of incubation as compared to time 0' in total GA and in secreted lipoprotein (Fig.1a, 1b).
Normally, in each hepatic fraction dolichol is contained in different concentrations. After chronic ethanol consumption, the levels of total dolichol decrease in whole homogenate (-25%), in cytosol (-20%) and in total microsomes, where a significant reduction of dolichol is observed (-36%).
The normal level of Dol-P is 59 ± 5.3 ng/mg protein and represents 45% of total microsomal dolichol (129 ± 15 ng/mg protein).
The quantitative determination of both Dol-free and Dol-P purified from microsomal extracts shows a significant rate of reduction in the chronic ethanol-treated rats (Fig.2).
While only 3% of Dol-P is present in the GA, this compartment has the highest content in total dolichol. In particular the secretory fraction F_1 shows the highest content in total dolichol (7510 ± 570 ng/mg protein); the enrichment in these membranes is approximately 60-fold with respect to total microsomes (131 ± 16 ng/mg proteins).
Chronic ethanol consumption is able to decrease the amount of total dolichol in both secretory (F_1, F_2) and formative (F_3) subfractions. The most marked decrease occurs in F_1 subfraction (Fig. 2b).

In order to evaluate the behaviour of the terminal glycosylation mechanisms, a study of UDP galactose: N-acetyl-glucosamine galactosyl-transferase (GT) and CMP-sialic acid: lactose sialyl transferase (ST) activities have been undertaken in the isolated Golgi subfractions. In isolated secretory sub-fractions (F_1 and F_2) and formative sub-fraction (F_3) of chronic ethanol-treated rats a significant reduction in GT and ST activity is observed (Tab.1).

Table 1. UDP-galactose:N-acetylglucosamine galactosyltransferase and CMP sialyc acid:lactose sialyltransferase activity in liver Golgi apparatus secretory (F_1, F_2) and formative (F_3) subfractions of rats chronically intoxicated with ethanol.

GOLGI APPARATUS	Galactosyltransferase units/mg protein		Sialyltransferase units/mg protein	
	Pair fed	Ethanol	Pair fed	Ethanol
GA F_1	220 ± 38	104 ± 19*	35 ± 6	21 ± 5*
GA F_2	110 ± 21	57 ± 10*	63 ± 13	44 ± 6*
GA F_3	39 ± 10	26 ± 4*	65 ± 12	32 ± 7*

Units referred to nm of galactose transfered to N-acetyl glucosamine/h/mg protein and nmol sialyc acid transfered to lactose/h/mg protein, and represent the means of 6-8 rats per groups. Other conditions as in Fig.1. Isolation of liver GA was carried out from total microsomal fraction of whole rat liver, by discontinuous sucrose density gradient ultracentrifugation as previously described by Nanni et al. (2, 3).The galactosyl and sialyl transferase specific activity were measured on aliquots of each Golgi fraction according to the method described by Fleischer (7).

* Significant as to corresponding pair fed group ($p<0.01$)

The technique of the feeding with ethanol as part of a totally liquid diet is considered the best standard modality to study the effects of chronic consumption in rats (15). In our model the pair-fed and ethanol treated rats reached comparable weights to those feeding of standard semisynthetic chow diet, suggesting that the animals did not modify their total caloric intake.

The significant and very remarkable increase of triglycerides in GA of chronic ethanol treated rats suggested the early implication of this compartment in lipoprotein accumulation during ethanol-induced fatty liver.The impairment of $[^{3}H]$-Na-palmitate and $[^{14}C]$-glucosamine dismission from liver GA produces a storage of the labelled precursors which may explain the liver steatosis observed in the chronic ethanol fed rats. Moreover, the marked retention of labelled lipoprotein at the level of GA correlates well with the impairment of secretion of labelled lipoprotein from hepatocytes isolated from chronic ethanol fed rats. The changes in labelled carbohydrate precursors of lipoprotein suggest that the chronic ethanol consumption may interfere with the glycosylation mechanisms of proteins and lipoproteins.

In order to study the possible alterations of glycoprotein metabolism at each level of glycosylation processes (5, 16), the patterns of dolichols and the terminal glycosylation were investigated in the liver ER and GA.

The high enrichment of microsomes in Dol-P correlates with its involvement in the biosynthesis of N-linked glycoproteins (17). The quantitative determination of Dol-P purified from microsomal extracts shows a significant rate of reduction in the chronic ethanol-treated rats.

Since the concentration of Dol-P appears to be rate-limiting for the synthesis of glycoproteins (18), these results indicate that ethanol is able to impair the established functions of microsomal Dol-P.

The high concentration of total dolichol in the GA suggests a possible role either in terminal glycosylation processing or in movements of lipoglycoproteins through the Golgi secretory region by controlling the permeability properties of membranes (6). The decrease of total dolichol in all Golgi fractions may modify the permeability of these membranes impairing glycoprotein maturation and secretion.

Terminal glycosylation of proteins and lipoproteins is performed by glycosyltransferases, particularly galactosyl- and sialyltransferase. These enzymes are present in the formative and secretory regions of the GA, mainly orientated towards the luminal side of Golgi membranes (7). The results observed indicate that glycosyltransferases are accessible and sensitive to toxic action of diffusible products of ethanol oxidation, that might disturb the microenvironment where the enzymes are located. This suggestion is in agreement with other investigations showing that chronic ethanol ingestion affects the activity of glycosyltransferase which in plasma membrane are able to transfer carbohydrates to lipid endogenous acceptors (19, 20).

The impairment of glycoprotein biosynthesis may be a consequence of ethanol metabolism. In fact, an amount of experimental evidence indicates that during its metabolism, ethanol produces radical compounds (21). Previous results have demonstrated that dolichol is sensitive to attack by free radicals (22). Therefore it is possible to correlate the already observed changes of dolichol content both in microsomes and in GA to prooxidant events. Moreover, acetaldehyde, the main product of ethanol oxidation, covalently bind to proteins of Golgi membranes, particularly to the protein of secretory fraction F_1 which contains the highest amount of glycosyltransferase enzymes (23).
The ability of acetaldehyde to covalently binds to these enzymes may explain the impairment of terminal glycosylation at the level of the GA. Preliminary data suggest that the supplementation of Lieber-De Carli diet with Vitamin E is able to protect against the prooxidant effect of ethanol, the peroxidative damage on dolichol levels and glycosylation processes.

Acnowledgements

This work has been supported by MURST, National Project "Liver Cirrhosis".The excellent technical assistance of Mr. Claudio Canepa and Mr. Giuseppe Catalano is greatly appreciated.

References

1) Nanni, G., Pronzato, M.A., Averame, M.M., Gambella, G.R., Cottalasso, D. and Marinari, U.M. (1978) Influence of acute ethanol intoxication on rat liver Golgi apparatus glycosylation activities, FEBS Lett. 92, 242-246.

2) Nanni, G., Cottalasso, D., Cetta, G., Pronzato, M.A., Marinari, U.M. (1986) Ethanol-induced impairment of glycoprotein metabolism in liver Golgi apparatus, Frontiers in Gastrointestinal Research 9, 50-69.

3) Cottalasso, D., Pronzato, M.A., Domenicotti, C., Nanni, G. and Marinari, U.M. (1990) Ethanol-induced decrease of dolichol levels in the rat liver microsome and Golgi apparatus. In M.U. Dianzani and P.Gentilini (eds), Chronic Liver Damage,. Elsevier Science Publishers, Amsterdam, pp. 39-50

4) Tollbom, O., Valtersson, C., Chojnachi, T. and Dallner, G. (1988) Esterification of dolichol in rat liver, J. Biol. Chem. 263, 1347-1352.

5) Hirschberg, G.B. and Snider, M.D. (1987) Topography of glycosylation in the rough endoplasmic reticulum and Golgi apparatus, Annual Review of Biochemistry 56, 63-87.

6) Monti, J.A., Christian, S.T. and Schutzbach, J.S. (1987) Effects of dolichol on membrane permeability, Biochimica et Biophysica Acta 905, 133-142.
7) Fleischer, B. (1981) Orientation of glycoproteins galactosyltransferase and sialyltransferase enzymes in vesicles derived from liver Golgi apparatus, Journal of Cell Biology 89, 246- 255.
8) Cottalasso, D., Barisione, G., Fontana, L., Domenicotti, C., Pronzato, M.A. and Nanni, G. (1994) Impairment of lipoglycoprotein metabolism in rat liver cells induced by 1,2-dichloroethane, Ocupational and Environmental Medicine 51, 281-285.
9) Edlund, C., Soderberg, M., Dallner, G. (1992) Ubiqiuinone, dolichol metabolism in aging and Alzheimer's disease, Biochem. Cell. Biol. 70, 422-428.
10) Tollbon, O, Chojnacki, T, Dallner, G. (1992) Transfer of Liposomes Containing Dolichol into Isolated Hepatocytes, Lipids. 27, 248-254.
11) Roine, R.P., Turpeinen, U, Ylikahri, R, Salaspuro, M.,MD. (1987) Urinary Dolichol-A New Marker of Alcholism, Alcohol. Clin. Exp. Res. 11, 525-527.
12) Stetter, F., Gaertner, H.J., Mann, G., Breyer-Plaff, U. (1991) Urinary Dolichol- A Doubtful Marker of Alcoholism, Alcohol. Clin. Exp. Res. 15, 938-941.
13) Marino, M, Bruscalupi, G., Manzi, P., Rivabene, R., Trentalance, A. (1994) Changes in Plasma Dolichol Levels, Transport, and Hepatic Delivery During Rat Liver Regeneration, Metabolism. 43, 677-680.
14) Edlund, C., Ericsson, J., Dallner, G. (1987) Change in hepatic dolichol and dolichyl monophosphate caused by treatment of rats with inducers of the endoplasmic reticulum and peroxisomes and during ontogeny, Chem.Biol. Interact. 62, 191-208.
15) Lieber, C.S. and De Carli, L.M. (1989) Liquid diet technique of ethanol administration: 1989 update, Alcohol and Alcoholism 24, 197-211.
16) Rip, J.W., Rupar, C.A., Ravi, K.and Carroll, K.K. (1985) Distribution, metabolism and function of dolichol and polyprenols, Progress in Lipid Research 24, 269-309.
17) Chojnacki, T. and Dallner, G. (1988) The biological role of dolichol, Biochemical Journal 251, 1-9.
18) Eggens, I., Eriksson, L.C., Chojnacki, T. and Dallner, G. (1984) Role of dolichyl phosphate in regulation of protein glycosylation in 2-acetylaminofluorene-induced carcinogenesis in rat liver, Cancer Research 44, 799-805.
19) Guasch, R., Renau-Piqueras, J., and Guerri, C. (1992) Chronic ethanol consumption induces accumulation of proteins in the liver Golgi apparatus and decreases galactosyltransferase activity, Alcoholism. Clinical & Experimental Research 16, 942- 948.
20) Ghosh, P., Liu, Q.H. and Laskhman, M.R., (1995) Long-term ethanol exposure impairs glycosylation of both N- and O- glycosylated proteins in rat liver, Metabolism, 44, 890-898.

21) Ingelman-Sundberg, M., Johansson, I., Yin, H., Terelius, Y., Eliasson, E., Clot, P. and Albano, E. (1993) Ethanol-inducible Cytochrome P4502E1: genetic polymorphism, regulation, and possible role in the etiology of alcohol-induced liver disease, Alcohol 10, 447-452.

22) Pronzato, M.A., Cottalasso, D., Domenicotti, C., Tenca, C., Traverso, N., Nanni, G. and Marinari, U. M. (1990) Effects of CCl4 poisoning on metabolism of dolichol in rat liver microsomes and Golgi apparatus, Free Radical Research Communications 11, 267-277.

23) Marinari, U.M., Pronzato, M.A., Pizzorno, R., Cottalasso, D., Maloberti, G., Domenicotti, C., Gazzo, P. and Nanni, G. (1993) Acetaldehyde-induced impairment of protein glycosylation in rat liver Golgi apparatus, Biochemistry and Molecular Biology International 29, 1131-1138.

CHAPTER 5

COMPARTMENTATION AND REDOX STATE OF THIOLS AND PROTEINS DURING ACUTE ETHANOL INTOXICATION IN RATS

E. ALTOMARE, G. VENDEMIALE, I. GRATTAGLIANO, A. SIGNORILE, A. PISTONE, M. CASSANO, O. ALBANO

Dipartimento di Medicina Interna, Università di Bari

SUMMARY

Ethanol is known to affect the cellular content of glutathione and to enhance the lipid peroxidation of biological membranes. However, little is known on intracellular thiol distribution during alcohol intoxication. We report the effect of acute alcohol intoxication on the intracellular compartmentation of free and protein sulfhydryls and the protein redox status in the rat. Oral administration of 25% ethanol (4g/kg) significantly decreased the hepatic concentration of glutathione in cytosol, mitochondria and nuclei. Also, significant changes in the content of sulfhydryl proteins and glutathione bound to proteins were noticed in liver mitochondria, while an enhanced rate of carbonyl protein formation was observed in all the subcellular fractions. The inhibition of acetaldehyde metabolism, but not that of ethanol, exaggerated the observed alterations; in particular, thiols and proteins resulted both oxidatively damaged to a higher extent especially in the mitochondrial compartment. These data indicate that acute ethanol administration differently impairs the redox status of thiols and proteins in the subcellular fractions of rat liver; these alterations seem to depend on acetaldehyde rather than ethanol itself and may be included among the mechanisms underlying alcoholic liver injury.

Introduction

Changes of the redox status and metabolism of endogenous sulfhydryls have been involved in several mechanisms of hepatocellular injury following metabolic activation of xenobiotics (1,2). However, the effect of acute ethanol exposure on the status of hepatic thiols and proteins have not been completely clarified. In fact, while high dose of ethanol depletes hepatic glutathione (GSH) by impairing the synthesis or forming adducts with acetaldehyde (2,3), little is known about the effect of ethanol on intracellular sulfhydryl proteins (P-SH), which are representative of major cell functions. As well, not much is reported on the effect of

P. Gentilini and M. U. Dianzani. New Trends in Hepatology, 42-47

ethanol on nuclear thiols, known to be effective in repair of DNA sequences from oxygen and chemical radical attack (4). Indeed, ethyl radicals can damage cellular molecules including proteins and DNA; this may be of clinical interest, since alcohol intoxication is thought to cause nucleic base mutation and impairment of the repair and surveillance systems (5,6).

Acute ethanol intoxication

In recent experiments in our laboratory, we evaluated the effect of acute alcohol intoxication on the intracellular compartmentation of free and protein sulfhydryls and on the protein redox status; moreover, the effect of the inhibition of ethanol/acetaldehyde metabolisms on the above parameters was also investigated. Male Sprague-Dawley rats, overnight fasting, received 25% ethanol solution (4g/kg) or an isocaloric carbohydrate. After 6h animals were decapitated and the livers removed. Another group of animals received, by intraperitoneal injection, 1 mmol/kg of 4-methylpyrazole (4-MP), an inhibitor of alcohol dehydrogenase (ADH), in a neutralized 0.1 M saline, 30 min prior to ethanol, or cyanamide (15 mg/kg), an aldehyde dehydrogenase (ALDH) inhibitor, as a 0.15% saline solution, 60 min prior to ethanol. From liver homogenate, mitochondria and nuclei were separately isolated.
The determination of glutathione bound to proteins (PS-SG) was performed on proteins and the intracellular content of oxidized proteins was evaluated by measuring the carbonyl protein concentration.

Results

Acute ethanol intoxication significantly decreased the GSH concentration in all the subcellular fractions of the liver (Tab.1).

Table 1: Total glutathione (GSH) concentrations in liver cytosol, mitochondria and nuclei of rats receiving: carbohydrate (controls), 4g/kg of 25% ethanol p.os, 1 mmol/kg 4-methylpyrazole (4-MP) i.p. 30 min prior to ethanol administration, 15 mg/kg cyanamide i.p. 60 min prior to ethanol administration. GSH is expressed as nmol/mg protein.

	Cytosol	Mitochondria	Nuclei
Controls	33.4±4.1	7.1±1.3	35.2±3.1
Ethanol	21.5±4.1*	4.3±1.0*	22.4±3.1*
Ethanol + 4-MP	32.1±6.1	6.9±1.2	31.6±5.1
Ethanol + Cyanamide	14.6±3.1**^	2.1±0.6**^	16.2±4.0**^

* $p<0.01$ and ** $p<0.001$ compared to controls; ^ $p<0.01$ compared to ethanol

Animals receiving ethanol also showed decreased P-SH and increased PS-SG contents in mitochondria and nuclei compared to controls; no such alterations were noticed in the cytosol (Tab.2 and Tab.3, respectively).

Table 2: Sulfhydryl protein (P-SH) concentrations in liver cytosol, mitochondria and nuclei of rats receiving: carbohydrate (controls), 4g/kg of 25% ethanol p.os, 1 mmol/kg 4-methylpyrazole (4-MP) i.p. 30 min prior to ethanol administration, 15 mg/kg cyanamide i.p. 60 min prior to ethanol administration. P-SH is expressed as nmol/mg protein.

	Cytosol	Mitochondria	Nuclei
Controls	40.7±5.1	38.4±3.8	37.9±3.8
Ethanol	33.1±4.1*	20.5±4.1*	30.7±4.3*
Ethanol + 4-MP	37.2±4.3	36.2±5.6	34.2±5.1
Ethanol + Cyanamide	19.8±3.5**^	13.4±3.8**^	21.2±4.8**^

* p<0.01 and ** p<0.001 compared to controls; ^ p<0.01 compared to ethanol

Table 3: Glutathione bound to proteins (PS-SG) concentrations in liver cytosol, mitochondria and nuclei of rats receiving: carbohydrate (controls), 4g/kg of 25% ethanol p.os, 1 mmol/kg 4-methylpyrazole (4-MP) i.p. 30 min prior to ethanol administration, 15 mg/kg cyanamide i.p. 60 min prior to ethanol administration. PS-SG is expressed as pmol -SH/mg protein.

	Cytosol	Mitochondria	Nuclei
Controls	98±7	102±6	104±7
Ethanol	159±17*	179±20*	136±20
Ethanol + 4-MP	107±12	105±11	110±16
Ethanol + Cyanamide	194±22**^	211±21**^	186±21**

* p<0.01 and ** p<0.001 compared to controls; ^ p<0.01 compared to ethanol

Moreover, acute ethanol administration significantly enhanced the rate of carbonyl protein formation in cytosol, mitochondria and nuclei (Tab.4).

Table 4: Carbonyl protein concentrations in liver cytosol, mitochondria and nuclei of rats receiving: carbohydrate (controls), 4g/kg of 25% ethanol p.os, 1 mmol/kg 4-methylpyrazole (4-MP) i.p. 30 min prior to ethanol administration, 15 mg/kg cyanamide i.p. 60 min prior to ethanol administration. Data are expressed as nmol carbonyl groups/mg protein.

	Cytosol	**Mitochondria**	**Nuclei**
Controls	1.68±0.21	1.26±0.12	1.54±0.18
Ethanol	2.08±0.22	1.87±0.19	2.20±0.21
Ethanol + 4-MP	1.76±0.17	1.38±0.17	1.66±0.22
Ethanol + Cyanamide	2.41±0.28**	2.79±0.36**^	2.31±0.26**

** $p<0.001$ compared to controls and ^ $p<0.01$ compared to ethanol

Administration of 4-MP prior to ethanol slightly decreased the concentrations of GSH (Tab.1) and P-SH (Tab.2), showing a protective effect against ethanol toxicity. By contrast, pretreatment with cyanamide significantly enhanced the effect of ethanol; in fact, the cytosolic, mitochondrial and nuclear contents of GSH and P-SH (Tab.1 and Tab.2, respectively) were further decreased in cyanamide pretreated animals.

As reported in Tab.2 and Tab.4 the levels of PS-SG and carbonyl proteins were subjected to a further significant increase after ethanol only in animals pretreated with cyanamide; 4-MP administration appeared to be devoid of any effect.

Considerations

Ethanol administration has been reported to impair the antioxidant defence of the cell and to induce lipid peroxidation both in humans (7) and experimental animals (8,9). Acute ethanol intoxication resulted in a significant fall of cytosolic, mitochondrial and nuclear concentrations of GSH and P-SH. Recently, acute ethanol severely impaired the protein and DNA redox state in mitochondria (10), these being more important than those to lipids (7). Also, alterations in the mitochondrial levels of GSH, have been recently associated to structural and functional changes of mitochondrial ATP synthase (11).

Ethanol is known to exert selective mitochondrial toxicity (12) and GSH depletion has been reportad to increase the mitochondrial susceptibility to oxidant stress (13). In agreement with these observations, the fall of GSH and P-SH, after acute ethanol adiministration, was closely related with increased formation of oxidized proteins, as shown by the increased concentrations of PS-SG and carbonyl proteins. The enhanced oxidation rate of proteins by cyanamide pretreatment suggests that acetaldehyde, and not directly ethanol, is responsible for the reported effects. The delayed mitochondrial oxidation of acetaldehyde, due to the inhibition of its metabolism, selectively enhanced the ethanol-induced damage to mitochondria by decreasing the GSH content and increasing protein oxidation. In conditions of free thiol deficiency, it is likely that free radicals attack P-SH, thus transforming them in radicalic proteins, which promptly react to form disulfide bridges with free or protein sulfhydryls. In this view, the rate of GSH bound to proteins may account also for a part of GSH oxidation.

The existence of a nuclear compartmentation of GSH is currently under investigation. The reported results did not show any nuclear/cytoplasmic concentration gradient for GSH; in fact, the rate of nuclear GSH depletion by acute ethanol seems to parallel that of cytosolic one. Also in the nucleus, the loss of GSH was associated to a fall of P-SH content and to increased protein oxidation; the latter is of clinical interest since proteins are normally bound to DNA and they also serve for activation of DNA sequences (14).

In conclusion, acute ethanol intoxication severely affects the intracellular distribution and redox status of sulfhydryl compounds; these changes appear to depend on acetaldehyde rather than ethanol toxicity and are closely associated with the production of oxidized proteins.

REFERENCES

1. Sood C, O'Brien PJ. Molecular mechanisms of chloroacetaldehyde-induced cytotoxicity in isolated rat hepatocytes. Biochem Pharmacol 1993;46:1621-1626.

2. Lauterburg BH, Davies S, Mitchell JR. Ethanol suppresses hepatic glutathione synthesis in rat in vivo. J Pharmacol Exp Ther 1984;230:7-11.

3. Strubelt O, Younes M, Urch T, Breining H, Pentz R. Hepatotoxicity of acetaldehyde in rats. Toxicol Lett 1987;39:77-84.

4. Smoluk GD, Fahey RC, Ward JF. Interaction of glutathione and other low molecular weight thiols with DNA: evidence for counterion condensation and coion depletion near DNA: Radiat Res 1988;114:3-10.

5. Diehl AM, Bisgaard HC, Kren BT, Steer CJ. Ethanol interferes with regeneration-associated changes in biotransforming enzymes: a potential mechanism underlying ethanol's carcinogenicity? Hepatology 1991;13:722-727.
6. Farinati F, Zhou ZC, Bellah J, Lieber CS, Garro AJ. Effect of chronic ethanol consumption on activation of nitrosopyrrolidine to a mutagen by rat upper alimentary tract, lung and hepatic tissue. Drug Met Disp 1985;13:210-214.
7. Vendemiale G, Altomare E, Grattagliano I, Albano O. Increased plasma levels of glutathione and malondialdehyde after acute ethanol ingestion in humans. J Hepatol 1989;9:359-365.
8. Shaw S, Jayatilleke E, Ross WA, Gordon ER, Lieber CS. Ethanol-induced lipid peroxidation potentiation by long-term alcohol feeding and attenuation by methionine. J Lab Clin Med 1981;98:417-424.
9. Kawase T, Kato S, Lieber CS. Lipid peroxidation and antioxidant defence systems in rat liver after chronic ethanol feeding. Hepatology 1989;10:815-821.
10. Wieland P, Lauterburg BH. Oxidation of mitochondrial proteins and DNA following administration of ethanol. Biochem Biophys Res Commun 1995;213:815-819.
11. Vendemiale G, Guerrieri F, Grattagliano I, Didonna I, Muolo L, Altomare E. Mitochondrial oxidative phosphorylation and intracellular glutathione compartmentation during rat liver regeneration. Hepatology 1995;21:1450-1454.
12. Rottenberg H, Robertson DE, Rubin E. The effect of ethanol on the temperature dependence of respiration and ATPase activities of rat liver mitochondria. Lab Invest 1980;42:318-326.
13. Fernandez-Checa JC, Garcia-Ruiz C, Ookthens M, Kaplowitz N. Impaired uptake of glutathione by hepatic mitochondria from chronic ethanol-fed rats. Tracer kinetic studies in vitro and in vivo and susceptibility to oxidant stress. J Clin Invest 1991;87:397-405.
14. Tan KH, Meyer DJ, Gillies N, Ketterer B. Detoxification of DNA hydroperoxide by glutathione transferases and the purification and characterization of glutathione transferases of the rat liver nucleous. Biochem J 1988;254:841-845.

CHAPTER 6

POSSIBLE ROLE OF ETHANOL-DERIVED FREE RADICALS IN THE PATHOGENESIS OF ALCOHOL-INDUCED LIVER DAMAGE

E. ALBANO, P. CLOT, M. PAROLA[#], and M. U. DIANZANI[#].

Department of Medical Sciences and [#]Experimental Medicine and Oncology, University of Turin, Turin, Italy.

Summary

In spite of decades of researches the biochemical mechanisms responsible for the hepatotoxic action consequent to alcohol abuse have not yet been completely elucidated [1]. Acetaldehyde, the main product of ethanol oxidation, is generally considered to be main responsible for the damaging effects associated to alcohol abuse [1]. In recent years, however, an increasing number of studies have suggested that, beside acetaldehyde, free radical intermediates might be involved in the pathogenesis of alcohol toxicity.

1. Evidences for the formation of ethanol-derived free radical metabolites.

1.1 EXPERIMENTAL EVIDENCES FOR THE FORMATION OF HYDROXY-ETHYL FREE RADICALS DURING ETHANOL METABOLISM

The possible role of free radicals in causing alcohol-induced liver injury has received an important experimental support by the use of Electron Spin Resonance (ESR) spectroscopy, in combination with spin trapping technique, which has shown that a free radical intermediate originates during the hepatic metabolism of ethanol [3]. This radical species, identified as 1-hydroxyethyl radical, is produced *in vitro* by both rat and human liver microsomes incubated in the presence of ethanol and NADPH [3] and its formation is associated with the activity of the ethanol-inducible form of cytochrome P450, known as CYP2E1 isozyme [4]. Although the generation of hydroxyethyl radicals represents a minor pathway in the

P. Gentilini and M. U. Dianzani. New Trends in Hepatology, 48-55

metabolism of ethanol, these radicals have also been detected *in vivo* in the bile of experimental animals following an acute ethanol treatment [5,6]. Further evidence supporting the *in vivo* generation of hydroxyethyl radical during chronic ethanol intake have come from experiments conducted in intragastrically ethanol-fed rats. In these animals we have observed that the formation of hydroxyethyl free radicals increases 7 folds during chronic ethanol-treatment [7]. Such an effect is completely prevented by the simultaneous treatment of the rats with diallysulphide or phenylethylthiocyanate, two compounds that interfere with the induction of CYP2E1 by ethanol [8]. The role of CYP2E1 in the generation of hydroxyethyl radicals during ethanol feeding is further supported by the presence of a linear correlation ($r = 0.732$; $p<0.002$) between the individual liver content of CYP2E1 and the amount of hydroxyethyl radicals detected in the same liver preparations [7].

1.2 CLINICAL EVIDENCE FOR THE FORMATION OF HYDROXY- ETHYL FREE RADICALS IN HUMANS

Since ethical reasons whould not allow the use of spin trapping technique in humans, the possible formation of hydroxyethyl radicals in drinkers has been recently investigated by immunological methods taking advantage of the fact that hydroxyethyl radicals are able to interact with proteins forming stable adducts [9]. Preliminary studies have shown that, when injected into rabbits, hydroxyethyl-proteins adducts are immunogenic and lead to the formation of IgGs that specifically recognize the hydroxyethyl epitope independently from the carrier protein [10]. Similar antibodies were also observed in rat chronically exposed to alcohol [7] suggesting the possibility of using the presence of anti-hydroxyethyl radical antibodies as a marker for the formation of ethanol-derived radicals in subjects abusing of alcohol. To investigate this point a microplate enzyme linked immunoabsorbent assay (ELISA) has been developed employing as antigen human serum albumin reacted with chemically produced hydroxyethyl radicals.

Using this assay we have observed that sera of alcoholic cirrhotics contain both IgGs and IgAs which recognize proteins modified by hydroxyethyl radicals, while practically no reaction is present with the sera of healthy controls or cirrhotics without evidence of alcohol abuse (Fig. 1)[11]. The antibodies detected in the sera of alcoholic patients are specific for hydroxyethyl radical-derived epitopes and do not cross react with acetaldehyde-modified albumin [11]. The presence of IgGs reacting with hydroxyethyl radical epitopes has been observed not only among patients with alcoholic liver disease (about 90% positivity), but also in heavy drinkers without clinical signs of hepatic damage (78-84% positivity). In both these groups anti-hydroxyethyl radical IgGs titres slowly declined upon abstinence and rapidly rise again, while drinking is resumed.

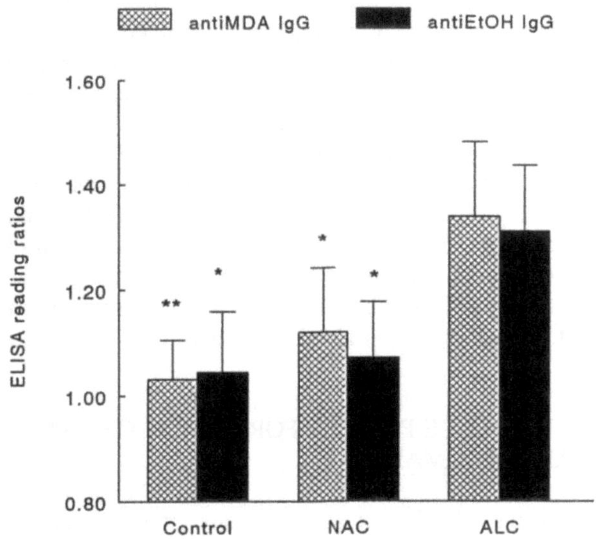

Levels of IgGs against hydroxyethy radicals (antiEtOH) or MDA (antiMDA) adducts with human serum albumin detected in the sera of healthy controls (n° 20), alcoholic cirrhotics (ALC) (n° 30) or cirrhotics without alcohol abuse (NAC) (n°20). The values are expressed as ratios between the spectrophotometric readings in the ELISA wells containing modified or native albumin, respectively. Statistical significance versus ALC * $p<0.05$; ** $p< 0.01$.

These observations not only confirm that hydroxyethyl radicals are actually produced in humans as consequence of excessive alcohol intake, but also demonstrate that alcohol abuse stimulates a specific immunoreaction against radical species derived from ethanol.

Studies aimed to characterize the proteins involved in the stimulation of immune reactions towards hydroxyethyl radicals have shown that anti-hydroxyethyl radical IgGs from alcoholics have higher affinity for hydroxyethyl radical adducts produced in liver microsomes during ethanol metabolism. By immunoblotting procedures it has been possible to demonstrate that at least four microsomal proteins with molecular weights of 78 kD, 60 kD, 52 kD and 40 kD, respectively, can be targets of anti-hydroxyethyl radical antibodies. The band at 52 kD is recognized by 86% of the sera examined, whereas immunoreactivity towards the other bands is observed in 30-48 % of the cases. The 52 kD protein has been identified by combined immunoblotting and immunoprecipitation techniques as ethanol-inducible CYP2E1 [12].

2. Possible involvement of hydroxyethyl free radicals in causing immuno-mediated liver injury

It has been demonstrated that alcoholic liver disease is associated with the presence of circulating antibodies directed against antigenic determinants in Mallory bodies and hepatocyte plasma membranes as well as by the detection of lymphocyte-mediated reactions against liver cells [13]. These immunological reactions have been ascribed to the binding of acetaldehyde to several proteins, since either experimental animals exposed to alcohols and alcoholic patients have high titers of immunoglobulins reacting with acetaldehyde-protein adducts [14]. However, in humans the formation of anti-acetaldehyde antibodies is not fully specific for alcoholic damage, since these antibodies can also be found in patients with liver diseases unrelated to alcohol [15]. Whether the development of antibodies directed against liver proteins modified by hydroxyethyl radicals might contribute to the pathogenesis of alcoholic liver lesions is still unknown, but the use of intragastrically alcohol-fed rats would probably help in clarifying this question. This experimental model consists in the administration to rats of high amounts of alcohol in association with a liquid diet through a permanent intragastric cannula and allows to reproduce in the rodents some of the histological features of human alcoholic hepatic injury in the form of steatosis, inflammation, focal necrosis and fibrosis [16]. We have recently observed that rats fed intragastrically with ethanol have increased levels of hydroxyethyl radical-derived antigens as well as of IgGs directed against these latter epitopes [7]. CYP2E1 inhibitors diallylsulphide and phenylethylthiocyanate completely prevent the formation of these antigenic determinants and of the relative antibodies [7]. Moreover, the levels of hydroxyethyl radical-derived epitopes in the microsomes of these rats are positively correlated to the extent of liver damage ($r = 0.626$; $p < 0.02$) [7].

Several studies have demonstrated that immune reactions are involved in the pathogenesis of hepatic damage induced drugs such as halothane, tienilic acid, dihydralazine, methyldopa and clometacin [17,18]. In the case of hepatitis caused by tienilic acid and dihydralazine the immune reaction appears to be directed against microsomal proteins and particularly the cytochrome P450 isoenzymes CYP2C9 and CYP1A2 [12]. However, differently from autoantibodies interacting with CYP2C9 and CYP1A2 [12], the antibodies here described mainly recognize CYP2E1 that has been modified by the binding of hydroxyethyl radicals. In this respect, the antibodies towards hydroxyethyl radical adducts share some analogies with those directed against trifluoroacetylated proteins that have been described in patients undergoing halothane-induced hepatitis [17]. By analogy, we can postulate that the formation of anti-hydroxyethyl radical antibodies in alcoholic patients might involve the oxidation of ethanol in the endoplasmic reticulum by the action of CYP2E1 with the generation of hydroxyethyl radicals which can then bind to the cytochrome itself and neighbouring proteins. Following cell death, the degradation of the modified proteins by macrophages might lead to the presentation of the peptides containing the hydroxyethyl moieties in association with major histocompatibility complex (MHC) class II molecules to $CD4^+$ helper T lymphocytes that can stimulate immature B lymphocytes to clonal expansion and differentiate into plasmocytes able to secrete anti-hydroxyethyl radical antibodies.

Early studies have shown that the incubation of hepatocytes from untreated or ethanol-fed rabbits with the sera of alcoholic patients, followed by the addition of peripheral blood mononuclear cells from normal subjects, leads to the destruction of ethanol-treated hepatocytes, but not of the cells from control animals [19]. The antigens involved in the above reactions have not been characterized. However, experiments in our laboratory using immunofluorescence and confocal microscopy have recently shown that anti-hydroxyethyl radical IgGs from alcoholic patients react with the outer side of the plasma membrane of intact hepatocytes incubated in the presence of alcohol, but not with control cells [20]. Moreover, the immunofluorescence due to anti-hydroxyethyl radical antibodies appear to co-localize on the cell surface with that of CYP2E1 [20]. Thus, the alkylation of plasma membrane CYP2E1 by hydroxyethyl radicals might be important in causing antibody-dependent cell-mediated cytotoxicity reactions toward the hepatocytes. Alternatively, the presentation on the hepatocytes surface of peptides containing the hydroxyethyl radical epitopes in association with MCH class I molecules can be postulated to trigger a $CD8^+$ cytotoxic T lymphocyte-mediated reaction towards the cells where hydroxyethyl radicals are formed.

3. Role of hydroxyethyl free radicals in causing oxidative injury associated with alcohol abuse.

Several authors have reported that both acute and chronic alcohol administration to rats increases the formation of lipid peroxidation products, such as lipoperoxides, conjugated dienes and malonildialdehyde (MDA) and decreases tissue levels of antioxidants [2]. Similar studies performed in humans demonstrate that markers of lipid peroxidation are higher in liver biopsies obtained from heavy drinkers than in specimens from non drinkers [2]. An increased breath exhalation of pentane, an other indicator of peroxidative damage, can also be observed in patients with alcoholic liver disease [21]. We have recently reported that in alcoholic cirrhotics blood levels of MDA and lipid hydroperoxides are about five fold higher than in cirrhotics without alcohol abuse or healthy controls [22]. Moreover, among

alcohol abusers, those with a daily alcohol intake above 200 g have amounts of peroxidation products 2-3 fold higher than those drinking daily less than 200 g of alcohol, irrespectively to the extent of liver injury [22]. The occurence of lipid peroxidation in alcoholic cirrhotics is further supported by the detection of antibodies towards MDA protein adducts in the sera of alcoholic patients (Fig. 1).
The mechanisms responsible for the stimulation of lipid peroxidation by alcohol might involve the generation of reactive oxygen species, such as superoxide anion (O_2^-) and hydrogen peroxide (H_2O_2) from several sources including mitochondrial respiratory chain, xanthine oxidase or aldehyde oxidase, microsomal monoxygenase enzymes and activated phagocytic cells, mostly infiltrating granulocytes and Kuppfer cells [2]. In the presence of trace amount of transition metals, in particular iron, O_2^- and H_2O_2 generated from these sources lead to the formation of highly reactive hydroxyl radicals ($OH\cdot$), which are responsible for the oxidation of biological constituents [2]. The contribution of iron in the genesis of oxidative alcohol damage is supported by the recent observation that supplementation with iron of intragastrically ethanol-fed rats greatly potentiates the prooxidant action of ethanol [23]. The possibility that the interaction of hydroxyethyl radicals with lipid might also be responsible for the stimulation of lipid peroxidation is suggested by the observation that either in ethanol-fed rats and in alcoholic patients there is a positive correlation between the titres of antibodies against hydroxyethyl radicals and those against MDA-protein adducts ($r = 0.528$; $p < 0.01$).
The interest for the role played by lipid peroxidation in the pathogenesis of alcohol toxicity has received new impulse by the observation that in intragastrically ethanol-fed rats lipid peroxidation follows the chronic administration of alcohol and there is a good correlation between the levels of peroxidative products, detectable in the liver and in the blood of these animals, and the extent of histological liver lesions, particularly hepatic fibrosis [24-26]. The mechanisms responsible for the fibrogenic action of lipid peroxidation appear to involve the stimulation by aldehydic end-products of lipid peroxidation of collagen synthesis by hepatic stellate cells [27] as well as the release of fibrogenetic cytochines from Kuppfer cells [28].

4. Conclusions

The results of combined experimental and clinical studies demonstrate that hydroxyethyl free radical intermediates are produced during ethanol metabolism by microsomal CYP2E1-dependent monoxygenase system. These free radical metabolites can be involved in the pathogenesis of alcoholic liver injury by triggering immunoallergic reaction towards hepatocytes. Furthermore, hydroxyethyl radicals can play a role in promoting lipid peroxidation reactions which appear to represent an important stimulus for the development of liver fibrosis.

References

1. Lieber, C.S.: Alcohol and the liver: 1994 update. *Gastroenterol* **106** (1994), 1085-1105.
2. Nordmann, R., Ribière, C., and Rouach, H.: Implication of free radical mechanisms in ethanol induced cellular injury. *Free Rad. Biol. Med.,* **12** (1992), 219-240.
3. Albano, E., Tomasi, A., Goria-Gatti, L., and Dianzani, M.U.: Spin trapping of free radical species produced during the microsomal metabolism of ethanol. *Chem-Biol Interact* **65** (1988), 223-234.
4. Albano, E., Tomasi, A., Goria-Gatti, L., Persson, J.O., Terelius, Y., Ingelman-Sundberg, M., Dianzani, M.U.: Role of ethanol-inducible cytochrome P-450 (P450IIE1) in catalysing the free radical activation of aliphatic alcohols. *Biochem Pharmacol* **41** (1991), 1895-1902.
5. Knecht, K.T., Bradfort, B.U., Mason, R.P. and Thurman, G.R.: In vivo formation of free radical metabolite of ethanol, *Mol Pharmacol* **38** (1990), 26-30.
6. Comoglio, A., Tomasi, A., Malandrino, S., Poli, G., and Albano, E.: Scavenging effect of silipide, a new silybin-phospholipid complex, on ethanol-derived free radicals. *Biochem Pharmacol* **50** (1995), 1313-1316.
7. Albano, E., Clot, P., Morimoto, M., Tomasi, A., Ingelman-Sundberg, M., and French, S.W.: Role of cytochrome P4502E1-dependent formation of hydroxyethyl free radicals in the development of liver damage in rats intragastrically fed with ethanol. *Hepatol* **23** (1996), 155-163.
8. Morimoto, M., Hagbjvrk, A-L., Wan, Y.J.Y., Fu, P.C., Ingelman-Sundberg, M., Albano, E., Clot, P., and French, S.W.: Modulation of alcoholic liver disease by cytochrome P4502E1 inhibitors. *Hepatol* **21** (1995), 11610-1617.
9. Albano, E., Parola, M., Comoglio, A., and Dianzani, M.U.: Evidence for the covalent binding of hydroxyethyl radicals to rat liver microsomal proteins. *Alcohol Alcohol* **28** (1993), 453-459.
10. Moncada, C., Torres, V., Vargese, E., Albano, E., and Israel, Y.: Ethanol-derived immuno-reactive species formed by free radical mechanisms. *Mol Pharmacol* **46** (1994), 786-791.
11. Clot, P., Bellomo, G., Tabone, M., Aricò, S., and Albano, E.: Detection of antibodies against proteins modified by hydroxyethyl free radicals in patients with alcoholic cirrhosis. *Gastroentrol* **108** (1995), 201-207.
12. Clot, P., Albano, E., Elliasson, E., Tabone, M., Aricò, S., Israel, Y., Moncada, C., and Ingelman-Sundberg, M.: Cytochrome P4502E1 hydroxyethyl radical adducts as the major antigenic determinant for autoantibody formation among alcoholics. *Gastroenterol* (submitted)
13. Klassen, L.W., Tuma, D., and Sorrell, M.F.: Immune mechanisms of alcohol-induced liver disease. *Hepatol* **22** (1995), 355-357.
14. Tuma, D., and Klassen, L.W.: Immune response to acetaldehyde-protein adducts in alcoholic liver disease. *Gastroenterol* **103** (1992), 1969-1973.
15. Worral, S., De Jersey, J., Shanley, B.C., and Wilce, P.A.: Antibodies against acetaldehyde-modified epitopes: presence in alcoholic, non-alcoholic liver disease and control subjects. *Alcohol Alcohol* **25** (1990), 509-517.
16. Tsukamoto, H., Towner, S.J., Ciofalo, L.M., and French, S.W.: Ethanol-induced liver fibrosis in rats fed high fat diet. *Hepatol* **6** (1986), 814-822.
17. Baune, P., Pessayre, D., Dansette, P., Mansuy, D., and Manns, M.: Autoantibodies against cytochrome P450: role in human diseases. *Adv Pharmacol* **30** (1994), 199-245.

18. Pessayre, D.: Role of reactive metabolites in drug-induced hepatitis. *J Hepatol* **23** (1995), (suppl. 1), 16-24.
19. Izumi, N., Hasumura, Y., and Tacheuchi, J.: Lymphocyte cytotoxicity for autologous human hepatocytes in alcoholic liver disease. *Clin Exp Immunol* **53** (1983), 219-224.
20. Clot, P., Parola, M., Bellomo, G., Tabone, M., Aricò, S., Ingelman-Sundberg, M., and Albano, E.: Human antibodies versus hydroxyethyl radical recognizes specific epitopes on the plasma membrane of isolated hepatocytes exposed to ethanol. *Hepatol* **22** (1995), 227A.1
21. Letteron, P., Duchettelle, V., Berson, A., Fromenty, B., Fish, C., Degott, C., Benhamou, P.J., and Pessayre, D.: Increased ethane exhalation, an in vivo index of lipid peroxidation, in alcohol abusers. *Gut* **34** (1993), 409-414.
22. Clot, P., Tabone, M., Aricò, S., and Albano, E.: Monitoring oxidative damage in patients with liver cirrhosis and different daily alcohol intake, *Gut* **35** (1994), 1637-1643.
23. Tzukamoto, H., Horne, W., Kamimura, S., Niemelä, O., Parkkila, S., Ylä-Herttuala, S., and Brittenham, G.M.: Experimental liver cirrhosis induced by alcohol and iron. *J Clin Invest* **96** (1995), 620-630.
24. French, S.W., Wong, K., Jui, L., Albano, E., Hagbjörk, A.-L., and Ingelman-Sundberg, M.: Effect of ethanol on cytochrome P-450 (CYP2E1), lipid peroxidation and serum protein adduct formation in relation to liver pathology pathogenesis. *Exp Mol Pathol* **58** (1993), 61-75.
25. Kamimura, S., Gaal, K., Britton, S.R., Bacon, B.R., Tridafilopoulos, G. and Tsukamoto, H.: Increased 4-hydroxynonenal levels in experimental alcoholic liver disease: Association of lipid peroxidation with liver fibrogenesis. *Hepatol* **16** (1992), 448-453.
26. Nanji, A.A., Khwaja, S., Tahan, S.R., and Sadrzadeh, H.S.M.: Plasma levels of a novel noncyclooxygenase-derived prostanoid (8-isoprostane) correlate with severity of liver injury in experimental alcoholic liver disease. *J Pharmacol Exp Ther* **269** (1994), 1280-1285.
27. Parola, M., Pinzani, M., Casini, A., Albano, E., Poli, G., Gentilini, A., Gentilini, P., and Dianzani, M.U.: Stimulation of lipid peroxidation or 4-hydroxynonenal treatment increases procollagen α-1(I) gene expression in humal liver fat-storing cells. *Biochem Biophys Res Commun* **194** (1993), 1044-1050.
28. Kamimura, S., and Tsukamoto, H.: Cytokine gene expression by Kupffer cells in experimental alcoholic liver disease. *Hepatol* **21** (1995), 1304-1309.

CHAPTER 7

HEPATIC IRON OVERLOAD INDUCED BY PHENYLHYDRAZINE: RELEASE OF IRON IN A FREE FORM AND DNA DAMAGE

M. COMPORTI, C. SIGNORINI, L. SUGHERINI, A. POMPELLA, L. CICCOLI & M. FERRALI

Istituto di Patologia Generale dell'Università di Siena - Via Aldo Moro, Siena

Summary

Incubation of mouse erythrocytes (RBC) with phenylhydrazine (Phz) and other oxidants induces release of redox-active iron from macromolecular complexes. This also occurs during *in vitro* RBC aging (24-48 hr aerobic incubation), and is accompanied by oxidation of membrane proteins, giving rise to the senescent cell antigen (SCA), a signal for the binding of IgG and removal by phagocytes. SCA formation (autologous IgG binding) also occur after incubation with Phz. Intracellular chelation of the released iron by ferrozine during the aerobic incubation prevents both membrane protein oxidation and SCA formation. Subchronic Phz intoxication of rats causes a striking increase in hepatic free iron; agarose-gel electrophoresis of liver DNA reveals a marked fragmentation, which is likely due to the release of reactive iron. The appearance of small γ-glutamyl transpeptidase-positive *foci* was also observed in the livers of the intoxicated animals. This may be of interest in view of the relationships between hemochromatosis and hepatocarcinogenesis.

As is known, iron plays a central role in generating harmful oxygen species. Its redox cycling, in fact, promotes the Fenton reaction which produces the potent oxidant, hydroxyl radical. Normally iron is transported and stored in specific proteins (1, 2) that prevent its reaction with reduced oxygen species. Thus to be redox cycling active iron has to be released from these complexes (3, 4).

Oxidant-induced iron release in erythrocytes. Our studies (5-7) have shown that iron is released in a free (desferrioxamine (DFO) chelatable) form when mouse erythrocytes are incubated with oxidizing agents such as phenylhydrazine, divicine, isouramil, acrolein, phenyl-hydroxylamine and others. In the experiments carried out with phenylhydrazine (analogous results were also obtained with the other toxins) we found that in native erythrocytes this drug (1 mM) induces iron release and methemoglobin formation, but not lipid peroxidation or hemolysis; while in erythrocytes previously depleted of GSH (by a short preincubation (10 min) with diethylmaleate, 1 mM), iron release and methemoglobin formation are accompanied by lipid peroxidation and hemolysis (5). It seems therefore that, only when the GSH level is severely

P. Gentilini and M. U. Dianzani. New Trends in Hepatology, 56-64

decreased, the phenylhydrazine-induced iron release is followed by lipid peroxidation and lysis.

The release of iron preceedes lipid peroxidation. The latter in turn precedes hemolysis (5). It seems therefore that the release of iron initiates a chain of reactions leading ultimately to lipid peroxidation and consequent hemolysis.

Intracellular iron chelation. Iron is released from hemoglobin (as we have observed (7) in experiments with reconstituited systems) and acts from the inside of the cell. In fact in experiments in which the released iron was chelated at intracellular level (in desferrioxamine preloaded cells) lipid peroxidation and hemolysis were prevented, which did not occur with extracellularly added desferrioxamine. The experimental design was the following (5): erythrocytes were preincubated with 0.1 or 10 mM DFO for 90 min. The cells were then recovered and extensively washed. The level of intracellular DFO was measured in a ghost-free hemolysate. The cells were then preincubated with DEM for 10 min, and finally incubated with phenylhydrazine.

Preincubation with 0.1 mM DFO resulted in an intracellular level of DFO (5.0 $\pm$ 0.5 μM) which was lower than that of the released iron (13.6 $\pm$ 0.6 μM). In this condition, lipid peroxidation and hemolysis still occurred. On the other hand, preincubation with 10 mM DFO resulted in an intracellular level of DFO (37.8 $\pm$ 4.0 μM) which was higher than that of the released iron (22.8 $\pm$ 2.5 μM). In this condition, lipid peroxidation and hemolysis were prevented (5).

In an additional experiment (5) erythrocytes were preincubated with 0.1 mM DFO for 15 min only. The intracellular concentration of DFO was relatively low (1.2 μM). DFO was not removed from the incubation medium; diethylmaleate and phenylhydrazine were subsequently added. The presence of DFO in the incubation medium did not prevent lipid peroxidation and hemolysis. It seems therefore that DFO is not acting from the outside of the cell, and that, only when DFO is present in the intracellular compartment in amounts equivalent to those of the released iron, are lipid peroxidation and hemolysis prevented.

As it is known (8, 9), DFO penetrates cells in minimal amounts only (it cannot penetrate at all human or calf erythrocytes). Therefore additional studies were carried out with substances capable of penetrating the cell and chelating iron. One of these substances is the flavonoid quercetin, which, contrary to its glucoside rutin, can cross the cell membrane. As shown by the absorption spectra, quercetin binds iron (shift of the absorption maximum from 377 to 423 nm upon the addition of increasing amounts of iron sulphate) and DFO extracts iron from the iron-quercetin complex (restoration of the quercetin spectrum). Therefore, in view of the iron-chelating capacity and of its capacity to enter cells, quercetin was tested for its ability to prevent the effects induced by phenylhydrazine on erythrocytes (10).

As mentioned above, incubation of GSH-depleted erythrocytes with phenylhydrazine (1 mM) produced, as usual, together with iron release and methemoglobin formation, also lipid peroxidation and hemolysis. The addition of quercetin in an amount (15 μM) lower than that of the released iron (27.7 ± 0.7 μM) did not prevent lipid peroxidation and hemolysis. On the other hand, the addition of quercetin in an amount (50 μM) higher than that of the released iron (26.8 ± 2.0 μM) completely prevented lipid peroxidation and hemolysis. The molar ratio of quercetin: iron is 2:1 in the complex, and therefore 50 μM of quercetin appears, in these experiments, able to chelate all the released iron (27 μM) in a semi-stoichiometric manner.

Results similar to those seen with phenylhydrazine were obtained (5) with the pyrimidine aglycones, divicine and isouramil, derived from vicine and convicine respectively, the potentially toxic glucosides contained in fava beans *(Vicia faba)*. Again, in erythrocytes previously depleted of GSH, divicin (1 mM) or isouramil (1 mM) induced, together with iron release and methemoglobin formation, also lipid peroxidation and hemolysis. Again, quercetin was able, when added in sufficient amounts (100 μM), to prevent lipid peroxidation and hemolysis.

With human erythrocytes divicine plus isouramil (0.5 plus 0.5 mM, respectively) did not induce lipid peroxidation or hemolysis even when the cells were depleted of GSH (10). However, they produced dramatic alterations of membrane proteins, such as an almost complete disappearance of a and b spectrin and band 3 (alterations known to occur, although to a lower extent, in glucose-6-phosphate dehydrogenase-deficient humans). The addition of quercetin (100 μM) completely prevented such membrane protein alterations, suggesting again that the latter ones are related to the release of iron.

Iron release and erythrocyte aging. A similar release of iron also occurs (11) during erythrocyte aging, induced experimentally by an aerobic incubation in buffer for 24-60 hr of erythrocytes (calf erythrocytes, in these experiments), and is accompanied by methemoglobin formation; whereas no substantial iron release nor massive methemoglobin production occurs when the incubation is carried out under anaerobic conditions, suggesting again the involvement of an oxidative stress in the release of iron. The release of iron is also accompanied by oxidative alterations of membrane proteins (11) and these alterations have been detected with both PAGE electrophoresis and infrared spectroscopy. PAGE electrophoresis shows the appearance of new bands in the range of 66-45 kDal and other alterations. These bands, which are not seen after the anaerobic incubation, are considered as an index of erythrocyte aging and are thought to originate from the oxidative degradation of protein band 3. The oxidative alterations of membrane proteins have also been observed with infrared spectrometry, which shows a consistent increase of carbonyl groups (absorption increase in the 1685-1650 cm^{-1} range), and other alterations of the spectrum, all related to protein oxidation.

It is generally accepted (12-15) that the senescent cell antigen is generated by the oxidative degradation of some membrane proteins (expecially band 3) and acts as a specific signal for the termination of old cells by initiating the binding of autologous IgG and subsequent removal by phagocytes. In order to investigate whether the protein alterations seen during the aerobic incubation give rise to the appearance of senescent cell antigen, the membranes of erythrocytes incubated under aerobic or anaerobic conditions were challenged with autologous IgG. We found (11) that the membranes from aerobically incubated cells bind an extremely higher amount of autologous Ig than those from anaerobically incubated ones, indicating that the aerobic incubation gives rise to the senescent antigen.

Further studies were carried out in order to investigate whether the release of iron seen during the aerobic incubation coud be related to the appearance of senescent antigen (11). It was found that the incubation of erythrocytes with phenylhydrazine, which, as mentioned above, induces a marked release of iron, also promotes a considerable binding of autologous IgG to the erythrocyte membranes, that is senescent antigen formation. Also, divicin and isouramil, which, like phenylhydrazine, induce iron release, promote autologous IgG binding (10). Therefore, in three conditions in which a marked release or iron occurs - namely prolonged aerobic incubation, incubation with phenylhydrazine and incubation with divicine plus isouramil - the formation of senescent antigen also occurs.

Additional support for the hypothesis that the release of iron is indeed causally related to the formation of senescent antigen was offered by experiments in which iron chelators able to enter cells were used in the attempt to chelate intracellularly the iron released during the aerobic incubation. We found (11) that the addition of the iron chelator ferrozine during the aerobic incubation prevents the formation of senescent cell antigen, that is the binding of autologous IgG (which is identical to that seen after the anaerobic incubation and well below that occurring after the aerobic incubation in the absence of ferrozine), in spite of the fact that the amount of the released iron is nearly equal to that seen in the absence of the chelator. The addition of ferrozine also prevents all the oxidative alterations of membrane proteins seen with infrared spectroscopy.

These results strongly suggest that ferrozine, which freely enters the cells, is capable of chelating at intracellular level all the released iron and preventing in such way the alterations of membrane protein, probably produced by redox cycling of the released iron and related to the formation of senescent cell antigen.

Quercetin which, as shown above, enters the erythrocytes and binds iron, is able, when added during the aerobic incubation, to prevent partially but significantly the binding of autologous IgG (10), that is the formation of senescent cell antigen.

Finally, a progressive iron release occurs in human erythrocytes incubated aerobically for 40 and 60 hr in saline phosphate buffer or stored in their own plasma at 4°C for 15 and 35 days (11). Therefore an iron release seems to be really related to the aging of red blood cells and it is likely to occur even under physiological conditions.

In summary, these results suggest the possibility that a metal-catalyzed oxidation of membrane proteins underlies erythrocyte aging. A cation capable of redox-cycling, such as iron released from its complexes, would bind to a divalent cation binding site on the protein. Reaction with O_2 or H_2O_2 would generate active oxygen species which would oxidize amino acid residues near that cation binding site. The overall scheme would be the following: an oxidative stress in the erythrocytes will promote iron release which in turn will promote oxidation of membrane proteins and the consequent formation of senescent cell antigen, that is the aging of erythrocytes.

Since iron is also released in the erythrocytes during blood storing, chelation of iron at intracellular level could represent a means to prolong the storage time of blood in blood stores.

Action at a distance of the released iron. Further studies (16) have shown that iron released from an erythrocyte lysate under conditions of oxidative stress is able to induce oxidative reactions and membrane damage even at a distance. In these studies the incubation system was represented by a ghost-free erythrocyte lysate into which a dialysis tube containing the only buffer was dipped. The incubation was carried out aerobically in the presence of phenylhydrazine (1 mM) as an oxidizing agent. Phenylhydrazine induces iron release in the lysate. Free iron is capable crossing the dialysis membrane, since it can be recovered into the dialysis tube. At the end of the incubation the content of the dialysis tube was added to the ghosts of the same erythrocytes, or to microsomes from liver or brain. It was found that free iron, released in the lysate and diffused into the dialysis tube, is capable of inducing oxidative alterations, that is lipid peroxidation and protein aggregation, in ghosts or microsomes.

TABLE 1. Total and free iron in livers and spleens of rats treated with phenylhydrazine (Phz) or saline (controls) for 6 days.

	Liver total iron (nmol/g)	Liver free iron (nmol/g)	Liver ferritin (pmol/g)	Ferritin iron (nmol Fe/ /mol ferritin)	Spleen total iron (nmol/g)	Spleen free iron (nmol/g)
Controls	410 ± 100	7.15 ± 0.30	50.0 ± 10.2	1376 ± 248	1450 ± 150	7.6 ± 0.1
Phz	3240 ± 320	50.07 ± 7.40	85.5 ± 17.8	2393 ± 573	7760 ± 430	19.5 ± 2.2

Phenylhydrazine was given s.c. at the dose of 0.1 mmol/kg body wt. for 6 days. The animals were kept without treatment on the 7th and 8th day, and were sacrificed on the 9th day. Results are means ± S.E. of 4 animals (Ferrali *et al.,* unpublished results).

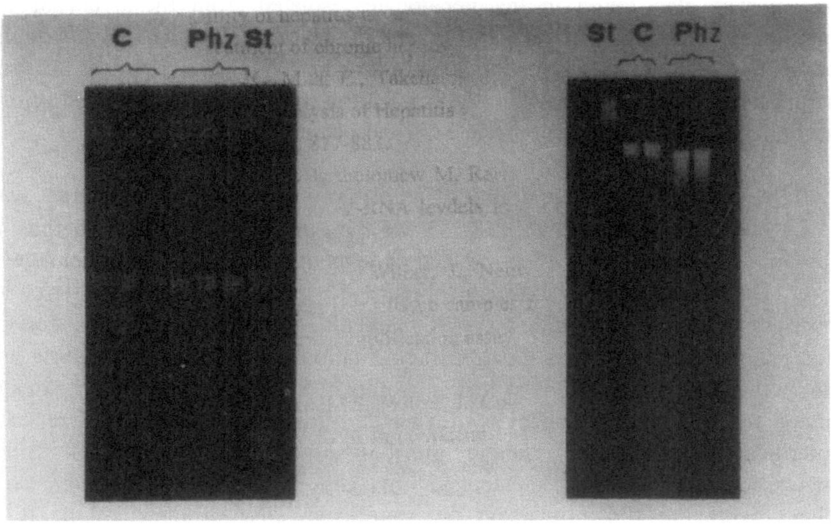

Figure 1. Agarose-gel electrophoresis of liver DNA from phenylhydrazine (Phz)-treated rats and corresponding controls. Phz treatment was performed as reported in Table 1. Liver DNA was prepared from either the whole tissue (left) or the isolated nuclear fraction (right). Electrophoresis was performed on 0.8% agarose gel and DNA was revealed with ethydium bromide under UV light. C, controls; Phz, phenylhydrazine-treated rats; St, DNA standards (top to bottom: 23, 9.4, 6.5, 4.4, 2.3, 2.0 Kbase-pairs).

These experiments clearly show that iron, once released from hemoglobin, is capable of activating oxidative reactions at a distance. In an *in vivo* situation, this may mean, for istance, that iron released from hemoglobin oxidation, as it occurs after extravascular hemolysis, can induce oxidative alterations in nearby cells, thus amplifying the hemorrhagic damage to a great extent.

Phenylhydrazine intoxication *in vivo* and iron release in the liver. The results of our experiments concerning phenylhydrazine intoxication *in vivo* are related to this phenomenon (17). We followed the model of subchronic intoxication with phenylhydrazine commonly used to obtain reticulocytosis. The intoxication resulted in a marked anemia and methemo-globinemia accompanied by a marked increase in spleen weight, obviously due to the increased hemocatheresis. The most interesting finding was that a striking increase (about 7 fold) in free iron occurs in the liver (Table 1). Such an increase was found in the ultrafiltered (protein-free) soluble fraction of the homogenate, and it was also found in the hepatocytes isolated from the livers of the intoxicated animals. Therefore it can be attributed to the hepatocellular component of the liver. Hepatic ferritin was also increased, as was its iron saturation (Table 1). The erythrocytes from the intoxicated rats showed on the second day of treatment the presence of senescent cell antigen.

DNA damage. Since the ability of redox cycling active iron to interact with DNA has been widely shown (18-21), we then investigated to see whether, in this model of phenylhydrazine-induced endogenous iron overload, a damage to liver DNA occurs. As shown in Figure 1, the DNA from the liver of phenylhydrazine-treated animals was markedly fragmented, as evidenced by agarose gel electrophoresis. Such a fragmentation appeared quite aspecific and not in the ladder-like pattern typical of apoptosis. Such a damage could be due to either reactive iron or phenylhydrazine (for instance formation of reactive intermediates from the hepatic metabolism of phenylhydrazine). Since incubation of isolated hepatocytes in culture or in suspension with phenylhydrazine did not result in significant DNA fragmentation, it is conceivable that the DNA damage seen after phenylhydrazine *in vivo* is due to the release of reactive iron in the liver cell rather than to hepatic metabolism of phenylhydrazine.

γ-Glutamyl transpeptidase (γ-GT)-positive *foci.* In view of the well known relationships between hepatic hemochromatosis and hepatocarcino-genesis, it appeared not unlikely that the capacity of iron to react with DNA represented a link between chronic iron overload and tumor initiation. In additional studies we have observed the appearance of little γ-GT-positive *foci* in the livers of animals treated with phenylhydrazine for various weeks. Although the appearance of γ-GT-positive *foci* is quite far from tumor formation, this result may open a new prospective in the studies of the relationships between iron release and tumor initiation.

In conclusion, the suggested pathway is the following: phenylhydrazine induces, through an oxidative stress, iron release in the erythrocyte. Free iron would promote, through oxidation of some membrane proteins, the formation of senescent antigen to which autologous Ig bind. The cells opsonized in such way are removed by the phagocyte system, which thus becomes iron overloaded. A general redistribution of iron, *via* transferrin, leads to an iron increase in the hepatocytes, and when the capacity of hepatocytes to maintain iron in a storage form (through ferritin) is overwhelmed, an increase in the free iron pool occurs, that is in the pool of iron present in low molecular weight molecules and catalytically active (22-24). Such free iron would interact with DNA causing an oxidative damage.

References

1. Crichton RR (1987) Iron metabolism and oxygen toxicity. Bioelectrochem. Bioenerg. 18: 105-116.

2. Crichton RR, Charloteaux-Wauters M (1987) Iron transport and storage. Eur. J. Biochem. 164: 485-506.

3. Halliwell B, Gutteridge JMC (1984) Oxygen toxicity, oxygen radicals, transition metals and disease. Biochem. J. 219: 1-14.

4. Halliwell B, Gutteridge JMC (1989) Free Radicals in biology and Medicine. 2nd Edition, Oxford: Clarendon Press.

5. Ferrali M, Signorini C, Ciccoli L, Comporti M (1992) Iron release and membrane damage in erythrocytes exposed to oxidizing agents, phenylhydrazine, divicine and isouramil. Biochem. J. 285: 295-301.

6. Ferrali M, Ciccoli L, Comporti M (1989) Allyl alcohol-induced hemolysis and its relation to iron release and lipid peroxidation. Biochem. Pharmacol. 38: 1819-1825.

7. Ferrali M, Ciccoli L, Signorini C, Comporti M (1990) Iron release and erythrocyte damage in allyl alcohol intoxication in mice. Biochem. Pharmacol. 40: 1485-1490.

8. Rice-Evans C, Baysal E, Singh S, Jones SA, Jones JG (1989) The interactions of desferrioxamine and hydroxypyridone compounds with haemoglobin and erythrocytes. FEBS Lett. 256: 17-20.

9. Lloyd JB, Cable H, Rice-Evans C (1991) Evidence that desferrioxamine cannot enter cells by passive diffusion. Biochem. Pharmacol. 41: 1361-1363.

10. Comporti M, Signorini C, Sugherini L, Caciotti B, Ciccoli L, Ferrali M (1995) Iron release, membrane protein oxidation, erythrocyte aging and effects of iron-chelation. Summer Meeting of the S.F.R.R., Budapest, July 27-29.

11. Signorini C, Ferrali M, Ciccoli L, Sugherini L, Magnani A, Comporti M (1995) Iron release, membrane protein oxidation and erythrocyte aging. FEBS Lett. 362: 165-170.

12. Kay MMB (1975) Mechanism of removal of senescent cells by human macrophages *in situ*. Proc. Nat. Acad. Sci. USA 72: 3521-3525.
13. Kay MMB (1981) Isolation of the phagocytosis-inducing IgG-binding antigen on senescent somatic cells. Nature 289: 491-494.
14. Kay MMB, Goodman SR, Sorensen K, Whitfield CF, Wong P, Zaki L, Rudloff V (1983) Senescent cell antigen is immunologically related to band 3. Proc. Nat. Acad. Sci. USA 80: 1631-1635.
15. Beppu M, Mizukami A, Nagoya M, Kikugawa K (1990) Binding of anti-band 3 autoantibody to oxidatively damaged erythrocytes. J. Biol. Chem. 265: 3226-3233.
16. Ferrali M, Signorini C, Ciccoli L, Comporti M (1993) Iron released from an erythrocyte lysate by oxidative stress is diffusible and in redox active form. FEBS Lett. 319: 40-44.
17. Comporti M, Signorini C, Sugherini L, Caciotti B, Pompella A, Ciccoli L, Ferrali M (1996) Hepatic iron overload induced by phenylhydrazine: release of iron in a free form and DNA damage. 5th Int. Symposium on Orthomolecular Medicine, Sao Paulo, March 20-22.
18. Loeb LA, James EA, Waltersdorph AM, Klebanoff SJ (1988) Mutagenesis by the autoxidation of iron with isolated DNA. Proc. Nat. Acad. Sci. USA 85: 3918-3922.
19. Dizdaroglu M, Rao G, Halliwell B, Gajewski E (1991) Damage to the DNA bases in mammalian chromatin by hydrogen peroxide in the presence of ferric and cupric ions. Arch. Bioch. Biophys. 285: 317-324.
20. Imlay JA, Chin SM, Linn S (1988) Toxic DNA damage by hydrogen peroxide through the Fenton reaction *in vivo* and *in vitro*. Science 240: 640-642.
21. Toyokuni S, Sagripanti J-L (1993) DNA single- and double-strand breaks produced by ferric nitrilotriacetate in relation to renal tubular carcinogenesis. Carcinogenesis 14: 223-227.
22. Miller JPG, Perkins DJ (1969) Model experiments for the study of iron transfer from transferrin to ferritin. Eur. J. Biochem. 10: 146-151.
23. Jacobs A (1977) Low molecular weight intracellular iron transport compounds. Blood 50: 433-439.
24. Weaver J, Pollack S (1989) Low-M_r iron isolated from guinea pig reticulocytes as AMP-Fe and ATP-Fe complexes. Biochem. J. 261: 787-792.

CHAPTER 8

THE EFFECTS OF DEVELOPMENT OF THE MDR1 PHENOTYPE ON CELL SUSCEPTIBILITY TO UNDERGOING LIPID PEROXIDATION AND IONIZING RADIATION.

ROBERTO MAZZANTI*§, ORNELLA FANTAPPIÈ*, PAOLA FABRIZIO*.

* *Istituto di Medicina Interna, Facoltà di Medicina e Chirurgia dell'Università di Firenze ed Istituto di Semeiotica Medica, Università di Parma, viale Gramsci, 14, Italy.*

SUMMARY

Resistance to anticancer drugs is frequently observed in cancer treatment. Cancer cells expressing the multiple drug resistant (MDR1) phenotype may be resistant to ionizing radiation used in radiotherapy as well as to cells with cytotoxic effect. We postulated that the common mechanism to explain these three different types of cell resistance to damaging agents is mediated by resistance to the toxic effect of free radicals. Experiments made to address this point showed that the MDR1 phenotype is not invariably associated with resistance to free radicals measured as susceptibility to undergoing lipid peroxidation or dying of ionizing radiation. Cancer cells can be resistant to free radical effects independently from the expression of the MDR1 phenotype. The induction of this phenotype by the transfection of the MDR1 gene in non transformed cells actually increases susceptibility to ionizing radiation and undergoing lipid peroxidation.

P-glycoprotein (P-gp) is a plasma membrane protein that is associated with the development of the so called multidrug resistant (mdr) phenotype . This characterizes several cancer cells that intrinsically possess or rapidly acquire drug resistance to chemically unrelated drugs. P-gp is a large protein that forms channels and transports drugs and other compounds such as cations , polypeptides and ATP, outside of cells. This protein is encoded by a small family of genes (mdr1, mdr2 and mdr3 in rodents and MDR1 and MDR2 in humans) that have been described in several organisms, from unicellular ones such as Plasmodium Falciparum or Saccharomyces Cerevisiae to primates (1). P-gps share a great part of their aminoacid sequence with some transport proteins of eukariotes and bacteria, suggesting that they are involved in the trasport of compounds that play a key role in the life of cells expressing this protein. Nomenclature of P-gp and correlated genes has been confusing because of the different names that have been given by different Author(s). More recently, considerable agreement has been achieved concerning the mdr1 (mouse) or MDR1 (human) gene, suggesting its involvement in conferring the drug resistant phenotype in cells and on mdr2, which seems to be involved in coding for the biliary protein transporter

P. Gentilini and M.U. Dianzani. New Trends in Hepatology, 65-73

of phospholipids in rats (2). The gene known as mdr3 in the mouse can be considered the human MDR1, whereas the mdr2 in the mouse is MDR3 in man. These three genes have strong homology and encode proteins that have similar but not identical sequences of amino acids suggesting similar but not identical characteristics and functions. Analysis of sequences of aminoacids that constitute P-gp has shown that the protein is constituted by two almost identical halves, each with 6 transmembrane spanning regions (hydrophobic region) and one ATP binding site.

P-gps, once they have been synthesized are phosphorilated, thereby activating their function. It has been proposed that the minimal functionally active P-gp consists in two identical parts, but in some cases, dimers or even tetramers of the proteins are formed to exert some function (3). If this hypothesis were true, the tetramers would have 48 transmembrane spanning domains with considerable influence, in our opinion , on membrane fluidity or susceptibility to ionizing radiation and membrane perturbing agents.

P-gp is an ATPase pump and the presence of ATP is essential to maintaining its function to transport drugs. Anything that inhibits ATP degradation also inhibits P-gp function. For this reason P-gp belongs to a superfamily of proteins called ATP -binding cassette (ABC) family or Traffic ATPases (4). One of the most important and known members of this family , the CFTR or cystic fybrosis gene product, has recently been cloned and sequenced. The mdr2 gene has been cloned and sequenced as well and it was found that its main function in the mouse was that of transporting biliary phospholipids (2).

In man, the MDR1 P-gp is expressed normally in many tissues where intense secretive process occurs. The adrenal cortex, intestine, kidney, liver, as well as brain endothelial cells, hematopoietic staminal cells, mucosa of gravid uterus and other tissues express P-gp in normal conditions. Its position in these cells is apical, suggesting that P-gp is involved in the process of active secretion such as detoxification from endogen and exogen xenobiotics (1).

In the liver, P-gp is mainly expressed in the biliary domain of the hepatocyte where the trasport of several conpounds is involved. It seems that both mdr1 and the mdr2 gene products are also expressed in the biliary domain. The former exports drugs, cations, steroids, cyclosporine and ATP from the hepatocyte, whereas the latter is responsible for secreting phospholipids.

The mdr1 phenotype can be inhibited in vitro by several drugs which inhibit the P-gp mediated transport. It has not been fully elucidated whether the inhibition of the mdr1 phenotype is a consequence of competition between P-gp substrates and inhibitors or whether inhibitors can act through other mechanisms. It is likely that both mechanisms are involved since it has been shown that some compounds such as steroids are not transported by P-gp, nevertheless they can inhibit its function. On the other hand, there are compounds that are transported but do not inhibit the P-gp function (5).

The fact that P-gp is expressed in both cancer cells with the mdr1 phenotype and in normal cells raises several questions. What is its physiological role in these different cell types? Why does P-gp expression increase in proliferating cells such as hepatocytes after hepatectomy? Furthermore, if the main function of P-gp in cancer cells is that of conferring drug resistance, what is the effect of its overexpression in cells that are not transformed? Recently, data obtained in patients with colon cancer or osteosarcoma treated with drugs that are not substrates for P-gp have pointed out that P-gp, although involved in mechanisms of drug resistance, may be a marker of prognosis rather than resistance to drugs (6). Does this mean that P-gp is a marker for malign tumors, but has a different meaning in cells that are not transformed? This issue has not been clarified.

Cells that express the MDR1 phenotype are resistant to several drugs whose metabolism leads to the production of oxygen and non oxygen free radicals. Furthermore, several cancer cells possess some resistance to ionizing radiation. MDR1 cells may be "resistant" to the killing effect of the host's immunocompetent cells that also act through the production of oxygen free radicals (ROS). Thus, it is possible to suggest that MDR1 cells become resistant to ROS. This hypothesis , if true, could represent a common mechanism in explaining resistance to different cell damaging agents such as ionizing radiation, drugs and cells with a natural killing effect.

In recent years, our studies have tried to determine whether the development of the mdr1 phenotype in cancer and non cancer cells can be associated with resistance to the cytotoxic effect of ROS. To address this point we studied the effects of the development of the MDR1 phenotype in a human hepatocellular carcinoma cell line (PLC/PRF/5), also known as the Alexander cell line. The MDR1 phenotype was induced in parental drug sensitive cells (P5) by progressive selective pressure using doxorubicin (Dox) as a selective agent. A clone (P1) with the expression of the full phenotype of MDR1 was selected and maintained in 0.1 μg/ml dox. A second subclone of MDR1 cells [P1(0.5)] was generated, progressively increasing dox concentration up to 0.5 μg/ml. This cell subclone was 100 fold more resistant to dox than P5 and expressed much greater amounts of P-gp than P1 (7).

To test whether the development of differential degrees of MDR1 phenotype lead to different susceptibility to free radicals, P5, P1 and [P1 (0.5)] cells were exposed to solutions containing mixtures of ADP-Fe or ascorbate-Fe. Susceptibility to undergoing lipid peroxidation was assessed by the determination of the formation of TBA reacting substances (TBARS) at the beginning of the exposure and after 60 min of incubation. Results showed that production of TBARS is much lower in the highly resistant cell subclone, [P1(0.5)] in comparison to parental drug sensitive P5 or the moderate MDR1 P1 cell suclone. The [P1(0.5)] clone was almost insensitive to the peroxidative effect of iron stimulated free radicals. The metabolism of malondialdheyde (MDA) was also measured in these experiments, showing that the highly resistant cell subclone was not able to metabolize MDA which constitutes most, if not all, of the TBA reacting substances in these conditions. Interestingly, [P1(0.5)] cells were found to have an increased content of vitamin E, a powerful scavenger of free radicals, in comparison to parental drug sensitive or moderate drug resistant cells. Glutathione content, glutathione-S-transferase activity, total and Se-dependent glutathione peroxidase activity were not significantly different in the two MDR1 cell subclones (8). These findings therefore suggested that an increased amount of cell vitamin E plays a crucial role in protecting the highly MDR1 cells from undergoing lipid peroxidation in there cells.

Vitamin E, or α-tocopherol , is a well known antioxidant, but has other and not yet fully elucidated functions. It has been shown recently, for instance, that it is involved in modulating cell proliferation, and that this phenomenon is not due to its antioxidant effect. In fact, β-tocopherol, although an antioxidant as strong as α-tocopherol, has no effect on cell proliferation and competes with vitamin E for a cytosol receptor (9). For these reasons, experiments were made to investigate whether vitamin E cell content could affect drug resistance to dox in drug sensitive cells by affecting resistance to free radicals. P5 cells were cultured in the presence of vitamin E (α-tocopherol succinate 5 μM) for 24 h , then cells were exposed for another 48 h to dox in increasing concentrations. Enrichment in vitamin E decreased cell susceptibility to undergoing lipid peroxidation, but did not affect cell survival in comparison to controls cultured in the presence of DMSO used to solubilize vitamin E. Thus, vitamin E did not appear able to increase drug resistance to dox, though it enhanced resistance to lipid peroxidation in this condition (R. Mazzanti et al., unpublished data).

Since the loss of susceptibility to undergoing lipid peroxidation is an early marker for malignant transformation in the liver and cancer cells are intrinsically less susceptible to undergoing lipid peroxidation (10), it was possible to hypothesize that the degree of resistance to iron stimulated lipid peroxidation in P1 could be related to the fact that they are cancer cells, independent from the MDR1 phenotype and expression of P-gp on plasma membrane. For these reasons, susceptibility to undergoing lipid peroxidation was studied in drug sensitive and drug resistant leukemia cells which do not express P-gp. Resistance to undergoing lipid peroxidation was observed in both leukemia cell lines that do not express P-gp (Figure 1) after exposing these cells to ADP-iron and ascorbate-iron mixtures. This observation suggests that less susceptibility to undergoing lipid peroxidation is a marker of proliferating cells rather than drug resistance.

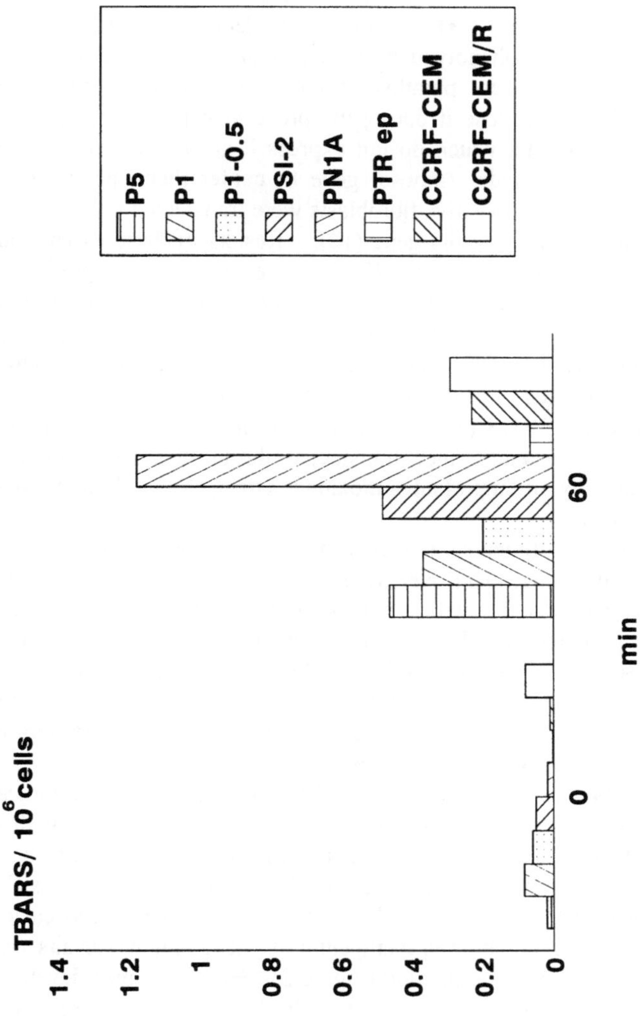

Figure 1. Susceptibility to undergoing lipid peroxidation in different cell lines (see text, for details)

One of the main problems in studying these phenomena is that most experiments are performed in cells that are transformed, therefore it is not possibe to exclude that the observation is due to a combination of effects caused by oncogénes or antioncogénes overexpressed or altered in these cells. To further improve our knowledge of the possible role of the MDR1 phenotype on susceptibility to free radicals we decided to investigate the effects of inducing this phenotype in cells that are not transformed. Two different models were chosen: parathyroid iperplastic cells that express P-gp in normal conditions and lose it during the process of transformation (11), and NIH 3T3 fibroblasts, which do not express P-gp but were transfected with the cDNA of the mdr1 (mouse) gene to confer them the mdr1 full phenotype. Parental drug sensitive fibroblasts were transfected only with the vector that was not carrying the gene (12). Results of these experiments showed that these two cell lines differed in regards to susceptibility to undergoing iron stimulated lipid peroxidation. Parathyroid cells were resistant to undergoing lipid peroxidation and acted similarly to HCC cancer cells with mdr1 phenotype (R. Mazzanti et al., unpublished data), whereas mdr1 gene transfected fibroblasts resulted more vulnerable to the peroxidative action of ROS (13). This last phenomenon was not due to a reduction in cell antioxidants, since transfected fibroblasts showed a normal or increased activity of important antioxidant enzymes, similarly to what occurs in mdr1 cells.

From all these experiments, it seems that the development of the mdr1 phenotype with the consequent overexpression of P-gp in plasma membrane is not always associated with resistance to ROS. On the contrary, susceptibility to undergoing lipid peroxidation may not be different from parental drug sensitive cancer cells (P1 as P5) or it may even be increased in fibroblasts. Resistance to free radicals, measured at least as lipid peroxidation, seems to be more related to transformation and/or proliferative status of the cells rather than to drug resistance.

Ionizing radiation is known to damage DNA by generating free radicals (14). For this reason experiments were done on different cells with or without the mdr1 phenotype to test their susceptibility to the damaging action of ionizing radiation. Human hepatocellular carcinoma cell lines [P5, P1, P1(0.5)] and NIH fibroblasts (3T3, PSI-2, PN1A) were exposed to a dose of 2.00 Gy/min. common in therapeutic use of radiation. Results were similar to those on lipid peroxidation (Figure 2). HCC cell lines developed resistance to ionizing radiation only at high degrees of drug resistance [P1(0.5)], whereas drug resistant fibroblasts (PN1A) were more vulnerable to radiation with a significant reduction of survival in comparison to parental drug sensitive or control fibroblasts. In other words, these observations suggest that a type of collateral toxicity to ionizing radiation in 3T3 drug resistant cells exists.

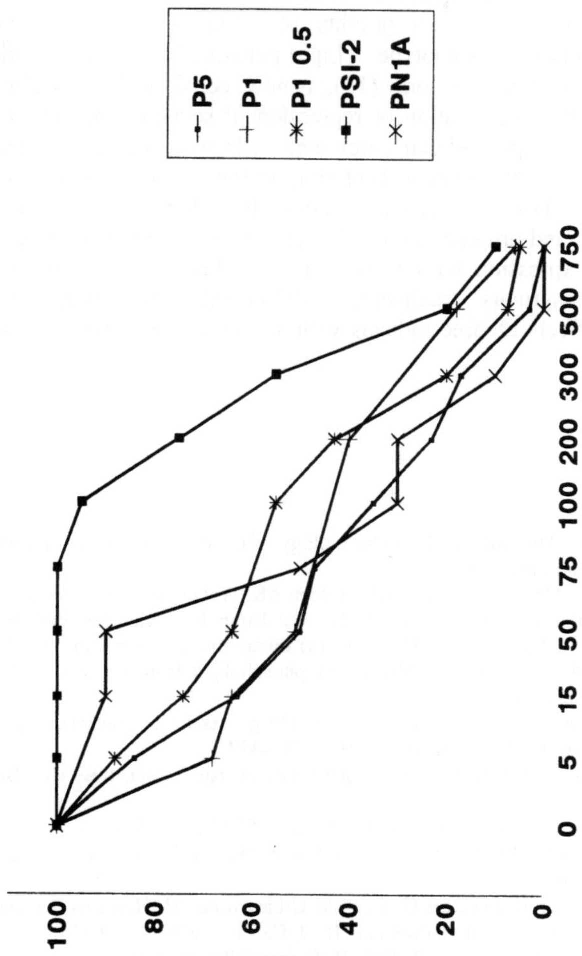

Figure 2. Curves of survival in HCC and 3T3 cells exposed to ionizing radiation.

In considering the combination of these studies, it is possible to hypothesize that the development of mdr1 phenotype per se might lead to increased susceptibility to the damaging effects of ROS or at least to an increased production of secondary by-products of lipid peroxidation. The common increase in cell antioxidants observed in mdr1 cells may be secondary to the increased susceptibility of drug resistant cells with moderate expression of the phenotype. Lipid peroxidation, once regarded as a mechanism of cell damage only (15), is now considered a key player in cell signalling by the activation or repression of several genes (16-18). The fact that human hepatocellular carcinoma cells with moderate MDR1 phenotype expression maintain susceptibility to the peroxidative action of ROS on membrane phospholipids may indicate that there is no difference between these cells and drug sensitive cells. However, once high degrees of MDR1 phenotype expression has occurred in cancer because of the delay in diagnosing or incongruous treatment, MDR1 cells may become very resistant to the effects of free radicals with a consequent increase in the malignity of cancer.

REFERENCES

1) Roninson IB, editor. Molecular and cellular biology of multidrug resistance in tumor cells. New York: Plenum Press, 1991.

2) Smith JJM, Schinkel AH, Oude Elferink RPJ, Groen AK, Wagenaar E, van Deemter L, Mol CAAM, Ottenhoff R, van der Lugt NMT, van Roon MA, van der Valk MA, Offerhaus GJA, Berns AJM, Borst P. Homozygous disruption of the murine mdr2 P-glycoprotein gene leads to a complete absence of phospholipid from bile and to liver disease. Cell. 1993;75:451-462.

3) Gottesman MM, Pastan I. Biochemistry of multidrug resistance mediated by the multidrug transperter. Annu. Rev. Biochem. 1993;62:385-427.

4) Higgins CF. ABC transporters: from microorganisms to man. Annu. Rev. Cell Biol. 1992;8:67-113.

5) Beck WT. Multidrug resistance and its circumvention. 1990;26:513-515.

6) Pinedo HM, Giaccone G. P-glycoprotein - a marker of cancer-cell behavior. N. Engl. J. Med. 1995;333:1380-1385.

7) Macnab GM, Alexander JJ, Lecatsas G, Bey EM Urbanowicz JM. Hepatitis B surface antigen produced by a human hepatoma cell line. Br. J. Cancer. 1976;34:509-515.

8) Mazzanti R, Fantappiè O, Fabrizio P, Relli P. Susceptibility to lipid peroxidation of human hepatocellular carcinoma cell lines with different levels of multiple drug-resistant phenotype. Lab. Invest. 1995;73:419-423.

9) Chatelain E, Boscoboinik DO, Bartoli GM, Kagan VE, Gey FK, Packer L, Azzi A. Inhibition of smooth muscle cell proliferation and protein kinase C activity by tocopherols and tocotrienols. Biochim. Biophys. Acta 1993;1176:83-89.

10) Dianzani MU. Lipid peroxidation and cancer: a Critical reconsideration. Tumori. 1989;75:351-356.

11) Sakaguchi K, Santora A, Zimering M, Curcio F, Aurbach GD, Brandi ML. Functional epithelial cell line cloned from rat parathyroid glands. Proc. Natl. Acad. Sci. USA 1987;84:3269-3273.

12) Croop JM, Guild BC, Gros P, Housman DE. Genetics of multidrug resistance: relationship of a cloned gene to the complete multidrug resistant phenotype. Cancer Res. 1987;47:5982-5988.

13) Mazzanti R, Fantappiè O, Fabrizio P, Pacini S, Relli P, Casamassima F, Milano F, Ruggiero M. Conferring drug resistance by the MDR1 gene transfection increases susceptibility to irradiation and lipid peroxidation in 3T3 cell line. Free Rad. Biol. & Med. in press.

14) Withers HR. Biological basis of radiation therapy for cancer. Lancet 1992;339: 156-163.

15) Sevian A, Hochstein P. Mechanisms and consequences of lipid peroxidation in biological systems. Ann. Rev. Nutr. 1985;5:365-390.

16) Ammendola R, Fiore F, Esposito F, Caserta G, Mesuraca M, Russo T, Cimino F. Differentially expressed mRNAs as a consequence of oxidative stress in intact cells. FEBS Letter 1995,371:209-213.

17) Fornace Jr AJ. Mammalian genes induced by radiation; activation of genes associated with growth control. Annu. Rev. Genet. 1992;26:507-526.

18) Keyse SM, Emslie EA. Oxidative stress and heat shock induced a human gene encoding a protein-tyrosine phosphatase. Nature. 1992;359:644-647.

CHAPTER 9

MOLECULAR AND CELLULAR ASPECTS OF IRON-MEDIATED LIVER TOXICITY

ANTONELLO PIETRANGELO, GIULIANA MONTOSI,
ROSSANA GUALDI, CINZIA GARUTI AND EZIO VENTURA

Dipartimento di Medicina Interna, Università degli Studi di Modena, Modena , Italy

Summary
Iron is essential for all living organisms. However, if present in excess or in molecular forms able to catalyze free radical reactions, toxicity arises. The paradigm of iron-induced organ disease is genetic hemochromatosis (GH), in which fibrosis, cirrhosis and cancer of the liver are common findings. Iron-toxicity is mainly due to its ability to catalyze free radical reactions which lead to membrane damage, enzyme inactivation and genotoxicity. In fact, high incidence of liver cancer has been reported in hemochromatosis, while the molecular basis for this carcinogenic effect is still elusive. Fibrosis is quite common in patients with iron overload. Recent experimental studies have shown that iron exert a fibrogenic and mitogenic effect on hepatic stellate cells (HSC), the ultimate effectors of liver fibrogenesis. Through direct or indirect mechanisms, iron-generated free-radical species and/or by-products of peroxidative oxidation of biological membranes may lead to hepatocyte damage or direct stimulation of HSC. Finally, iron, in conjunction with other hepatotoxins (e.g. alcohol, viruses, etc.) may dramatically enhance liver damage and accelerate progression of liver disease.

With the exceptions of certain species of bacteria, all living organisms require environmental iron for growth and for a variety of metabolic pathways. In fact, the flexible coordination chemistry and favorable redox potential of iron account for its use as an ideal cofactor for many structural and metabolic functions. However, in an oxygen-containing environment, if present in amount that exceeds the detoxifying cellular systems, iron is a generator of hydroxyl radicals, which have a

P. Gentilini and M. U. Dianzani. New Trends in Hepatology, 74-84

variety of toxic effects on cells. The liver, as a main site of iron deposition, is also a special target for iron toxicity This review mainly focuses on two aspect of iron toxicity: i) iron as a direct hepatotoxin; ii) iron as a co-factor of liver toxicity.

In humans, the paradigm of iron-associated organ disease is genetic (hereditary or idiopathic) hemochromatosis (GH). This term distinguishes a primary derangement of iron metabolisms from secondary causes of siderosis as found in thalassemia, transfusional siderosis, porphyrias, alcoholic cirrhosis.

In GH, increased amounts of iron are absorbed from the diet and deposited mainly in parenchymal cell of the liver, pancreas, heart and other organs. This leads to cell toxicity, organ failure and cancer. In GH, the feed-back control normally exerted by body iron stores on iron absorption is lost, and it is only partially restored at later stages of the disease. Fibrosis, micronodular cirrhosis and cancer are the most common hepatic manifestations in GH. Hepatic iron concentration is greatly increased in the majority of homozygous GH subjects reaching as much as 40-60,000 μg/g dry wt (reference value: below 1,000 μg/g dry wt), with little overlap with the other secondary hemochomatosis groups. Iron accumulates mainly into parenchymal cells while reticuloendothelial cells are stained for iron only in late GH. In the absence of alcoholism, fibrosis or cirrhosis in hemochromatosis appears to be present only with hepatic iron concentration above a threshold of 22,000 μg/g dry wt.

An increased incidence of hepatoma is a major cause of death in GH, with an incidence estimated to be 220 times that in a control population (1). Whether this is a direct consequence of iron toxicity or simply reflects the relatively indolent nature of the cirrhosis and hence a prolonged risk of hepatoma is not clear. Hepatocellular carcinoma usually develops on the basis of preexisting cirrhosis. The pathogenesis of hepatocellular carcinoma in hemochromatosis and the precise role of hepatic iron overload are still uncertain. The usual speculation is that iron overload in any cell exposes that cell to injury from noxious oxygen species the formation of which is catalyzed by reactive "free-iron". Iron has been shown to be mutagenic *in vitro,* and may therefore initiate hepatocarcinogenesis. Yet, in iron loaded and chemically induced cancerous rats, early neoplastic lesions are characterized by their inability to stain for iron (2). In a recent study, hepatic "iron-free" foci have been found in 83% of patients with GH (3). During a 15 yr follow-up period, 50% developed liver cancer (4). Thus, these lesions seem to represent proliferative areas that correspond to preneoplastic foci. Clearly, the finding of such foci on the initial biopsy from a patient with hemochromatosis should lead to regular screening for hepatocellular carcinoma by ultrasound examination and serum α–fetoprotein.

Early studies reported signs of fibrosis in young individuals with GH in the absence of necro-inflammatory events (5). Occasionally, GH patients with extensive cirrhosis or signs of portal hypertension have been found without significant hepatic biochemical abnormalities. These findings emphasized the possible role of iron as a profibrogenic agent itself. In recent years, investigators have tried to give experimental support to these early clinical observations and understand the cellular pathways mediating the hepatotoxic and fibrogenic effects of iron. A major difficulty in approaching this issue experimentally has been the lack of an animal model producing the full pathological picture of the cirrhotic liver seen in GH. In fact, in animal models of iron toxicity, in spite of significant increase in liver iron content, occasionally approaching that seen in human disease, necrotic events are limited and fibrotic response minimal. In GH, in the absence of other inciting insults, the hepatic disease is rather "mild" and usually slowly progresses over a long-time period to the micronodular cirrhosis. This may depend on the fact that, under physiological conditions, iron and iron-generated free radical species are quite well tolerated in the cellular microenvironment. During evolution, indeed, finely-tuned and phylogenetically highly preserved defensive systems have developed against iron toxicity in eukaryotic cells. The best example of such systems is the cytoplasmic "sensor"of iron (and presumably of the cellular redox state), the iron regulatory protein (IRP), which rapidly and consistently controls minimal perturbations of iron (and possibly ROS) equilibrium in the cell (Figure 1).

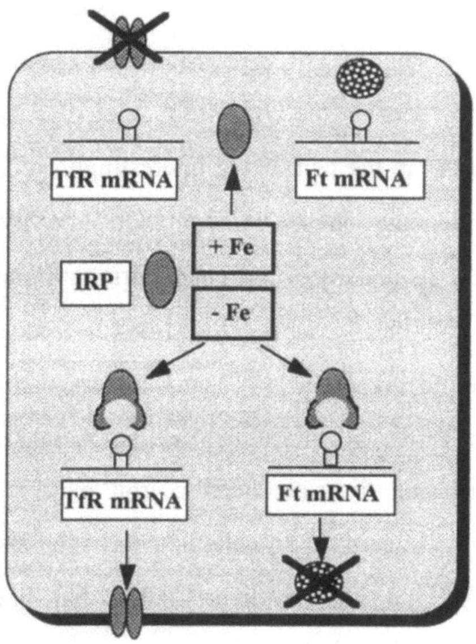

Figure 1. The iron regulatory protein model. TfR=transferrin receptor; Ft=ferritin.

IRP is able to control in the opposite direction uptake and storage of iron in the cell (6). In fact, during iron starvation IRP is activated and binds specific iron responsive elements (IRE) in the untranslated region (UTR) of the ferritin (5' UTR) and transferrin receptor (3'UTR) messenger RNA (mRNA). Upon binding, opposite effects are exerted on the fate of these mRNAs: translation of ferritin mRNA is hindered, while stabilization of TfR mRNA is achieved by protection toward nuclease attack. The net result of these molecular interactions is that less iron is stored due to inhibition of ferritin synthesis while more iron is extracted from the extracellular milieu by virtue of enhanced TfR expression. The opposite occurs during cell iron overload. Thus, by sensing the "free iron" pool, IRP can rapidly equilibrate the total amount of iron in the cell. More interestingly, redox switching control IRP activation and oxidant stress, inflammation and liver regeneration have been shown to modulate its activity (7,8). Thus, during all these pathobiological states, potentially toxic catalitically active "free iron" is freed in the cytoplasm where it may initiate free radical reactions.

To overwhelm this and other protective systems (such as the variety of "antioxidants" cellular defences) chronic and dramatic hepatic iron burden is necessary. This, may ultimately lead to cell necrosis, so-called "sideronecrosis", and focal inflammation (9). Although in the past GH liver disease has been commonly defined as an "inflammation-free" pathological entity, this concept should be probably now reconsidered. In fact, the hepatic inflammatory component in GH is not overwhelming, but appreciable, and limited to areas of maximal deposition of iron. As recently reported, microinflammatory foci are invariably encountered in GH patients showing evident signs of fibrosis (10). Yet, the qualitative aspect of the inflammatory reaction is certainly different from other chronic liver disease, such as alcoholic liver disease, in which granulocytes may predominate. In GH, most likely, monocytic population of proliferating resident predominate. In GH, most likely, monocytic population of proliferating resident Kupffer cells or incoming mononuclear cells and, in some instances, periportal myofibroblasts and fibroblasts, may prevail.

As mentioned, a common pathological finding in GH livers is fibrosis. Experimentally, it has been shown that HSC are major effectors of liver fibrogenesis during chronic iron overload. In fact, by using *in situ* hybridization techniques combined with immunohistochemistry against desmin, a marker of HSC, and collagen mRNA analysis on isolated hepatic cell fractions, expression of collagen gene is invariably located into HSC (11). Moreover, upon iron treatment and *in vivo* thymidine labeling, it has also been shown that HSC do proliferate (12). Thus, the main features of HSC activation (i.e. enhanced collagen type I expression and proliferation) have been found during iron intoxication.

Interestingly, in humans with GH, fibrosis is present only when sinusoidal cell iron overload is appreciable (3). Mechanistically, in stages of advanced GH, the drive to fibrogenesis may be due to iron-induced hepatocellular necrosis, and sinusoidal cell iron overload is a mere consequence of phagocitic activity of sideronecrotic hepatocytes (Figure 2).

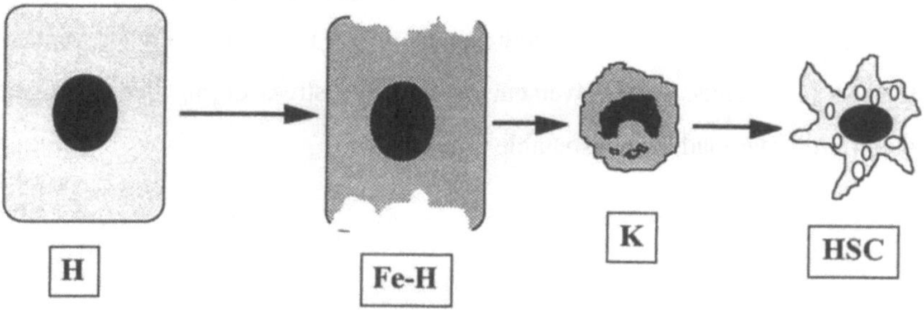

Figure 2. Iron-mediated hepatocellular necrosis (sideronecrosis) leads to Kupffer cell activation and stimulation of hepatic stellate cells. H=hepatocyte; Fe-H=iron-loaded hepatocyte; K=Kupffer cell; HSC=hepatic stellate cell.

In fact, selective targeting of considerable amount of iron to Kupffer cells by parenteral treatment with iron-salts did not induce activation of collagen mRNA into HSC as assessed by *in situ* hybridization (13). On the other hand, comparable hepatocellular iron loading in iron-fed rats led to HSC activation. In the latter, focal sideronecrosis was found. Activation of Kupffer cells due to the necrogenic event may induce the release of fibrogenic cytokines ultimately responsible for HSC activation. Indeed, enhanced expression of TGF-β has been detected into Kupffer cell aggregates of iron-treated gerbils (12).

Seemingly, in young individuals with GH and normal liver histology, activation of collagen gene has been found over smooth-muscle α-actin positive cells in areas where mononuclear cell aggregates are present (14). This suggest that a fibrogenic stimulus of iron can be exerted also at a "pre-necrosis" stage. In fact, fibrogenesis might be also sustained by an oxidant-stress-mediated iron-induced cell damage, or by the release of additional fibrogenic factors such as free-radical species or lipid-peroxidation by products. The latter, which are potentially fibrogenic have been found into lobular areas of iron-loading during experimental siderosis (9)(15). More interestingly, antioxidant treatment in vivo counteracts the toxic effects mediated by iron (15) and totally prevents liver fibrosis (12). Thus, an involvement of oxidative stress during liver fibrogenesis due to iron overload is undesputable (Figure 3).

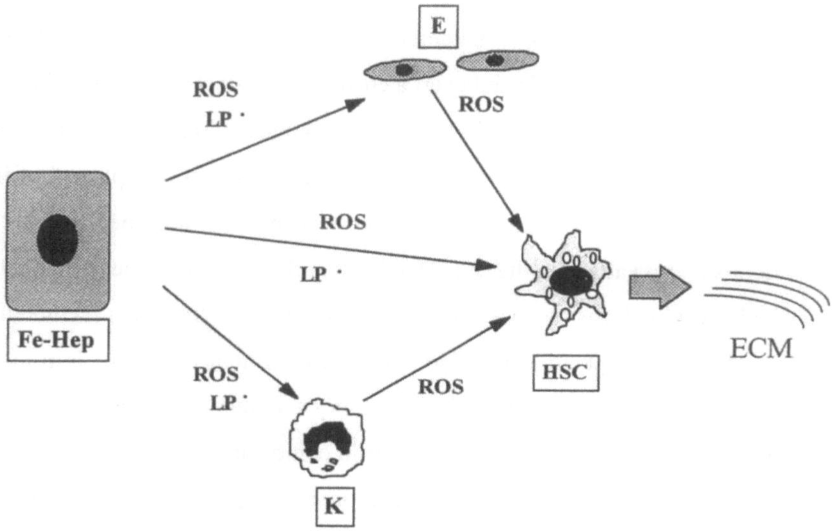

Figure 3. Possible pathways of iron-mediated fibrogenesis through oxidative stress. Fe-H=iron-loaded hepatocyte; K=Kupffer cell; HSC=hepatic stellate cell; E=endothelial cell; ECM=extracellular matrix; ROS=reactive oxygen species; LP·= lipid-peroxidation by-products.

The molecular basis of such an effect of iron remains to be elucidated.

Of greater clinical impact is the potential "fibrogenicity" of iron when acting in concert with other hepatotoxins (e.g. viruses, alcohol, and other xenobiotics). In these instances, even at low level of tissue iron burden, dramatic toxicity may arise, with rapid acceleration of the liver disease. This is probably due to the fact that in the presence of a damaging event, regardless of its nature, the prooxidant action of iron may amplify and propagate the initial toxic effect or contribute to its cytotoxicity. Even a slight increase in the highly reactive "free iron pool" may favour these events by offering an optimal catalyst for free radical reactions and cell toxicity. Of course, besides a direct toxic effect on hepatocytes, a "free radical" microenvironment favoured by iron excess would contribute to activation of Kupffer cells and exert a chemotactic effect on mononuclear cells toward the area of primary damage. In this context, iron may be, in certain instances, "co-initiator", or, mostly, best "propagator" and "amplifier" of liver toxicity, even if the initiating damaging event was not mediated by an oxidative stress attack to the cell. The fact that the only experimental models in which liver cirrhosis has been obtained following iron treatment include iron-loaded animals treated with ethionine or low protein diet (16), iron-loaded gerbils with pre-existing micro-inflammatory foci due to gut endotoxins (12), iron-treated rats with CCl_4 alone (17) or in combination with alcohol (18) and iron-treated rats with alcohol intoxication and high-fat diet (19), strongly support the above concepts. Common to many of these experimental models of hepatic fibrosis is a necro-inflammatory event which, pre-existing or concomitant to iron load, is exacerbated by iron excess in the liver.

In conclusion, iron has the potential of inducing liver damage, fibrosis and cancer. Its ability of serving as catalyst of free-radical reactions also dramatically enhances its toxic potential when operating in conjunction with other inciting hepatotoxins (alcohol, viruses et al.). These concepts emphasize the importance of early diagnosis of liver siderosis and prompt removal of excess iron in primary as well as secondary human iron storage diseases.

References

1. Niederau, C., Fisher, R., Sonnenberg, A., Stremmel, W., Trampish, H.J., and Strohmeyer, G. (1985) Survival and causes of death in cirrhotic and noncirrhotic patients with primary hemochromatosis. N Engl J Med 313, 1256-1262.

2. Williams, G.M. and Yamamoto, R.S. (1972) Absence of stainable iron from preneoplastic and neoplastic lesions in rat liver with 8-Hydroxyquinalone induced siderosis. *J Natl Cancer* 49, 685-692.

3. Deugnier, Y.M., Guyader, D., Crantock, L., Lopez, J.M., Turlin, B., Yaouanq, J., Jouanolle, H., Campion, J.P., Launois, B., Halliday JW, Powell LW. (1993) Primary liver cancer in genetic hemochromatosis: a clinical, pathological, and pathogenetic study of 54 cases. Gastroenterology 104, 228-234.

4. Deugnier, Y.M., Charalambours, P., Le Quilleuc, D., Turlin, B., Searle, J., Brissot, P., Powell, L.W. and Halliday, J.W. (1993) Preneoplastic significance of hepatic iron-free foci in genetic hemochromatosis: a study of 185 patients. Hepatology 18, 1363-1369.

5. Finch, S.C., and Finch, C.A. (1955) Idiopathic hemochromatosis: an iron storage diseaase. Medicine 34, 381-430,.

6. Klausner, R. D., Rouault, T. A. and Harford, J. B: Regulating the fate of mRNA: the control of cellular iron metabolism. Cell 72:19-28, 1993

7. Cairo, G. and Pietrangelo, A. (1994) Transferrin-receptor gene expression during rat liver regeneration: evidence for posttranscriptional regulation by IRF_B, a second IRE binding protein. J Biol Chem 269, 6405-6409.

8. Cairo, G. and Pietrangelo, A. (1995) Nitric-oxide-mediated activation of iron-regulatory ptotein controls hepatic metabolism during acute inflammation. Eur J Biochem 233, 358-363,.

9. Pietrangelo, A. (1996) Metals, oxidative stress and liver fibrogenesis. Sem Liv Dis 16, 13-30.

10. Stal, P., Broome, U., Sheynius, A., Befritz, R. and Hultcrantz, R. (1995) Kupffer cell iron overload induces intercellular adhesion molecule-1 expression on hepatocytes in genetic hemochromatosis. Hepatology 21, 1308-1316.

11. Pietrangelo, A., Gualdi, R., Casalgrandi, Geerts, A., De Bleser, P., Montosi, G. and Ventura, E. (1994). Enhanced hepatic collagen type I mRNA expression into fat-storing cells in a rodent model of hemochromatosis. Hepatology 19, 714-721.

12. Pietrangelo, A., Gualdi, R., Casalgrandi, G., Montosi, G., and Ventura, E. (1995) Molecular and cellular aspects of iron-induced hepatic cirrhosis in rodents. J Clin Invest 95, 1824-1831.

13. Gualdi, R., Casalgrandi, G., Montosi, G., Ventura, E. and Pietrangelo, A. (1994) Excess iron into hepatocytes is required for activation of collagen type I gene during experimental siderosis. Gastroenterology 107, 1118-1124.

14. Pietrangelo, A., Montosi, G., Garuti, C., Stal, P., Hultcrantz, R. (1995) Molecular and cellular aspects of liver disease in genetic hemochromatosis. Hepatology 22,1057A.

15. Pietrangelo, A., Borella, F., Casalgrandi, G., Montosi, G., Ceccarelli, D., Gallesi, D., Giovannini, F., Gasparetto, A., Masini, A. (1995) Antioxidant activity of silybin in vivo during long-term iron overload in rats. Gastroenterology 109:1941-1949.

16. Goldberg, L. and Smith, J.P. (1955) Iron overloading and hepatic vulnerability. Am J Clin Pathol 25, 514-542.

17. Kent, G., Volini, F.I., Minick, O.T., Orfei, O. and De la Huerga, J. (1964) Effect of iron loading upon the formation of collagen in the hepatic injury induced by carbon tetrachloride. Am J Pathol 45, 7=29-155.

18. Mackinnon, M., Clayton, C., Plummer, J., Ahern, M., Cmielewski, P., Ilsley,A. and Hall, P. (1995) Iron overload facilitates hepatic fibrosis in the rat alcohol/low-dose carbon tetrachloride model. Hepatology 21, 1083-1088.

19. Tsukamoto H, Horne W, Kamimura S, Kamimura, S., Niemela, O., Parkkila, S., Ylaherttuala, S. and Brittenham, G.M. (1995) Experimental liver cirrhosis induced by alcohol and iron. J Clin Invest 96, 620-630.

CHAPTER 10

THE CELLULAR AND MOLECULAR BASIS OF LIVER FIBROGENESIS

Massimo PINZANI, Fabio MARRA, Vinicio CARLONI, Alessandra CALIGIURI, Raffaella DE FRANCO, Alessandra GENTILINI, Paolo MONTALTO, Chiara SALI, Roberto Giulio ROMANELLI, and Paolo GENTILINI

Istituto di Medicina Interna-Centro Interuniversitario di Fisiopatologia Epatica, Università degli Studi di Firenze, I-50134 Firenze, Italia

Summary

Hepatic stellate cells (HSC), perisinusoidal mesenchymal elements with possible pericytic functions within the liver, have recently been shown to play multiple physiological and pathophysiological roles. In particular, several *in vivo* and *in vitro* studies have clearly indicated that HSC play a relevant role in the progression of liver fibrogenesis. More recently, the attention has been focused on the mechanisms leading to HSC activation, proliferation and synthesis of extracellular matrix components. Among other soluble factors potentially involved in these processes, transforming growth factor-ß1 and platelet-derived growth factor have been shown to act in a paracrine, and possibly autocrine, fashion on HSC, thus perpetuating their activated state.

Studies performed in the last decade have greatly contributed to clarify the characteristics and functions of liver nonparenchymal cells, both in physiological and pathophysiological conditions. In particular, much attention has recently been focused on the biology of hepatic stellate cells (HSC, also referred to as fat-storing cells, Ito cells, hepatic lipocytes), especially concerning the possible implication of this cell type in the development of hepatic fibrogenesis following chronic liver tissue injury (1). Fibrogenesis is currently viewed as a dynamic process strictly related to the extent and duration of parenchymal injury. This modern view implies that several fibrogenic disorders, including atherosclerosis, once identified as "degenerative", are today considered as the result of events such as reiterative tissue damage and chronic

P. Gentilini and M. U. Dianzani. New Trends in Hepatology, 85-92

inflammation. In general, the process leading to liver fibrosis, similarly to the process of normal wound healing, includes three phases following tissue injury: acute inflammation, synthesis of collagenous and noncollagenous extracellular matrix (ECM) components, tissue remodeling. This latter phase includes ECM remodeling and organized parenchymal regeneration. According to this scheme, a single liver tissue injury eventually results in an almost complete resolution. On the contrary, the persistence of the original insult causes the prolonged activation of the tissue repair mechanisms, thus leading to tissue fibrosis rather than to effective tissue repair. In other words, ECM accumulation predominates over hepatocellular regeneration. Qualitatively, the ECM components of the fibrotic matrix are similar to those already present in normal liver. However, in fibrotic liver all ECM components are dramatically increased in quantity, redistributed in different anatomical areas, and possibly varied in their relative ratios (2). In particular, collagen types I and III constitute the main framework of the so-called "fibrillar matrix" that gradually substitute the basal membrane-like structures present along the sinusoids and in between hepatocellular plates. These quantitative and qualitative changes in the composition of ECM, in addition to their mechanical and physical implications, contribute to the formation of a new biochemical environment. Indeed, each ECM component has the ability to modulate cell growth, migration, gene expression, and other important cellular functions directly by interaction with cell adhesion molecules and, indirectly, by trapping mitogenic biomolecules in their active or inactive forms (3).

The cellular source of connective tissue components in fibrotic liver has been controversial for many years. Surprisingly and uniquely in human pathology, the role of mesenchymal cells in the development of hepatic fibrosis was greatly underestimated until recent years. This was due to the lack of *in vivo* molecular studies and/or to the observation that primary cultures of hepatocytes produce considerable amounts of collagens. However, the demonstration of a significant contamination of hepatocyte cultures with HSC (4) and the *in vivo* identification of the cell type(s) responsible for the synthesis of ECM components in rat and human fibrotic liver (5-7), finally directed the efforts in the right perspective. Although different types of liver cells have the capacity to synthesize ECM components, HSC are currently considered the main connective tissue producing cells in fibrotic liver.

In conditions of chronic liver damage, as well as following prolonged culture on plastic, HSC undergo a process of activation from the quiescent "storing" phenotype to the highly proliferative "myofibroblast-like" phenotype. This transition is gradual and occurs through an intermediate stage defined as "transitional cell". This transformation is characterized by a dramatically increased synthesis of collagen types I and III, that appears predominant over the synthesis of collagen type IV (I>III>>IV) and other ECM components. The concept of a gradual phenotypical transformation is supported by studies *in vivo* documenting a shift in predominance from HSC to transitional cells following liver injury (8,9), although it is still uncertain whether further activation of transitional cells results in myofibroblast-like cells *in vivo*. Even though *in vitro* studies, utilizing HSC isolated from rat, mouse and human liver, tend to confirm the gradual transition to myofibroblast-like cells, the contribution of "genuine" myofibroblasts or fibroblasts to the production of fibrillar matrix is likely, particularly in selected areas such as fibrous septa and around the central vein (10).

Following a single, time-limited liver tissue injury (e.g., single administration of CCl_4 in rats, uncomplicated acute viral hepatitis in humans), the activation of HSC, as well as other liver nonparenchymal cells, is likely to play an important role in the tissue repair process. Similarly to the original injury, this activation is time-limited and implies proliferation of HSC (8) following a rather complex interplay with ECM components, cytokines, polypeptide growth factors and other soluble mediators. In this context, chemotaxis and proliferation of HSC and other ECM-producing cells is likely to represent a key event in the restoration of an ECM network indispensable for a correct tissue repair. At this "reversible" stage of activation, HSC may also contribute, together with sinusoidal endothelial cells, to hepatocellular regeneration by providing soluble factors such as hepatocyte growth factor (HGF) (11). Established experimental and clinical evidence indicates that restoration of the normal tissue characteristics is *per se* sufficient to determine the reversibility of this process. On the contrary, in chronic liver diseases, the presence of reiterative tissue damage associated with chronic inflammation is likely to represent a major cause leading to a complete phenotypical modulation of HSC. In other words, the reversibility or irreversibility of HSC activation seems to be largely due to the tissue microenvironment rather than to intrinsic properties of the cells. Studies performed in recent years have emphasized some important aspects potentially related to the initiation of HSC activation. A first important element concerns the disruption of the normal ECM pattern that follows liver tissue injury and acute inflammation. Analogously to what is observed by culturing HSC on plastic, loss of adhesion with the various elements constituting the basal membrane-like ECM of the space of Disse is likely to determine a marked increase of the proliferative and synthetic properties of HSC. This issue is becoming more and more important with the demonstration that the movement, shape and proliferation of cells is greatly influenced by the cooperation of ECM components and cell adhesion molecules. Along these lines, Carloni and coworkers (12) have recently provided important information on the complex interplay existing between activated HSC and the ECM through the expression of specific integrin receptors.

Another important aspect related to the initiation of activation concerns the exposure of HSC to soluble mediators that may potentially affect their proliferative attitude and/or synthetic ability. It is again important to stress that exposure to these mediators, generically defined as "inflammatory", may be time-limited or chronically present according to the nature, extent and reiteration of parenchymal damage. Following liver injury, several cell types, resident or infiltrating, could be involved in the synthesis and release of soluble factors playing a biological role on HSC. In this regard, it should be stressed that the term "inflammation" indicates a rather complex association of different cell types (i.e. lymphocytes, neutrophils, mononuclear cells, platelets) playing different roles. This distinction implies that clusters of soluble factors, specifically directed at different cell targets, are contemporaneously present in the tissue. It is likely that none of these factors work alone and that a complex network of interactions occurs between these mediators and their targets. *In vitro* studies have indicated that all these factors, taken singularly or in combination, have some effect on FSC proliferation, chemotaxis and/or ECM deposition. However, several studies performed in the past five years have suggested that two polypeptide growth factors, namely platelet-derived growth factor (PDGF) and transforming growth factor-β1 (TGF-ß), greatly contribute to the profibrogenic role of HSC. In this article we will focus on the role of PDGF in the progression of hepatic fibrogenesis because of the significant contribution provided by our group in this area of research.

PDGF, a key mitogen for mesenchymal cells, consists of two polypeptide chains, referred to as A- and B-chain, which can form three possible dimeric forms: AA, AB, and BB (13). Two PDGF receptor subunits, α or type A and ß or type B have been identified. The two subunits differ in their ability to bind different PDGF isoforms: the B-chain of PDGF can bind both α and ß subunits, whereas the A-chain can bind only α subunits. Dimerization of the receptor then results in the autophosphorylation and acquisition of the ability to phosphorylate other proteins regulating different intracellular signalling pathways (14).

A pathogenic role for PDGF has been demonstrated in several fibrogenic disorders, including glomerulosclerosis, pulmonary fibrosis, and atherosclerosis (15-18). Studies performed in our laboratory, utilizing a model of acute liver injury obtained by administering a single CCl_4 dose in rats, indicate that PDGF may play an important role in the process of liver tissue repair following acute injury by acting as a powerful chemotactic and mitogenic factor for resident and infiltrating mesenchymal cells (19). However, in chronic liver diseases, where the presence of reiterative tissue damage is associated with a persistent inflammatory state, the "pro-healing" action of PDGF may constitute a major element in the development of liver fibrosis. Our recent demonstration of a marked overexpression of the genes encoding for PDGF-A and B chains as well as α and ß receptor subunits in cirrhotic human liver, tends to confirm a functional role of this growth factor in the development of liver fibrosis (20).

Among other polypeptide growth factors potentially involved in chronic tissue inflammation, PDGF is the most potent mitogen for cultured HSC isolated from mouse or rat liver (21,22). Similarly to other potentially related mesenchymal cells (e.g., smooth muscle cells, type 1 astrocytes, glomerular mesangial cells), activated HSC have been shown to secrete a PDGF-like protein and to stimulate their own growth in an autocrine fashion (23).

When chronic liver injury is not clearly associated with an abundant inflammatory infiltrate, other soluble substances may sustain the activation of HSC through pathways that are specific for a particular type of damage. In alcoholic liver injury, for example, acetaldehyde, the main metabolite of ethanol, is able to increase gene transcription and synthesis of different ECM components in activated HSC (24,25). In addition to acetaldehyde, products of lipid peroxidation generated by exposure to ethanol or the production of iron overload (26) may also perpetuate HSC activation. Along these lines, Parola and coworkers have shown that stimulation of lipid peroxidation or exposure to 4-hydroxynonenal, a highly reactive aldehydic end-product of lipid peroxidation, increases procollagen I gene expression in activated human fat-storing cells (27).

The rapidly evolving knowledge in the field of liver fibrogenesis and the identification of HSC activation as a central event in the liver wound-healing response have greatly improved the possibility to devise pharmacological strategies aimed at interrupting the sequence of events resulting in massive liver fibrosis.

Acknowledgements. Research from the authors' laboratory quoted in this review was supported by grants from Ministero Italiano dell'Universita' e della Ricerca Scientifica e Tecnologica-Progetto Nazionale Cirrosi Epatica ed Epatiti Virali (Rome, Italy). Financial support was also provided by Fondazione Italiana per lo Studio del Fegato (Italian Liver Foundation, Florence, Italy).

References

(1) Pinzani M. (1995) Novel insights into the biology and physiology of the Ito cell. *Pharmac. Ther.* 66 :387-412.

(2) Schuppan, D. (1990) Structure of the extracellular matrix in normal and fibrotic liver: collagens and glycoproteins. *Sem. Liver Dis.* 10: 1-10.

(3) Schuppan, D., and Milani, S. (1993) Matrix, matrix synthesis, and molecular networks in hepatic fibrosis. In Zern, M.A. and Reid, L.M. (eds): *Extracellular Matrix. Chemistry, Biology, and Pathobiology with Emphasis on the Liver*, Marcel Dekker Inc., New York, pp. 201-254.

(4) Maher, J.J., Bissell, D.M., Friedman, S.L., and Roll, F.J. (1988) Collagen measured in primary cultures of normal rat hepatocytes derives from lipocytes within the monolayer. *J. Clin. Invest.* 82: 450-459.

(5) Milani, S., Herbst, H., Schuppan, D., Hahn, E.G., and Stein, H. (1989) In situ hybridization for procollagen types I, III and IV mRNA in normal and fibrotic rat liver: evidence for predominant expression in nonparenchymal liver cells. *Hepatology* 10: 84-92.

(6) Milani, S., Herbst, H., Schuppan, D., Riecken, E.O., and Stein, H. (1989) Cellular localization of laminin gene transcripts in normal and fibrotic human liver. *Am J Pathol* 134: 1175-1182.

(7) Maher, J.J., and McGuire, R.F. (1990) Extracellular matrix gene expression increases preferentially in rat lipocytes and sinusoidal endothelial cells during hepatic fibrosis in vivo. *J. Clin. Invest.* 86: 1641-1648.

(8) Burt, A.D., Robertson, J.L., Heir, J., and Macsween, R.N.M. (1986) Desmin-containing stellate cells in rat liver; distribution in normal animals and response to experimental acute liver injury. *J. Pathol.* 150: 29-35.

(9) Mak, K.M., and Lieber, C.S. (1988) Lipocytes and transitional cells in alcoholic liver disease: a morphometric study. *Hepatology* 8: 1027-1033.

(10) Bhunchet, E., and Wake, K. (1992) Role of mesenchymal cell populations in porcine serum-induced rat liver fibrosis. *Hepatology* 16: 1452-1473.

(11) Maher, J.J. (1993) Cell-specific expression of hepatocyte growth factor in liver. Upregulation in sinusoidal endothelial cells after carbon tetrachloride. *J. Clin. Invest.* 91: 2244-2252. .

(12) Carloni, V., Romanelli, R.G., Pinzani, M., Laffi, G., and Gentilini, P. (1996) Expression and function of integrin receptors for collagen and laminin in cultured human hepatic stellate cells. *Gastroenterology*, (in press).

(13) Ross, R. (1989) Platelet-derived growth factor. *Lancet* i: 1179-1182.

(14) Cadena, D.L., and Gill, G.N. (1992) Receptor tyrosine kinases. *FASEB J.* 6: 2332-2337.

(15) Nagaoka, I., Trapnell, B.C., and Crystal, R.G. (1990) Upregulation of platelet-derived growth factor-A and -B gene expression in alveolar macrophages of individual with idiopathic pulmonary fibrosis. *J. Clin. Invest.* 85: 2023-2027.

(16) Gesualdo, L., Pinzani, M., Floriano, J.J., Hassan, M.O., Nagy, N.U., Schena, F.P., Emancipator, S.N., and Abboud, H.E. (1991) Platelet-derived growth factor expression in mesangial proliferative glomerulonephritis. *Lab. Invest.* 65: 160-167.

(17) Gesualdo, L., Di Paolo, S., Milani, S., Pinzani, M., Grappone, C., Ranieri, E., Pannarale, G., and Schena, F.P. (1994) Expression of platelet-derived growth factor receptors in normal and diseased human kidney. *J. Clin. Invest.* 94 :50-58.

(18) Ross, R. (1993) The pathogenesis of atherosclerosis: a perspective for the 1990s. *Nature* 362: 801-809.

(19) Pinzani, M., Milani, S., Grappone, C., Weber, F.L. Jr., Gentilini, P., and Abboud, H.E. (1994) Expression of platelet-derived growth factor in a model of acute liver injury. *Hepatology* 19: 701-707.

(20) Pinzani, M., Milani, S., Herbst, H., De Franco, R., Grappone, C., Gentilini, A., Caligiuri, A., Pellegrini, G., Vinh Ngo, D., Romanelli, R.G., and Gentilini, P. (1996) Expression of platelet-derived growth factor (PDGF) and its receptors in normal human liver and during active hepatic fibrogenesis. *Am. J. Pathol.* 148 :785-800.

(21) Pinzani, M., Gesualdo, L., Sabbah, G.M., and Abboud, H.E. (1989) Effects of platelet-derived growth factor and other polypeptide mitogens on DNA synthesis and growth in cultured rat liver fat-storing cells. *J. Clin. Invest.* 84: 1786-1793.

(22) Pinzani, M., Abboud, H.E., Gesualdo, L., and Abboud, S.L. (1992) Regulation of macrophage-colony stimulating factor in liver fat-storing cells by peptide growth factors. *Am. J. Physiol.-Cell. Physiol.* 262: C876-C881

(23) Marra, F., Ghosh Choudhury, G., Pinzani, M., and Abboud, H.E. (1994) Regulation of platelet-derived growth factor secretion and gene expression in human fat-storing cells. *Gastroenterology* 107: 1110-1117.

(24) Moshage, H., Casini, A., and Lieber, C.S. (1990) Acetaldehyde selectively stimulates collagen production in cultured rat liver fat-storing cells but not in hepatocytes. *Hepatology* 12: 511-518.

(25) Casini, A., Cunningham, M., Rojkind, M., and Lieber, C.S. (1991) Acetaldehyde increases procollagen type I and fibronectin gene transcription in cultured rat fat-storing cells through a protein synthesis-dependent mechanism. *Hepatology* 13: 758-765.

(26) Pietrangelo, A., Gualdi, R., Casalgrandi, G., Geerts, A., De Bleser, P., Montosi, G., and Ventura, E. (1994) Enhanced hepatic collagen type I mRNA expression into fat-storing cells in a rodent model of hemochromatosis. Hepatology 19 :714-721.

(27) Parola, M., Pinzani, M., Casini, A., Albano, E., Poli, G., Gentilini, A., Gentilini, P., and Dianzani, M.U. Stimulation of lipid peroxidation or 4-hydroxynonenal treatment increases procollagen $\alpha 1(I)$ gene expression in human liver fat-storing cells. *Biochem. Biophys. Res. Comm.* 194: 1044-1050.

CHAPTER 11

PROLIFERATION OF HEPATIC STELLATE CELLS AND LIPID PEROXIDATION: CHANGES DUE TO POLYPHENOLS.

G. SVEGLIATI BARONI, L. D' AMBROSIO, G. FERRETTI^, P. BIONDI°, A. CASINI°, A. DI SARIO, S. SACCOMANNO*, A.M. JEZEQUEL*, A. BENEDETTI, F. ORLANDI.

*Department of Gastroenterology; ^ Department of Biochemistry; *Institute of Experimental Pathology, University of Ancona; ° Alcohol Research Center & Gastroenterology Unit, University of Florence*

Summary

Hepatic fibrosis represents the final steps of chronic liver injury and consists of excessive deposition of extracellular matrix components. Hepatic stellate cells (HSC) are responsible for this event when, through a process of activation, they proliferate and acquire a myofibroblatic phenotype. In this article, we review the role of oxidative stress in liver fibrosis. Moreover we also demonstrate that lipid peroxidation products, directly or released by damaged hepatocytes, stimulate HSC proliferation and collagen synthesis. This effect can be inhibited by resveratrol, a novel polyphenolic antioxidant.

Hepatic fibrosis is a common response to chronic liver injury of variable origin (viral, metabolic, toxic). Regardless of the aetiologic factor, liver fibrosis is characterized by increased production of extracellular matrix components which form the hepatic scars and consists of fibril-forming collagens, particularly collagen type I (1-4), and matrix glycoconjugates such as proteoglycans, fibronectins and hyaluronic acid (5). Hepatic stellate cells (HSC) (previously named fat-storing or Ito cells) have been identified as the primary source of excess extracellular matrix production in liver fibrosis (6). In normal rat liver, HSC are situated in the space of Disse and are characterized by the presence of vitamin A (7) and by their positivity for desmin (8). During the development of fibrosis, HSC proliferate (9) and undergo a process of activation, developing a myofibroblast-like appearance. Activated HSC are characterized by cell enlargement with increased rough endoplasmic reticulum and loss of retinoids (10), and expression of alpha

P. Gentilini and M. U. Dianzani. New Trends in Hepatology, 93-103

smooth-muscle actin (alpha-SM-actin) (6, 11-15). Activated HSC may be seen within scars in close contact with collagen fibrils positive for collagen types I and III (16, 17). Collagen specific transcripts have been detected in these cells by in situ hybridization (18-19).

As mentioned above, HSC proliferation seems to be an early event in chronic liver injury leading to liver fibrosis (6). This event has been clearly studied by Geerts et al in the carbon tetrachloride (CCl_4) model of liver injury (9). In fact they have demonstrated that the number of HSC increased in the pericentral zone, close to the area of necrosis, after a single injection of CCl_4 reaching a maximum at 96 hr. HSC were in fact observed in the pericentral area and in bands of tissue between adjacent central veins, simulating the septa seen in later stages of CCl_4 intoxication. The increased number was presumably due to increased cell proliferation, as shown by increased ^{3}H-thymidine uptake by desmin-positive cells showing a peak after 72 hr. To further study the fibrogenetic process, we have developed a low-mortality, reproducible model of liver fibrosis induced by repeated injections of dimethylnitrosamine (DMN) (20-23). As for CCL_4, this is characterized, in the early stage, by centrilobular injury followed by perivenular fibrosis and formation of septa with development of micronodular cirrhosis after 3 weeks of treatment. In this model, we have shown that collagen accumulation is precedeed by proliferation of HSC which tend to accumulate where fibrous septa will later appear (24), associated with increased expression of mRNAs for type I, III and IV procollagen (25). This model has also allowed us to test in vivo drugs such as interferon-gamma (IFN-γ), which have shown an antifibrotic effect in vitro (26). Using this cytokine in the DMN model of liver fibrosis, we were able to reduce the number of proliferating HSC and this was accompanied by a reduced deposition of extracellular matrix components (27).

HSC proliferation can thus be considered an important aspect of the involvement of HSC. Interestingly, the process of HSC activation in vivo can be mimicked in vitro by culturing HSC on uncoated plastic dishes (28). In fact it has been demonstrated that HSC isolated from normal rat liver undergo, between the third and the sixth day in culture, phenotypic changes in cells with ultrastructural characteristics of myofibroblasts. These morphological modifications are accompanied by differences in the amount and types of collagens synthesized (29): in fact freshly isolated HSC synthesize mainly collagen type IV, while on day seven the predominant types are collagen I and III which are the main isoforms in fibrotic livers (1-4).

In recent years, there has been a growing amount of data on the possible role of lipid peroxidation products in the fibrogenetic process, starting from the evidence that oxidative stress can modulate collagen gene expression in fibroblasts (30-32). Evidence coming from either experimental or clinical studies indicate that lipid peroxidation of biological membranes is associated with the development of liver fibrosis. For example, increased lipid peroxidation parameters (hepatic levels of malondialdehyde, conjugated diene and 4-hydroxynonenal) was associated with the early stage of fibrosis in experimental alcoholic liver disease (33) and aldehyde-protein adducts colocalized with excess iron deposition were detected in the cytosol of periportal hepatocytes in chronic iron overload (34). When the chronic iron overload was prolonged up to 6-8 months, a periportal fibrosis was observed together with enhanced signal for collagen type I mRNA into HSC only, while no signal was detected on iron-laden hepatocytes (19). Moreover iron overload (35) and CCL_4 injury (36) are colocalized with lipid peroxidation adducts (using immunohistochemistry) and increased collagen I and TGF-β transcripts (by in situ hybridization). This association between lipid peroxidation and enhanced collagen synthesis, observed also in two different models of experimental alcoholic liver disease (37-38), suggest a close link, independent from the etiologic factor, between oxidative stress and fibrogenesis.As indicated above, cultures of HSC are now considered a reliable model to study the regulation of ECM synthesis and have been used to confirm the association found in vivo between lipid peroxidation and active fibrogenesis. For example acetaldehyde, a potential pro-oxidant factor related to ethanol metabolism, has been shown to stimulate collagen gene transcription and synthesis in cultured rat HSC (39). Moreover, confirming the previous studies on fibroblasts, the direct exposure of human HSC to the pro-oxidant system ascorbate/iron results in the early induction of lipid peroxidation paralleled by a significant increase in the expression of procollagen type I mRNA and in the accumulation of the protein in the culture media (40). However, the direct effect of of oxidative stress in vivo has been questioned. In fact, Gualdi (41) et al. studied collagen gene expression in rats with either dietary overload from carbonyl iron or parenteral overload from iron dextran. Both groups of animals showed a comparable increase in hepatic iron compared to controls, with parenchymal accumulation in the dietary group and reticuloendothelial overload in the parenteral one. Interestingly a signal for collagen type mRNA was identified in nonparenchymal cells of iron-fed rats, while no activation was found in rats with parenteral overload suggesting a stimulatory pathway by hepatocytes-released products on HSC.

As demonstrated (27), an early response to chronic liver injury is HSC proliferation. This can be observed also in the CCL4 model, in which liver injury is due to oxidative stress. When HSC are activated, PDGF is the most potent mitogen (6). It has been recently shown that the PDGF-induced proliferation of rat vascular smooth muscle cells (VSMC) requires an increased intracellular concentration of lipid peroxidation products (42). In fact when VSMC were stimulated with PDGF an increased intracellular concentration of H_2O_2 was observed together with an increased amount of tyrosine-phosphorylated proteins (particularly of the p42 and p44 isoform of MAP-kinase) and of ^{3}H-thymidine incorporation. All these results suggest that lipid peroxidation products may act as an intracellular second messenger and thus be implicated also in proliferation of activated HSC, which have a phenotype similar to that of VSMC.In recent years, several investigators have focused their attention on the antioxidant properties of differrent compounds contained in alcoholic beverages and particularly on polyphenolic flavonoids. In in-vitro studies with phenolic substances and human low-density lipoprotein (LDL), it has been shown that these substances inhibited the copper-catalysed oxidation of LDL significantly more than α-tocopherol (43). In a recent epidemiological study (44) it has been shown that flavonoid intake was significantly inversely associated with mortality from coronary heart disease and with incidence of myocardial infarction. When the propensity of plasma and low-density lipoprotein (LDL) to undergo lipid peroxidation was studied, it was found that it was significantly reduced in subjects who consumed red compared to white wine (45). This effect is related to phenolic substances existing in red wine which are absorbed and elevate polyphenol concentration in plasma and LDL and may be responsible for the antioxidant properties of red wine.The effect of these substances on the liver has not yet been extensively studied. However, a preliminary report (46) seems to indicate an antioxidant effect of these polyphenolic compounds on lipid peroxidation in rat liver liposomes and microsomes. Moreover, resveratrol (3,5,4'-trihydroxystilbene) seems to be the most powerful of these compounds.

Considering these data, we have conducted experiments to evaluate if the oxidative stress could promote proliferation of HSC, either directly or through factors released by damaged hepatocytes, and if this effect could be modified by resveratrol.

Malondialdehyde levels were determined in hepatocytes (47) and HSC (39) medium after incubation with or without ferric iron nitrilotriacetate (FeNTA) complex (48). As expected, MDA levels significantly increased in hepatocytes incubated with FeNTA (HCM/Fe) compared to controls (HCM) (Fig. 1). A similar effect was noticed when HSC were incubated with FeNTA (Fig. 2). MDA levels in HSC medium increased already after 1 hr and were slightly higher at 5 hr. The simultaneous incubation with Res significantly reduced MDA levels close to control values in HSC medium. Various preparations of medium harvested from hepatocytes were then added to nonconfluent HSC cultures maintained in Iscove's medium supplemented with 0.5% FCS for 24 hr. Bromodeoxyuridine (BrdU, 5×10^{-5} final concentration), an analog of thymidine which incorporates in S-phase nuclei (27), was added in the last six hours of incubation. S-phase nuclei incorporating BrdU were detected by an immunoperoxidase staining using monoclonal IgG anti-BrdU as primary antibody (Dako, Italy). The addition, at 1:8 dilutions, of HCM/Fe was able to stimulate HSC proliferation after 24 hr of incubation at levels twofold higher compared to control or HCM cells (Fig. 3).

To confirm the role of lipid peroxidation products on the above results, nonconfluent cultures of HSC were also directly incubated with FeNTA (0.1 mM), in the presence or absence of Res (50 μM). Incubation with FeNTA significantly increased the LI of HSC already after 6 hr (34.6 ± 6.1) compared to FeNTA+Res (14.1 ± 2.55), which showed values similar to controls (16.6 ± 2.3). These significant differences were maintained also after 24 hr of incubation: 23.3 ± 5.9 vs 7.8 ± 2.3 vs 6.8 ± 1.8 for FeNTA, FeNTA+Res and controls respectively.

Because the final event in chronic liver injury is the development of fibrosis, we have also evaluated the effect of Res in reducing the oxidative stress-induced collagen synthesis. After 24 hr of incubation in serum- and insulin-free medium, cell medium was then used to evaluate procollagen type I accumulation by ELISA (39). Incubation with FeNTA significantly increased collagen accumulation as previously described (40), and this was reduced twofold by the simultaneous presence of Res (Fig. 4).

Thus our results suggest a cause-effect relationship betweeen lipid peroxidation and increased HSC proliferation, which represents an early event in chronic liver injury leading to hepatic fibrosis (6, 9, 27). Interestingly we have also demonstrated a mitogenic role of products released by lipid peroxidation-damaged hepatocytes on HSC, until now suggested only in vivo

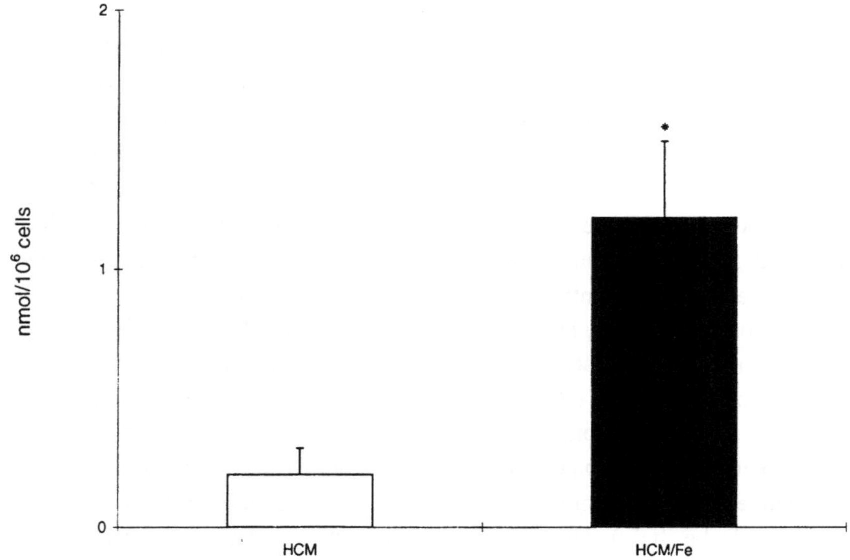

Figure 1. MDA levels in hepatocytes medium. Hepatocytes were incubated for 5 hr in Dulbecco's medium without (HCM) or with FeNTA (HCM/Fe) (100 μM). MDA levels were determined by the TBARS method.
* $p < 0.05$ vs HCM.

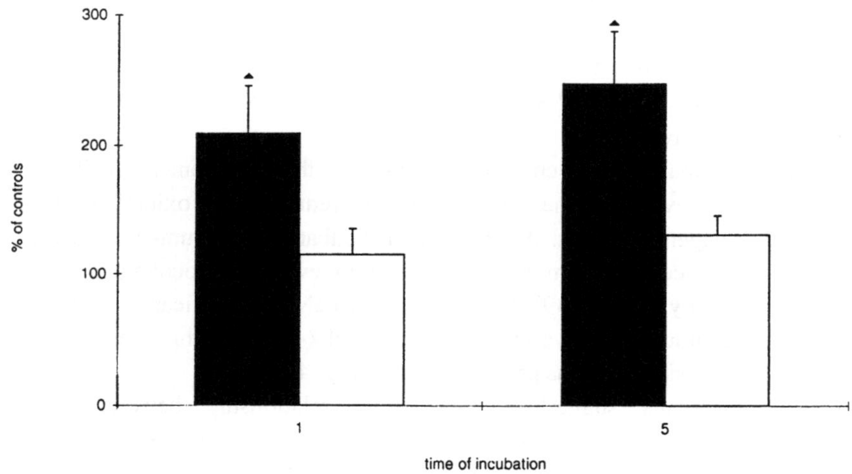

Figure 2. MDA levels in HSC medium. HSC (passage 1-3) were cultured for 24 hr in serum- and insulin-free medium and then incubated in Dulbecco's medium with FeNTA (black bars) or with FeNTA+Res (50 μM). MDA levels were determined by the TBARS method after 1 and 5 hr of incubation.
$p < 0.05$ vs FeNTA.

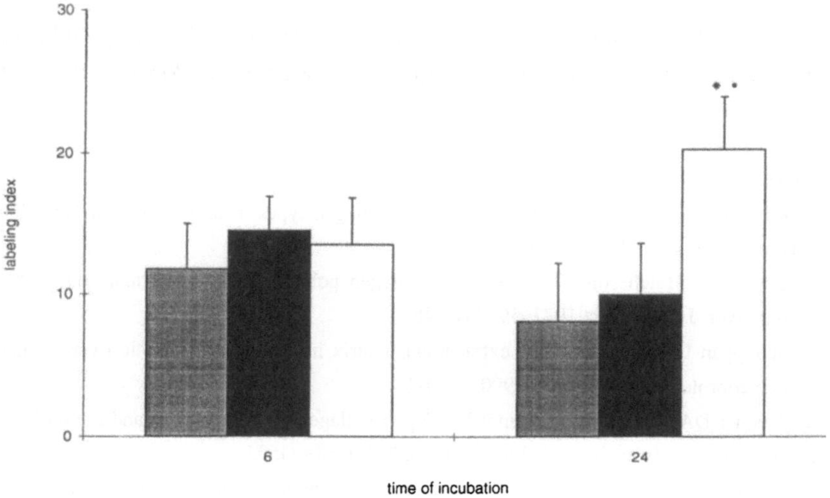

Figure 3. HSC proliferation after incubation with hepatocytes-conditioned medium. HSC were cultured for 24 hr in Iscove's medium containing 0.5% serum and then incubated with the same medium (grey bars) or supplemented with HCM (black bars) or HCM/Fe (white bars) for 6 and 24 hr. BrdU-positive (S-phase) nuclei were detected by immunostaining and expressed as labeling index (% positive nuclei).

• $p < 0.05$ vs controls; ● $p<0.05$ vs HCM.

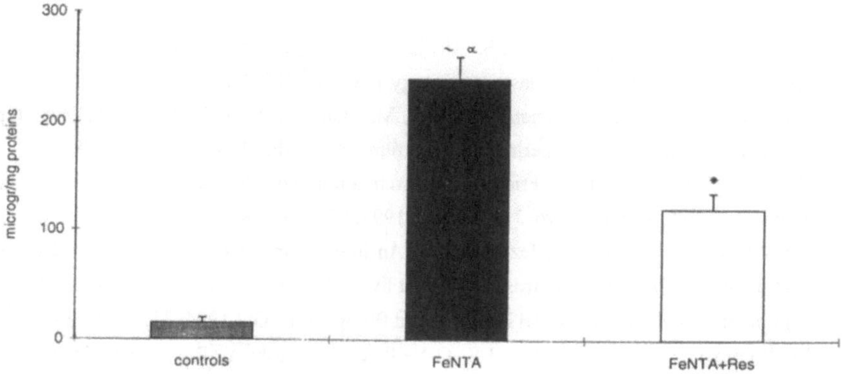

Figure 4. Procollagen type I accumulation in HSC medium. HSC were cultured in serum- and insulin-free medium for 24 hr and then incubated for an additional 24 hr with the same medium or supplemented with FeNTA (100 μM) or FeNTA+Res (50 μM). Procollagen type I was determined in cell medium by ELISA and expressed as μg/mg of total protein.

* $p < 0.05$ vs controls; ∝ $p < 0.005$ vs Fe; ≈ $p < 0.001$ vs controls.

(41). Finally this study indicates a possible role for resveratrol (a poliphenolic antioxidant) for the study of liver injury associated or due to oxidative stress, as indicated for diseases of different etiology (44).

References

1) Rojkind M, Giambrone MA, Biempica L. Collagen types in normal and cirrhotic liver. Gastroenterology 1979; 76: 710-719.

2) Seyer JM, Hutcheson ET, Kang AH. Collagen polymorphism in normal and cirrhotic human liver. J Clin Invest 1977; 59: 241-248.

3) Schuppan D. Structure of the extracellular matrix in normal and fibrotic liver: collagen and glycoproteins. Sem Liv Dis 1990; 10: 1-10.

4) Brenner DA, Westwick J, Breindl M. Type I collagen gene regulation and the molecular pathogenesis of cirrhosis. Am J Physiol 1993; 264: G589-G595.

5) Gressner AM, Bachem MG. Cellular sources of noncollagenous matrix proteins: role of fat-storing cells in fibrogenesis. Semin Liv Dis 1990; 10: 30-46.

6) Friedman SL. The cellular basis of hepatic fibrosis. N Engl J Med. 1993; 25:1828-1835.

7) Friedman SL, Roll JF, Boyles J, Bissell DM. Hepatic lipocytes: the principal collagen producing cells of normal rat liver. Proc Natl Acad Sci USA 1985; 82: 8681-8685.

8) Yokoi Y, Namihisa T, Kuroda H, Komatsu I, Miyazaki A, Watanabe S, Usui K. Immunocytochemical detection of desmin in fat-storing cells (Ito cells). Hepatology 1984; 4: 709-714.

9) Geerts A, Lazou JM, De Bleser P, Wisse E. Tissue distribution, quantitation and proliferation kinetics of fat-storing cells in carbon tetrachloride-injured rat liver. Hepatology 1991; 13: 1193-1202.

10) Mak KM, Leo MA, Lieber CS. Alcoholic liver injury in baboons: transformation of lipocytes to transitional cells. Gastroenterology 1984; 87: 188-200.

11) Tanaka Y, Nouchi T, Yamane M, Irie T, Miyakawa H, Sato C, Marumo F. Phenotypic modulation in lipocytes in experimental liver fibrosis. J Pathol 1991; 164: 273-278.

12) Rockey DC, Housset CN, Friedman SL. Activation-dependent contractility of rat hepatic lipocytes in culture and in vivo. J Clin Invest 1993; 92: 1795-1804.

13) Mancini R, Benedetti A, Jezequel AM. An interleukin-1 receptor antagonist decreases fibrosis induced by dimethylnitrosamine in rat liver. Virchows Archiv 1994; 424: 25-31.

14) Gressner AM. Perisinusoidal lipocytes and fibrogenesis. Gut 1994; 35: 1331-1333.

15) Ramm GA, Li SCY, Britton RS, O'Neill R, Kobayashi Y, Bacon BR. Chronic iron overload causes activation of rat lipocytes in vivo. Am J Physiol 1995: 268: G451-G458.

16) Clement B, Emonard H, Rissel M, Druguet M, Grimaud J-A, Herbage D, Bourel M, Guillouzo A. Cellular origin of collagen and fibronectin in the liver. Cell Mol Biol 1984; 30: 489-496.

17) Kent G, Gay S, Inohue T, Bahu R, Minick OT, Popper H. Vitamin-A containing lipocytes and formation of type III collagen in liver injury. Proc Natl Acad Sci USA 1976; 73: 3719-3722.

18) Milani S, Herbst H, Schuppan D, Kim KY, Riechen EO, Stein H. Cellular localization of type I, III, and IV procollagen gene transcripts in normal and fibrotic human liver. Am J Pathol 1990; 137: 59-70.

19) Pietrangelo A, Gualdi R, Casalgrandi G, Geerts A, De Bleser P, Montorsi G, Ventura E. Enhanced hepatic collagen type I mRNA expression into fat-storing cells in a rodent model of hemocromatosis. Hepatology 1994; 19: 714-721.

20) Tsukamoto H, Matsuoka M, French SW. Experimental models of hepatic fibrosis: a review. Sem Liv Dis 1990; 10: 56-65.

21) Ramadori G. The stellate cell of the liver. New insights into pathophysiology of an intriguing cell. Virchows Archiv B Cell Pathol 1991; 61: 147-158.

22) Fernandez-Munoz D, Caramelo C, Santos JC. Sistemic and splanchnic hemodynamic disturbances in conscious rats with experimental liver cirrhosis without ascites. Am J Physiol 1985; 249: G316-G320.

23) Baraona E, Liu W, Ma X-L, Svegliati Baroni G, Lieber CS. Acetaldehyde-collagen adducts in n-nitrosodimethylamine-induced liver cirrhosis. Life Sci 1993; 52: 1249-1255.

24) Mancini R, Jezequel AM, Benedetti A, Paolucci F, Trozzi L, Orlandi F. Quantitative analysis of proliferating sinusoidal cells in dimethylnitrosamine-induced cirrhosis. An immunohistochemical study. J Hepatol 1992; 15: 361-366.

25) Ala-Kokko L, Pihlajaniemi T, Myers CJ, Kivirikko KI, Savolainen ER. Gene expression of type I, III and IV collagens in hepatic fibrosis induced by dimethylnitrosamine in the rat. Biochem J 1987; 244: 75-79.

26) Rockey DC, Maher JJ, Jarnagin WR, Gabbiani G, Friedman SL. Inhibition of rat hepatic lipocytes activation in culture by interferon-gamma. Hepatology 1992; 16: 776-784.

27) Svegliati Baroni, G., D' Ambrosio, L., Curto, P., Casini, A., Mancini, R., Jezequel, A.M., Benedetti, A. (1996) Interferon-gamma decreases hepatic stellate cells activation and extracellular matrix deposition in rat liver fibrosis. Hepatology in press

28) Geerts A, Vrijsen R, Rauterberger J, Burt A, Schellink P, Wisse E. In vitro differentation of fat-storing cells parallels marked increase of collagen synthesis and secretion. J Hepatol 1989; 9: 59-68.

29) Knittel, T., Schuppan, D., Meyer Zum Buschenfelde, K-H., Ramadori G. 1992 Differential expression of collagen types I, III and IV by fat-storing (Ito) cells in vitro. Gastroenterology 102: 1724-1735.

30) Brenner, D.A., Chojkier, M. 1987 Acetaldehyde increases collagen gene transcription in cultured human fibroblasts. J Biol Chem 262: 1652-1658.

31) Chojkier, M., Houglum, K., Solis-Herruzo, J., Brenner, D.A. 1989 Stimulation of collagen gentile expression by ascorbic acid in cultured human fibroblasts. J Biol Chem 264: 16957-16962.

32) Houglum, K., Brenner, D.A., Chojkier, M. 1991 Inhibition of collagen gene expression by ascorbic acid in cultured human fibroblasts. J Clin Invest 87: 2230-2235.

33) Kamimura, S., Gaal, K., Britton, R.S., Bacon, B.R., Triadafilopoulos, G., Tsukamoto, H. 1992 Increased 4-hydroxynonenal levels in experimental alcoholic liver disease: association of lipid peroxidation with liver fibrogenesis. Hepatology 16: 448-453.

34) Houglum, K., Filip, M., Witztum, J.L., Chojkier, M. 1990 Malondialdehyde and 4-hydroxynonenal protein adducts in plasma and liver of rats with iron overload. J Clin Invest 86: 1991-1998.

35) Houglum, K., Bedossa, P., Chojkier, M. 1994 TGF-β and collagen-α 1 (I) gene expression are increased in hepatic acinar zone 1 of rats with iron overload. Am J Physiol 267: G908-G913.

36) Bedossa, P., Houglum, K., Trautwein, C., Holstege, A., Chojkier, M 1994 Stimulation of collagen-α 1(I) gene expression is associated with lipid peroxidation in hepatocellular injury: a link to tissue fibrosis? Hepatology 19: 1262-1271.

37) Albano, E., Clot, P., Morimoto, M., Tomasi, A., Ingelman-Sundberg, M., French, S.W. 1996 Role of cytochrome P4502E1-dependent formation of hydroxyethil free radical in the development of liver damage in rats intragstrically fed with ethanol. Hepatology 23: 155-163.

38) Niemela, O., Parkkila, S., Yla.Herttuala, S., Villanueva, J., Ruebner, B., Halsted, C.H. 1995 Sequential acetaldehyde production, lipid peroxidation and fibrogenesis in micropig model of alcohol-induced liver disease. Hepatology 22: 1208-1214.

39) Casini, A., Cunningham, M., Rojkind, M., Lieber, C.S. (1991) Acetaldehyde increases procollagen type I and fibronectin gene transcription in cultured rat fat-storing cells through a protein synthesis-dependent mechanism. Hepatology 13: 758-765.

40) Parola, M., Pinzani, M., Casini, A., Albano, E., Poli, G., Gentilini A., Gentilini P., Dianzani, M.U. (1993) Stimulation of lipid peroxidation or 4-hydroxynonenal treatment increases procollagen α 1(I) gene expression in human liver fat-storing cells. Biochem Biophys Res Comm 194: 1044-1050.

41) Gualdi, R., Casalgrandi, G., Montosi, G., Ventura, E., Pietrangelo, A. 1994 Excess iron into hepatocytes is required for activation of collagen type I gene during experimental siderosis. Gastroenterology 107: 1118-1124.

42) Sundaresan , M., Yu, Z.X., Ferrans, V.J., Irani, K., Finkel, T. (1995) Requirement for generation of H2O2 for platelet-derived growth factor signal transduction. Science 270: 296-299.

43) Frankel, E.N., Kanner, J., German, J.B., Parks, E., Kinsella, J.E. (1993) Inhibition of oxidation of human low-density lipoprotein by phenolic substances in red wine. Lancet 341: 454-456.

44) Hertog, M.G.L., Feskens, E.J.M., Hollman P.C.H., Katan, M.B., Kromhout D. 1993 Dietary antioxidant flavonoids and risk of coronary heart disease: the Zutphen Elderly Study. Lancet 342: 1007-1011.

45) Fuhrman, B., Lavy, A., Aviram, M. 1995 Consumption of red wine with meals reduces the susceptibility of human plasma and low-density liporptoein to lipid peroxidation. Am J Clin Nutr 61: 549-554.

46) Blond, J.P., Denis, M.P., Bezard, J. (1995) Action antioxydante du resveratrol sur la lipoperoxidation. Sci Alimen 15: 347-358.

47) Benedetti, A., Svegliati Baroni, G., Marucci, L., Mancini, R., Jezequel, A.M., Orlandi, F. (1993) Regulation of intracellular pH in isolated periportal and perivenular rat hepatocytes. Gastroenterology 105: 1797-1805.

48) Morel, I., Lescoat, G., Cillar, J., Pasdelop, N., Brissot, P., Cillard, P. (1990) Kinetic evaluation of free malondialdehyde and enzyme leakage as indices of iron damage in rat hepatocytes cultures: involvement of free radicals. Biochem Pharmacol 39: 1647-1655.

CHAPTER 12

REOXYGENATION INJURY IN ISOLATED RAT HEPATOCYTES

An experimental model system to study the mechanisms of oxidative stress

Paolo Caraceni, Antonio Gasbarrini, Franco Trevisani, Marco Domenicali, Giovanni Gasbarrini, David H. Van Thiel, and Mauro Bernardi.

Istituto di Patologia Medica, University of Bologna; Istituto di Clinica Medica, Catholic University of Rome; and Liver Disease Program, Oklahoma Medical Research Foundation, Oklahoma City, USA.

SUMMARY

Isolated rat hepatocytes generate large amounts of oxygen free radicals during post-anoxic reoxygenation and, consequently, experience a significant cell injury. Mitochondria and microsomes but not the cytosolic xanthine oxidase system appear to be the main intracellular sources of free radical production. Lipids and proteins rather than DNA are damaged by oxygen free radicals during the early phases of post-anoxic reoxygenation. Finally, protein oxidation appears to be temporally and causally related to the development of the cell injury.

1. Introduction

Ischemia-reperfusion injury is involved in the pathogenesis of liver damage occurring during several pathological conditions such as hepatic surgery, shock, and liver transplantation. Paradoxically, reperfusion and resupply of oxygen can exacerbate the liver damage caused by an ischemic insult. The mechanisms responsible for reperfusion injury are not clearly determined, but a considerable amount of evidences indicates that the generation of oxygen free radicals (OFR) plays an important pathogenetic role. First, OFR have been measured and identified during reperfusion using techniques such as electron spin resonance and chemiluminescence; second, indices of oxidative stress such as lipid peroxidation and glutathione disulfide release are increased during reperfusion; third, reperfusion injury can be prevented by antioxidants including superoxide dismutase, deferoxamine, gluthatione, and vitamin E.

Several *in vivo* experimental models have been used to investigate the role of the oxidative stress in hepatic reperfusion injury. Biological systems of isolated liver cells can provide valuable mechanistic information on the cellular

P. Gentilini and M. U. Dianzani. New Trends in Hepatology, 104-112

mechanisms underlying reoxygenation injury since the experimental protocol can be conducted under well-defined conditions. The data emerging from studies using isolated hepatocytes in suspension, in monolayer culture and, mostly, immobilized and perfused in agarose gel threads are herein reviewed.

2. Oxygen Free Radical Formation and Reoxygenation Injury

Isolated hepatocytes are capable of generating large amounts of OFR during reoxygenation following a prolonged period of anoxia as monitored in real time by using chemiluminescence techniques (1,2). The upper panel of Fig. 1 shows the lucigenin-enhanced chemiluminescence (LCL), which detects specifically superoxide anion ($O_2^{\bullet-}$)(1), emitted by perfused rat hepatocytes exposed to 2.5 h of anoxia and 2 h of reoxygenation. Immediately upon resupply of oxygen, the rate of $O_2^{\bullet-}$ formation increases about 12 fold above the basal aerobic levels within 15 min and, then, it returned progressively to control values. In these experiments, reoxygenation injury was temporally related to OFR generation.

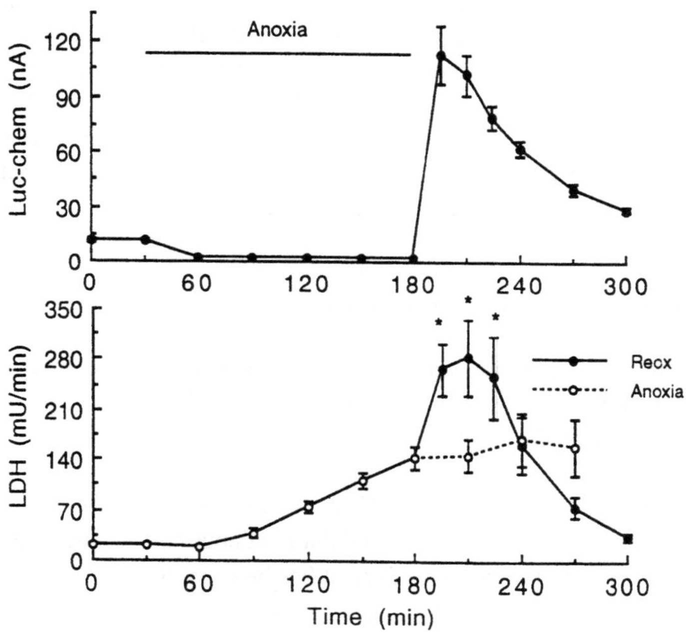

Fig. 1. LCL (upper panel) and LDH release (lower panel) in perfused rat hepatocytes exposed to 2.5 h of anoxia followed by 2 h of reoxygenation or to continuous anoxia.

As shown in the lower panel of Fig. 1, after the reintroduction of oxygen, the rate of LDH release increases reaching a value, which is almost double that observed in cells kept continuously under anaerobic conditions, indicating the occurrence of a significant reoxygenation injury. The fact that the increase of LDH release is delayed 15-30 min compared to the peak of chemiluminescence suggests that OFR formation occurs first and is followed by cell damage.

$O_2^{\bullet-}$ radicals are not highly reactive per se and their toxicity reside in the transformation to more toxic free radicals including hydrogen peroxide (H_2O_2) and hydroxyl radicals ($HO\bullet$) as described by the Haber-Weiss reaction. The formation of $HO\bullet$ from H_2O_2 is catalyzed by Fe^{2+} and, consequently, chelating the intracellular free iron can inhibit the formation of $HO\bullet$ radicals. Indeed, low concentrations of the iron-chelator Deferoxamine prevents reoxygenation injury without affecting $O_2^{\bullet-}$ formation (6).

In contrast, when the hepatocytes are reoxygenated after a shorter period of anoxia, OFR generation is lower and most of the cells remains viable without evidence for reoxygenation injury. This may be explained by the fact that hepatocytes are provided with very effective defense mechanisms and, therefore, OFR are capable of causing directly cell injury when their intracellular formation is several fold above the physiological level and the antioxidants reserves are impaired as it occurs during reoxygenation following a prolonged period of anoxia (1-4). Thus, the length of the anoxic period is crucial for the occurrence of the subsequent reoxygenation injury. Its exact length is variable and depends on many factors including the animal species, the nutritional status, the isolation method and the experimental model system (1-5).

3. Cellular Sources of Oxygen Free Radicals

The OFR produced by isolated hepatocytes during post-anoxic reoxygenation can be generated from several cellular sources including the cytosolic xanthine/xanthine oxidase, the mitochondria and the microsomes.

3.1. CYTOSOLIC XANTHINE/XANTHINE OXIDASE SYSTEM

Because the xanthine oxidase inhibitor allopurinol has been shown to protect the liver from reperfusion injury, it has been proposed that this enzyme, activated by the increase in cytosolic Ca^{++} induced by ischemia, would produce, at reperfusion, large amounts of $O_2^{\bullet-}$ from the xanthine and hypoxanthine accumulated in the liver during ischemia as a result of the ATP hydrolysis and purine degradation. However, studies using isolated hepatocytes have excluded that this reaction pathway occurs at a significant extent in liver parenchymal cells (1,2,7-9). Indeed, under these experimental conditions, allopurinol is not able either to reduce the $O_2^{\bullet-}$ and H_2O_2 formation or to prevent the cell injury during reoxygenation. Furthermore, in experiments with isolated hepatocytes in suspension, cell death precedes the conversion of xanthine dehydrogenase to the active form xanthine oxidase (9). Thus, in whole livers, the beneficial effect of allopurinol could be the result of its action on cells other than hepatocytes, such as Kupffer and endothelial cells.

3.2. MITOCHONDRIA

Several lines of evidences indicate that the mitochondrial respiratory chain is a major source of OFR during hepatic post-ischemic reperfusion. Mitochondria generate both $O_2^{\bullet-}$ and H_2O_2 in minimal quantities even under physiological conditions. The production of these reactive oxygen species is greatly enhanced on reoxygenation of previously hypoxic cells when the mitochondrial metabolic state is characterized by a reduction of the components of the respiratory chain. The role of mitochondria during reoxygenation is further supported by experiments with antimycin A (1,2,7,8,10), which is known to increase the availability of electrons for the formation of reactive oxygen species by inhibiting the electron transfer from cytochrome b_{562} to ubisemiquinone and ubiquinone. While antimycin A does not produce significant changes on OFR-induced chemiluminescence under normoxic conditions (2), it almost doubles the $O_2^{\bullet-}$ formation and the cell injury experienced by isolated rat hepatocytes during post-anoxic reoxygenation (8).

3.3. MICROSOMES

Liver microsomes catalyze a wide variety of biological oxidations which require molecular oxygen and NADPH with $O_2^{\bullet-}$ generation. Since treatment with diphenyliodinium, a NADPH oxidase inhibitor easily taken up by hepatic microsomes, reduces either lucigenin-enhanced chemiluminescence or LDH release, it is likely that microsomes contribute to $O_2^{\bullet-}$ generation and reoxygenation injury in parenchymal liver cells (8).

4. Molecular Targets of Oxygen Free Radical Attack

OFR can cause cell injury by attacking a great variety of cellular molecules including lipids, proteins, and nucleic acids. The occurrence of these alterations and their relative contribution to the pathogenesis of hepatic reoxygenation injury is not clearly determined as yet.

4.1. LIPID PEROXIDATION

Lipid peroxidation (LP) arising from the reaction of free radicals with lipids is considered an important feature of oxidative stress (11). A considerable amount of data indicates that LP occurs in liver cells during post-ischemic reperfusion; however, it is still debated whether the associated changes in membrane fluidity or permeability are necessary to cause cell death.

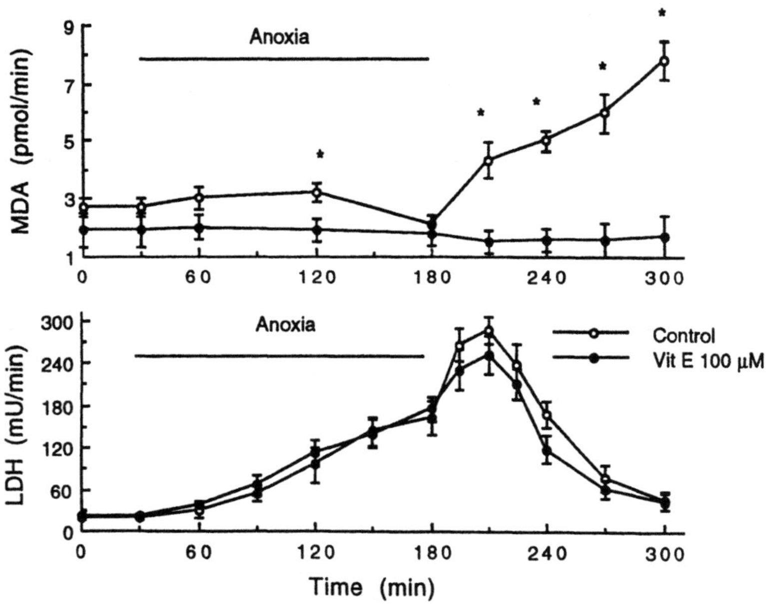

Fig. 2. MDA (upper panel) and LDH (lower panel) release with Vitamin E-treated and control rat hepatocytes exposed to 2.5 h of anoxia followed by 2 h of reoxygenation.

Recent studies using perfused rat hepatocytes have provided new insights on the temporal and causal relationship between OFR generation, LP and cell injury during post-anoxic reoxygenation (1,11). The production of malondialdehyde (MDA), a LP end-products, chronologically follows the burst in $O_2^{\bullet -}$ formation (1). LP ultimately results from the transformation of $O_2^{\bullet -}$ to more toxic species such as H_2O_2 and HO· through the Haber-Weiss reaction (12).

In contrast, LP does not occur in the proper sequence of events with regard to the cell injury. First, the MDA increase above the basal pre-anoxic rate reaches the statistical significance only during the second hour of reoxygenation when LDH is back to control levels and the majority of the cells have already lost viability (1). Thus, LP which occurs after cell death is not easily distinguished from that which may be causally related to cell injury. Second, the chain breaking anti-oxidant Vitamin E abolishes LP without affecting cell injury as shown in Fig. 2 (11).

The sum of these data clearly indicate that LP is not primarily responsible for the development of cell death during the early phases of reoxygenation in parenchymal liver cells. Nevertheless, a pathogenetic role for LP in a later phase of reperfusion injury cannot be excluded. At this regard, various end-products of LP, such as 4-hydroxynonenal, are chemoattractants for neutrophils, induce DNA damage and compromise detoxification systems.

4.2. PROTEIN OXIDATION

A considerable amount of proteins and enzymes have been shown to be particularly sensitive to the noxious effect of OFR. Oxidation of amino acid residues in proteins causes modification such as deamination, carbonyl group formation and cleavage of peptid bonds. These changes produce conformational and functional alterations in proteins leading to fragmentation, aggregation, loss of enzyme activity and susceptibility of proteolytic digestion (10,13).

Protein oxidation occurs during post-ischemic reperfusion in several organs including brain, lung and heart. Recent evidences indicate that oxidative damage to proteins is also an important feature of the hepatocyte injury during post-anoxic reoxygenation. Indeed, the increase of protein carbonyl content, index of protein oxidation, occurs early upon oxygen reintroduction and it is temporally related to the development of cell injury (14).

4.3. DNA OXIDATION

DNA is another target molecule in cellular oxidative injury. The reaction between DNA and OFR, in particular HO• radicals, leads to several alterations including damaged bases, inter- and intra-strand crosslinks, and single-strand breaks. The cells are protected against these lesions by repair mechanisms involving enzymes and other nuclear factors. However, when the repair systems are overwhelmed by the extent of oxidative injury, the persistence of the lesions induces a variety of biological consequences, such as mutation induction, blocking of transcription and replication, and chromosomal aberration (15).

A large number of studies have shown that DNA oxidation is associated with aging, carcinogenesis and exposure to ionizing radiation. In contrast, only indirect evidences of DNA damage by OFR have been shown to occur in the whole liver as a result of post-ischemic reperfusion. In isolated rat hepatocytes, preliminary observations indicate that the level of DNA oxidation, assessed by the content of 8-hydroxyguanosine (8-OHdG), which is formed by the reaction of guanine base with HO·, increases slightly during anoxia remaining elevated during reoxygenation. However, these changes are not statistically significant when compared to the basal pre-anoxic values suggesting that DNA oxidation may not be an important event in the early phases of reoxygenation (14).

Nevertheless, the effective role of DNA oxidation in the genesis of hepatic reperfusion injury is still to be determined for several reasons. First, the formation of 8-oxo-dG is only one of the many DNA base modifications caused by OFR and, therefore, it is possible that reoxygenation injury induces other types of DNA damage. Second, the biological effects of DNA oxidation result from the sum of the lesions caused by OFR and their repair by the specific cellular systems, but the relative importance of these alternative processes is unknown. Third, the extent of DNA oxidation should be quantitated in the mithocondrial fraction more than in the total cellular DNA since mitochondria are a main site of OFR generation and have poor repair processes.

5. Conclusions

The reoxygenation injury experienced by isolated rat hepatocytes is related to the occurrence of an important oxidative stress. Immediately upon the resupply of oxygen, liver parenchymal cells generate large amounts of superoxide anions which can be measured in real time using a lucigenin -enhanced chemiluminescence technique. However, since hepatocytes are provided of very effective defense mechanisms, oxygen free radicals are capable of causing directly cell injury when their intracellular formation is several fold above the physiological level and the antioxidants reserves are impaired as it occurs during reoxygenation following a prolonged period of anoxia.

Mitochondria and microsomes but not the cytosolic xanthine oxidase system appear to be the main intracellular sources of the $O_2^{\bullet-}$ generated during reoxygenation. Cell injury is not caused by $O_2^{\bullet-}$, which is not highly toxic per se, but ultimately results from the transformation of $O_2^{\bullet-}$ to more toxic species such as H_2O_2 and HO· through the iron-dependent Haber-Weiss reaction as indicated by the protection with the iron-chelator Deferoxamine.

Lipids and proteins rather than DNA are damaged by oxygen free radicals. However, only protein oxidation appears to be temporally and causally related to the development of the cell injury suffered by isolated rat hepatocytes during the early phases of post-anoxic reoxygenation.

References

1) Caraceni P, Rosenblum ER, Van Thiel DH, Borle AB. Reoxygenation injury in isolated rat hepatocytes: relation to oxygen free radicals and lipid peroxidation. Am J Physiol 266: G799-806, 1994.

2) Littauer A and De Groot H. Release of reactive oxygen by hepatocytes on reoxygenation: three phases and role of mitochondria. Am J Phys 1992; 262: G1015-1020.

3) De Groot H. Isolated cells in the study of the molecular mechanisms of reperfusion injury. Toxicol Lett 1992; 63: 111-125.

4) Caraceni P, Gasbarrini A, Van Thiel DH and Borle AB. Oxygen free radical formation by isolated hepatocytes during post-anoxic reoxygenation: scavenging effect of albumin. Am J Physiol 1994; 266: G451-G458.

5) Caraceni P, Gasbarrini A, Nussler A, Di Silvio M, Bartoli F, Borle AB and Van Thiel DH. Human hepatocytes are more resistant than rat hepatocytes to anoxia-reoxygenation injury. Hepatology 20: 1247-1254; 1994.

6) Caraceni P, Van Thiel DH, Borle AB. Dual effect of deferoxamine on free radical formation and reoxygenation injury in isolated hepatocytes. Am J Physiol 1995; 269: G132-G137.

7) De Groot H. and Brecht M. Reoxygenation injury in rat hepatocytes: mediation by O_2/H_2O_2 liberated by sources other than xanthine oxidase. Biol. Chem. Hoppe-Seyler 1991; 372:35-41.

8) Caraceni P, Ryu HS, Van Thiel DH, Borle AB. Source of oxygen free radicals produced by rat hepatocytes during post-anoxic reoxygenation. Biochim Bioph Acta 1995; 1268: 249-254.

9) De Groot H and Littauer A. Reoxygenation injury in isolated hepatocytes: cell death precedes the conversion of xanthine dehydogenase to xanthine oxidase. Bioch Biophys Res Comm 1988; 155: 278-282.

10) Dawson TL, Gores GJ, Nieminen AL, Herman B, Lemasters JJ. Mitochondria as a source of reactive oxygen species during reductive stress in rat hepatocytes. Am J Physiol 1992; 264: C961-C967

11) Yu BP. Cellular defenses against damage from reactive oxygen species. Physiol Rev 74: 137-161; 1994.

12) Caraceni P, Yao T, Gasbarrini A, Borle AB, Bowie BT, Zern M, Van Thiel DH and Degli Esposti S. Vitamin E prevents lipid peroxidation but does not reduce rat hepatocytes injury during the early phase of reoxygenation. Life Sci 55 (18): 1427-1432; 1994.

13) Stadtman ER. Protein oxidation and aging. Science. 1992; 257: 1220-1224.

14) Caraceni P, De Maria N, Ryu HS, Gasbarrini A, Maidt ML, Pye O, Floyd RA, Van Thiel DH. Cellular targets for free radical attack during reoxygenation injury in perfused hepatocytes. [Abstract] Hepatology 20 (4): 180A; 1994.

15) Satoh MS, and Lindhal T. Enzymatic repair of oxidative DNA Damage. Cancer Research (suppl.) 1994; 54: 1899-1901.

CHAPTER 13

OXIDATIVE STRESS AND CELL DAMAGE FOLLOWING ORTHOTOPIC LIVER TRANSPLANTATION.

E. CHIARPOTTO[1], F. BIASI[2], J. CUTRIN[1], M. SALIZZONI[3], G. LANFRANCO[4], M. RIZZETTO[3], A. BOVERIS[5] and G. POLI[1,2].

[1]*Department of Experimental Medicine and Oncology, University of Torino and Interuniversity Centre of Hepatic Physiopathology, Italy;* [2]*CNR Centre of Immunogenetics and Experimental Oncology, Italy;* [3] *Transplantation Unit and* [4] *"Baldi e Riberi" Laboratory, Azienda Ospedaliera Molinette, Torino, Italy;* [5] *Institute of Biological Chemistry and Physicochemistry, University of Buenos Aires, Argentina.*

Summary

Hepatic reperfusion injury in human orthotopic liver transplantation is associated with increased steady state levels of reactive oxygen species. Different hematic parameters of tissue redox balance can be analyzed in adult patients at the beginning of liver transplantation and at different times after reperfusion. A significant increase of oxidative stress parameters, i.e. red cell malonaldehyde and plasma lipoperoxides, is evident soon after reperfusion with respect to basal time and is accompanied by a decrease of plasma vitamin

P. Gentilini and M. U. Dianzani. New Trends in Hepatology, 113-121

E. This alteration of redox balance is paralelled by a significant increase of cytolysis evaluated in terms of alanine aminotransferase. The presence of a significant correlation between alterations of the redox status and irreversible cell damage after liver reperfusion supports the implication of oxidative reactions in the occurrence of ischemia- reperfusion tissue injury following orthotopic liver transplantation.

Introduction

Ischemia is a widely occurring event which can take place generally in an organ during surgery, under conditions of shock and with transplantation. Increasing periods of ischemia give rise to enhanced damage, which can be reversible or irreversible, depending on the length. Paradoxically, reoxygenation after a hypoxic period leads to exacerbation of the injury. The specific mechanisms responsible for reperfusion injury, are still unclear, but in recent years, there has been much evidence linking post-ischemic reperfusion tissue injury with overproduction of reactive oxygen species (ROS) [1]. In particular, ischemia-reperfusion injury is involved in the pathogenesis of liver damage that occurs during the above reported pathological conditions, i.e. hepatic surgery, circulatory shock and liver transplantation [2]. Liver transplantation surgery has been established as a common therapy for irreversible liver diseases. Early liver graft failure is, however, one of the most important complications [3]. A critical role in the genesis of such early impaired performance is ascribed to the liver insult consequent to reperfusion of the ischemic organ. The ischemia-reperfusion injury may result from several processes in the transplantation including donor organ harvesting, cold ischemic preservation of the graft, warm ischemia before anastomosis of the hepatic artery and the portal vein, and reperfusion after restoration of blood flow in recipients. Several *in vivo* and *in vitro* animal models have been used to study the ischemia reperfusion injury of liver [4-6], and in the experimental rat model clear evidence has been obtained of the pathogenetic involvement of free radical oxidative reactions in the reperfusion injury after liver transplantation (for a review see [7]). On the other hand, little is known about the sensitivity of human hepatocytes to anoxia-reoxygenation.

Oxidative damage and cytolysis

In the field of orthotopic human liver transplantation, the occurrence of oxidative damage, as well as its role in postoperative hepatic injury, urgently requires elucidation. Here we report data on oxidative damage occurring in humans in the early phases following orthotopic liver transplantation, in terms of blood indices of impaired tissue redox balance. In addition, we studied the possible relationship between the extent of oxidative damage and cytolysis. Nineteen adult patients underwent orthotopic liver transplantation (OLT) in the Transplantation Unit of the "Ospedale Maggiore di S. Giovanni Battista e della Citta' di Torino", Hospital. The mean age of the patients was 49 ± 6 years. The indications for organ transplantation (with the number of patients in parentheses) were: chronic active hepatitis with cirrhosis HCV+ or HBV+ (11), fulminant hepatitis (1), hepatocellular carcinoma (1), alcoholic cirrhosis (2), primary biliary cirrhosis (4). Orthotopic transplantation of liver preserved in UW solution (NPBI, The Netherlands) followed the standard procedure described by Tzakis et al. [8]. Ten adult subjects without any biochemical or clinical signs of disease were recruited as control group. Blood samples were collected immediately before general anesthesia and at different times after complete declamping up to 120 min; plasma and red blood cells were separated and analysed within two hours. Oxidative damage was assessed by evaluating the steady-state level of malonaldehyde (MDA) in erythrocytes [9] and of lipid peroxides (LPO) [10] and vitamin E in plasma [11]. Irreversible liver damage was evaluated in terms of alanine aminotransferase (ALT) plasma levels by commercial kit.

TABLE 1. Red blood cell malonaldehyde (MDA) content, plasma lipid peroxide (LPO), vitamin E (vit E) and alanine amino transferase (ALT) levels at basal time and 120 min after reperfusion in patients subjected to OLT.

	Basal	120 min Reperfusion
MDA (nmoles/ml pRBC)	3.4 ± 1.2	6.9 ± 2.9 [a]
LPO (nmoles/ml plasma)	1.6 ± 1.2	4.1 ± 1.6 [a]
Vit E (nmoles/ml plasma)	26.4 ± 4.3	20.9 ± 4.6 [a]
ALT (U/l)	42.0 ± 16.0	947.0 ± 533.0 [a]

Values are mean ± S.D.

[a] Significantly different from basal value ($p < 0.001$).

Normal subject values: MDA 1.3 ± 0.1; LPO 1.4 ± 0.3; Vit E 32.6 ± 4.4; ALT 30.4 ± 5.2.

pRBC: packed red blood cells.

The marked change towards oxidation of the tissue redox equilibrium, shown indirectly in the peripheral blood by the increase in levels of the two indicators of prooxidant condition (MDA and LPO), as well as by the decrease of vitamin E in all transplanted patients examined in the very early phases of reperfusion during OLT, underlines a condition of oxidative stress (Table 1).

In fact, in all patients we detected a significant increase of both erythrocyte MDA and plasma LPO at 120 min reperfusion time compared to basal values accompanied by a statistically significant consumption of plasma vitamin E as well as by a statistically significant increase of ALT. In particular, the significant difference of oxidative stress parameters between basal time and 120 minutes after reperfusion, confirms that reoxygenation is the triggering event in the pathogenesis of oxidative damage consequent on liver transplantation.

TABLE 2. Red blood cell malonaldehyde (MDA) content and plasma lipid peroxide (LPO) levels at basal time and at different times after reperfusion in OLT (typical trend).

Time	MDA (nmoles/ml pRBC)	LPO (nmoles/ml plasma)
Basal	2.2	1.2
1 min	4.2	1.9
10 min	6.1	3.6
60 min	7.1	7.1
120 min	9.3	4.8

pRBC: packed red blood cells.

This finding is further supported by the progressive increase of erythrocyte MDA and plasma LPO levels in the very early phases of reperfusion during OLT (1, 10, 60 and 120 min after portal vein declamping) (Table 2). Consistent results have been reported in our previous study on oxidative damage in human liver transplantation in which all patients were monitored for 20 days after surgery [12].

The good linear correlation, statistically significant, demonstrated among the different markers of oxidative damage as well as among oxidative damage and cytolysis markers as regards their variation from basal to post-reperfusion values in each patient (Table 3) strongly recommends their combined use to provide a reliable and comprehensive image of oxidative reactions going on after liver transplantation.

TABLE 3. Linear correlation among the different values of oxidative damage / cytolysis obtained in each liver transplanted patient at basal and 120 min reperfusion time.

	Correlation Coefficients (r)
MDA/LPO	0.54[a]
MDA/ALT	0.58[a]
MDA/VIT E	- 0.38[a]
LPO/ALT	0.64[a]
LPO/VIT E	- 0.37[a]
ALT/VIT E	- 0.43[a]

Spearman's rank correlation analysis was adopted. [a]Significance: $p<0.05$.

In any case, a more complete characterization of oxidative damage after reperfusion is necessary to evaluate its possible implication in the pathogenesis of events such as cytolysis or cholestasis, whose pharmaceutical down-modulation might be crucial. Only by means of antioxidant intervention it will be possible to confirm whether post-graft cytolysis and organ dysfunction are at least partly caused by the early burst of oxidative reactions. A randomized study of the effect of antioxidants in post-ischemic liver injury in transplant recipients is now in progress. However, a variety of findings are already indicative of a pathogenetic role of oxidative stress in liver dysfunction after transplantation: i) the statistically significant linear relation observed in the individual liver transplants between the increase of oxidative damage and cytolysis at post-reperfusion time (Table 3); ii) the experimental demonstration that lipid peroxidation can be the cause, but not a mere consequence of hepatocyte lysis [13,14]; iii) the ever-growing literature on the protective effect of antioxidants in other human surgical conditions of ischemia-reperfusion, e.g. kidney transplantation [15] and cardiopulmonary bypass [16].

Acknowledgements

The work has been carried out with grants from the Ministry of University, Rome, Italy, 60% funds and National Projects on Liver Cirrhosis and Viral Hepatitis and on Free Radicals and Redox Equilibrium.

Juan Cutrin is indebted to the Fondazione per le Biotecnologie, Torino, Italy, for the support of a fellowship.

References

1. Omar, B., McCord, J. and Downey, J. (1991) Ischemia-reperfusion, In: Sies, H., ed.*Oxidative stress: Oxidants and Antioxidants*, Academic Press, London, pp. 493-527.
2. Shibayama, Y., Asaka, S. and Nishijima, A. (1991) Mechanism of liver injury following ischemia, *Exp. Mol. Pathol.* **55,** 251-260.
3. Kakizoe, S., Yanaga, K., Starzl, T.E. and Demetris, A.J. (1990) Evaluation of protocol before transplantation and after reperfusion biopsies from human orthotopic liver allografts: considerations of preservation and early immunological injury, *Hepatology* **11,** 932-941.
4. Sakr, M.F., Zetti, G.M., Hassainen, T.I., Farghali, H., Nalesnik, M.A., Gavaler, J.S., Starzl, T.E., et al (1991) FK 506 ameliorates the hepatic injury associated with ische,ia and reperfusion in rats, *Hepatology* **13,** 947-951.
5. Wu, T.W., Hashimoto, N., Au, J.X., Wu, J., Mickle, D.A. and Carey, D. (1991) Trolox protects rat hepatocytes against oxyradical damage and the ischemic rat liver from reperfusion injury, *Hepatology* **13,** 575-580.
6. Littauer, A. and De Groot, H. (1992) Release of reactive oxygen by hepatocytes on reoxygenation: three phases and role of mitochondria, *Am. J. Physiol.* **262,** G1015-G1020.
7. Jaeschke, H. (1991) Reactive oxygen and ischemia-reperfusion injury of the liver, *Chem.-Biol. Interact.* **79,** 115-136.
8. Tzakis, A., Todo, S. and Starzl T.E. (1989) Orthotopic liver transplantation with preservation of the inferior vena cava, *Ann Surg* **210,** 649-652.
9. Bernheim, F., Bernheim, M.L.C. and Wilbur, K.M. (1948) The reaction between thiobarbituric acid and the oxidative products of certains lipids,*J.Biol. Chem.* **174,** 257-264.

10. Tateishi, T., Yoshimine, N. and Kuzuya, F. (1987) Serum lipid peroxide assayed by new colorimetric method *Exp. Gerontol.* **22,** 103-111.

11. Burton, G.W., Webb, A. and Ingold, K.U. (1985) A mild, rapid and efficient method of lipid extraction for use in determining vitamin E/lipid ratio, *Lipids* **20,** 29-39.

12. Biasi, F., Bosco, M., Chiappino, I., Chiarpotto, E., Lanfranco, G., Ottobrelli, A., Massano, G., Donadio, P.P., Vaj, M., Andorno, E., Rizzetto, M., Salizzoni, M. and Poli, G. (1995) Oxidative damage in human liver transplantation *Free Rad. Biol. Med.* **19,** 311-317.

13. Poli, G., Albano, E. and Dianzani, M.U. The role of lipid peroxidation in liver damage (1987) *Chem. Phys. Lipids* **45,** 117-142.

14. Biasi, F., Bosco, M., Lanfranco, G. and Poli, G. (1995) Cytolysis does not per se induce lipid peroxidation: evidence in man *Free Rad. Biol. Med.* **18,** 909-912.

15. Mayumi, T., Schiller, H.J. and Bulkley, G.B. (1993) Pharmaceutical intervention for the prevention of post-ischemic reperfusion injury, in: Poli G., Albano E. and Dianzani M.U. (eds.), *Free Radicals: From Basic Science to Medicine.* Birkhäuser Verlag, Basel, pp. 438-457.

16. Johnson, W.D., Kayser, K.L., Brenowitz, J.B, Saedi, S.F. (1991) A randomized controlled trial of allopurinol in coronary bypass surgery. *Am. Heart J.* **121,** 20-24.

CHAPTER 14

THE GENOMIC RESPONSE OF LIVER CELLS TO POST-ISCHEMIC REPERFUSION AND OXIDATIVE STRESS.

A. BERNELLI-ZAZZERA
Istituto di Patologia Generale dell'Università degli Studi di Milano; Centro di Studio sulla Patologia Cellulare del CNR, Milano, Italy.

Summary

The genomic response of liver cells has been studied during chemically-induced oxidative stress and in the course of reperfusion following ischemia. In addition to a core of common changes, some alterations in the expression, or in the time-course of activation, of particular genes seem to be peculiar to the ischemic-reperfused liver: under the latter circumstance oxidative damage caused by reperfusion is clearly superimposed on molecular injuries caused by ischemia, which are mainly responsible for the activation of the heat shock factor and the induction of the major heat shock gene hsp 70.

Work done in my laboratory in the last years was mainly aimed at the study of the biochemical events in the ischemic-reperfused liver. During investigations on protein synthesis, we found that post-ischemic reperfusion induced the synthesis of a particular set of proteins, identified as heat-shock proteins, widely studied and now more appropriately designated as stress proteins [1]. Later on we realized that oxidative events, occurring during reperfusion, could be involved in the induction of heat shock genes, in particular those of the major hsp 70 gene family, and we began a comparative study of gene reprogramming during oxidative stress and reperfusion stress.

In the following pages I will not try to be comprehensive, but I will essentially present the most relevant results obtained in my laboratory. Changes in gene expression have emerged as a common mechanism used by cells to respond, and possibly to adapt, to emergency situations that induce what is now broadly indicated as "cellular stress". Oxidative stress, a particular case of cellular stress, arises when the balance between oxidant species and antioxidant defenses is shifted in favour of the former [2]. The most convenient way of causing an experimental condition of oxidative stress is the production of an excess, or the direct treatment with oxidant species: and this we did, by exposing isolated hepatocytes or cultivated hepatoma cells to the ADP-iron couple, which triggers intracellular oxidative reactions, or to 4-hydroxynonenal (HNE), one of the products of lipoperoxidation. Under these conditions some proteins are induced,

P. Gentilini and M. U. Dianzani. New Trends in Hepatology, 122-129

which are different in the two cases but are always a subset of the proteins newly synthesized by each cell type upon heat shock. In particular a protein of 31 kDa, which can now be reasonably identified as heme oxygenase (Hox), is induced by HNE in a dose dependent manner, and the effects of heat and of HNE seem to be additive. From these results we concluded that lipoperoxidative events partially mimic the pattern of protein synthesis typical of heat shock, but do not induce proteins that are not included in the hsps group [3]. The pattern of protein synthesis occurring under peroxidative conditions does not overlap with heat shock, but is comprised in the latter: each of the peroxidative conditions tested in our experiments seemed to cover different areas of the overall induction of hsp. Concentrating on the effects of HNE on HepG2 hepatoblastoma cells, we could demonstrate the synthesis of hsp 70, the most conserved and widely studied among hsps. HNE acts mainly on transcription: in HepG2 cells the increase in the steady-state level of hsp 70 mRNA was detected by two different techniques of molecular hybridization [4]. By means of electrophoretic mobility shift analysis we then demonstrated that HSE has the same effect as heat shock in causing the appearance of a protein, known as heat shock factor (HSF), which binds to the consensus sequence called heat shock element (HSE) specific for induction of heat shock genes, and triggers the synthesis of hsp mRNAs [5].

Concurrently with these investigations, we made a series of observations on the induction of heat-shock proteins in ischemic-reperfused livers. The re-establishement of blood supply after a period (1 hour) of non-necrogenic ischemia of rat liver induces a host of changes that can be interpreted as adaptations or responses to the intracellular environment of ischemic cells. These changes comprise a reprogramming of gene expression, with appearance of polysomes coded by mRNAs for proteins similar to those present in the liver of hyperthermic rats [6]. Our observations were soon confirmed [7]. Restoration of circulation after ischemia increases the expression of the hsc 73 gene, the constitutive member of the rat hsp 70 gene family and induces another gene, the hsp 70, which is the main and best known heat-shock inducible gene [8]. For a few hours after blood reperfusion, high steady-state levels of hsp 70 and hsc 73 are maintained in rat livers: run on experiments demonstrate that the increased expression of these genes depends essentially on activation of transcription.

The synthesis of proteins of the hsp 70 family was also demonstrated with the use of post-ischemic rat liver slices [9].

To analyze in greater detail the mechanisms of induction of heat shock genes in post-ischemic livers we have studied the time course of induction and the effects of cycloheximide, an inhibitor of protein synthesis, on the expression of the c-fos and c-jun ("immediate-early response genes") and of the hsp 70 gene. We have then studied the binding of protein constituents of nuclear extracts to a synthetic nucleotide reproducing the sequence of the heat-shock element HSE, in order to detect the possible presence and activation in the ischemic-reperfused tissue of the specific transcription factor HSF which is the first step of the chain of events leading to the synthesis of heat shock proteins. The expression of hsp 70 gene appears only after a certain threshold of ischemic cell damage, that was quantified in 1 hour of ischemia, and only after a certain time of reperfusion, amounting to 2 hours of re-established blood flow. Induction of c-fos and c-jun requires a lower duration of ischemia (30 min), and has a shorter lag phase (1 hour): it is the most prompt change in gene expression caused by post-ischemic reperfusion.

On the whole, the induction of c-fos and c-jun in ischemic-reperfused livers follows the pattern common to the other circumstances where these genes are overexpressed, namely it is prompt but transient. The threshold for induction of the latter mRNAs seems to be lower than for hsp 70 induction, but short periods of ischemia (10-15 minutes) are equally ineffective. The products of c-fos and c-jun constitute the transcription factor AP-1, that operates in the activation of many inducible genes. To see if induction of hsp 70, which comes later than c-fos and c-jun, was in some way dependent on the action of AP-1 we performed some experiments in rats pretreated with cycloheximide, which inhibits protein synthesis.

High levels of hsp 70 mRNA are attained, and possibly anticipated, in ischemic-reperfused livers of rats pretreated with this drug which, at the dose used in our experiments, causes an inhibition of protein synthesis of about 90% and blocks the elongation of nascent peptide chains that resumes at reperfusion of previously ischemic rat liver [10]. This observation shows that induction of hsp 70, although it comes later than c-fos and c-jun, does not depend on the presence of the transcription factor AP-1, which is the product of these genes. More generally, experiments with cycloheximide show that the HSF, which preexists in the liver and only needs post-transcriptional changes - most probably dimerization - to bind to the HSE, does not require cooperative association with newly synthesized transcription factors [11]. On the other hand, the lack of effect of cycloheximide in inducing hsp 70 in normal rats further demonstrates that arrest of protein synthesis, such as occurs during ischemia [10, 12] is not sufficient for induction which seems to require additional factors, such as a damage to protein molecules, either preformed and present during ischemia or synthesized at the resumption of blood circulation. But the experiments of band shift analysis reveal another important fact.

The binding of HSF to the HSE-like oligonucleotide already starts during the period of ischemia, although the subsequent reperfusion increases the effect. ROS arising during reperfusion can act only when superimposed to other changes, occurring during the actual phase of ischemia: and the first phase of the process of activation seems to occur before the generation of ROS.

The idea that a condition of oxidative stress alone could not entirely explain the induction of the hsp 70 gene received further support from observations with transplanted livers. Experiments of protein synthesis by tissue slices from livers stored in the cold, in appropriate fluids designed for preserving explanted livers, indicate that these livers retain a good capacity for protein synthesis throughout the time of storage. Soon after transplantation, however, the livers undergo a profound impairment in the capacity for protein synthesis, which recovers slowly in the following hours. There is never any indication of synthesis of stress proteins, and of hsp 70 in particular. The steady-state level of mRNAs for albumin, transferrin and β-actin, which are well expressed in post-ischemic reperfused livers in vivo and are well maintained in donor livers preserved in U.W. solution, are reduced early after transplantation and recover only many hours later. Run-on analysis shows that an early defect in transcription, and a partial recovery of this process later on, are responsible for these changes. The behaviour of these mRNAs is, therefore, clearly different in reperfused and transplanted livers. On the whole, the early stages of liver transplantation, which can be envisioned as a reperfusion after well controlled ischemia in vitro, seem to be characterized by a depressed capacity of gene expression, without the reactive phenomenon of activation of stress protein genes that occur in reperfused post-ischemic livers [9].

Reperfusion seems to lead to different genomic responses depending on the kind of ischemia, warm or cold, that occurs before. Then the question is: what are the triggers of the heat shock gene response in ischemic-reperfused livers and why are they absent or ineffective in the cold-stored transplanted tissue. Two factors in particular have been emphasized as possible sparks of the induction of heat-shock genes; oxidative stress and/or protein malfolding. Reperfusion can cause generation of ROS, which can in turn be followed by lipoperoxidation. Warm ischemia can possibly lead to accumulation of improperly processed, misfolded or partially denatured proteins, that can set in motion the mechanism of induction of heat shock genes when the circulation is reestablished. If these changes do not occur, such as happens in cold ischemia, hsp 70 gene is not induced when the blood flow is re-established. This is in agreement with a fact that I have already mentioned before; the hsp 70 gene is not induced if the period of ischemia is too short, i.e. if the intracellular environment does not undergo an adequate level of change. Apparently, cold storage of the donor livers does not trigger the changes that are the prerequisite for the deleterious effects of reperfusion. This conclusion, taken from cold-stored transplanted livers, is reinforced by another observation. The amount of Hox mRNA increases after ischemia-reperfusion, heat shock and $CoCl_2$- produced oxidative stress: indeed the level of Hox is generally assumed to be a good indicator of oxidative stress. But the oxidative stress caused by $CoCl_2$ treatment does not induce the expression of the hsp 70 gene [10]: therefore chemically induced oxidative stress proved inadequate to activate hsp 70 gene expression as done by heat shock or post-ischemic reperfusion. ROS are certainly generated during post-ischemic reperfusion and, by overtaxing the antioxidant defences, they can cause oxidative stress, but the results of our experiments suggest a more complex relationship between oxidative stress and the induction of hsp 70 gene. To unravel these relationships we have studied some other types of chemically induced oxidative stress produced by drugs acting with different mechanisms of action. The drugs were (*a*) Buthionine sulphoximine (BSO) a selective inhibitor of glutathione synthesis through inhibition of the limiting enzyme γ-glutamylcysteine synthetase; (*b*) Phorone, which drastically depletes cellular glutathione, through the action of glutathione S-transferase; (*c*) Nitrofurantoin, which caused the formation of $O_2^{\bullet}$- and H_2O_2 by redox cycling and finally lowers glutathione concentration.

All these agents induce Hox, a marker of oxidative stress, although the intensity and time course of expression of the gene may vary a little, depending from the particular mechanism of action of any single agent. None of these agents, however, induces hsp 70 mRNA: on the contrary the expression of the cognate hsc 73 gene increases, albeit to a different extent and with different kinetics, in all the tested conditions of oxidative stress. The immediate early response genes c-fos and c-jun are also induced. Run-on experiments with isolated nuclei demonstrate that the increase in the steady-state levels of hsp 73, c-fos, c-jun and Hox mRNA depends on transcriptional activation, although we cannot exclude an associated increased stability of the mRNAs.

The results obtained with β-actin indicate that the increased transcription of hsc 73, fos, jun and Hox is selective and there is not a general activation of the transcriptional processes [13].

Differences between agents, and in particular the levels of expression of hsc 73 after different times of treatment, are likely to depend on how rapidly each agent can act on the liver cells of the animal. Activation of the constitutive cognate, rather than the inducible gene of the hsp 70 family under conditions of oxidative stress is not entirely novel although it was not clearly appreciated: it was reported by menadione treatment of CHO cells although discrimination between the two forms was not direct, and the failure of menadione to activate hsp 70 was also observed in NIH 3T3 cells [cit. in 13]. A high level of expression of hsc 73, such as occurs in fast-growing hepatomas [14] or in regenerating liver [15] is generally considered to be growth-related as opposed to the stress-related expression of hsp 70: but it is not entirely surprising in view of a possible role of ROS in the stimulation of cell growth.

As already done with HSF-HSE binding in ischemic-reperfused livers we performed EMSA experiments on nuclear extracts from livers subjected to chemically-produced oxidative stress, to study the binding of the transcriptional factors HSF, NFkB, AP-1 and AP-2 to oligonucleotides of the same base composition as their specific consensus sequences. HSF, the activator of heat-shock genes is also active, directly or indirectly, on the promoters of hsc 73 and HOx. NFkB, a mediator of inducible gene transcription is known to undergo redox regulation. NFkB binding activity has been demonstrated in highly purified hepatocytes and appears to be inducible both *in vivo* and *in vitro.* AP-1 is a dimer protein that activates gene expression in a redox-dependent way, under the influence of many agents. AP-2 is associated to NFkB in many cellular responses.

TABLE 1. Comparative summary of liver gene expression and transcription factors activation under the conditions of oxidative stress and ischemia-reperfusion described in the text.

	Oxidative stress	**Ischemia-riperfusion**
Genes		
hsp 70	not induced	induced
hsc 73	activated	slightly activated
Hox	induced	induced
c-jun	induced	induced (> fos)
c-fos	not induced	induced (< jun)
MT-1	induced	not determined
Transcription factors		
HSF	not activated	activated (see text)
NFkB	activated	activated
AP-1	not activated	not activated
AP-2	activated	activated

The oxidative stress induced by the above mentioned chemicals activates NFkB and AP-2, but not AP-1 and HSF transcription factors. The partial exception of phorone can be explained by the extreme reduction of glutathione caused by this drug: NFkB dissociates from its cytoplasmic inhibitor IkB but the reduction of a cysteine in a key position prevents its binding capacity, which cannot therefore be revealed by the usual band shift technique. Therefore, there is a difference in gene expression between oxidative stress and ischemia-reperfusion. Both these conditions are capable of increasing the expression of HOx, which is considered as a *bona fide* marker of oxidative stress: but chemicals causing oxidative stress, which in common with reperfusion enhance the expression of the cognate growth-related gene hsc 73, do not induce the stress-related gene hsp 70. Also the pattern of induction of the early-immediate response genes c-fos and c-jun observed during the chemically induced oxidative stress differs from that found in ischemia-reperfusion. Therefore a "pure" prooxidant cellular environment is not sufficient to cause activation of hsp 70 gene, and induction of the latter by heat-shock and post-ischemic reperfusion is not likely to originate from the oxidative-stress components present in both these circumstances. There is a growing consensus on the idea that the molecular signal acting on the induction of hsp 70 is protein misfolding and/or denaturation [14].

The agents of oxidative stress that we have studied do not activate the heat shock factor HSF involved in the response to heat shock and post-ischemic reperfusion. Heat shock consensus sequences have been reported in the promoter of the HOx gene but apparently are not the targets of the oxidative stress-induced activation of this gene, which seems rather to occur concurrently with an activation of the transcriptional factors NFkB and AP-2. The same transcription factors are likely to be involved, most probably in co-operation with other factors, in the associated increased expression of the hsc 73 gene.

Acknowledgements. These studies were supported by Consiglio Nazionale delle Ricerche (CNR) and by Ministero dell'Università e della Ricerca Scientifica e Tecnologica (MURST) in the context of the National Project "Liver Cirrosis and Chronic Hepatitis". I thank Ms. M.G. Bombonato for typing the manuscript.

References.

1. Morimoto, R.I., Tissieres, A., and Georgopoulos, C. *The biology of heat shock proteins and molecular chaperones.* New York Academic Press, 1994.
2. Ahmad, S. *Oxidative stress and antioxidant defenses in biology.* New York Chapman and Hall, 1995.
3. Cajone, F., and Bernelli-Zazzera, A. Oxidative stress induces a subset of heat shock proteins in rat hepatocytes and MH_1C_1 cells. *Chem-Biol Interactions.* **65** (1988), 235-246.
4. Cajone, F., and Bernelli-Zazzera, A. The action of 4-hydroxynonenal on heat shock gene expression in cultured hepatoma cells. *Free Rad. Res. Comms.* **7** (1989), 189-194.
5. Cajone, F., Salina, M., and Bernelli-Zazzera, A. 4-hydroxynonenal induces a DNA-binding protein similar to the heat-shock factor. *Biochem. J.* **262** (1989), 977-979.
6. Cairo, G., Schiaffonati, L., Bardella, L., and Bernelli-Zazzera, A. Synthesis of heat shock proteins in rat liver after ischemia and hyperthermia. *Hepatology* **5** (1985), 357-361.
7. Fujio, N., Hatajama, T., Kinoshita, H., and Yukista, M. Induction of mRNAs for heat shock proteins in livers of rats after ischemia and partial hepatectomy. *Mol. Cell. Biochem.* **77** (1987), 173-177.

8. Schiaffonati, L., Rappocciolo, E., Tacchini, L., Cairo, G., and Bernelli-Zazzera, A. Reprogramming of gene expression in post-ischemic rat liver: induction of protooncogenes and hsp 70 gene family. *J. Cell. Physiol.* **143** (1990), 79-87.
9. Schiaffonati, L., Cairo, G., Tacchini, L., Pappalardo, C., Gatti, S., Piazzini-Albani, A., and Bernelli-Zazzera, A. Protein synthesis and gene expression in transplanted and post-ischemic livers. *Transplantation* **55** (1993), 977-982.
10. Cajone, F., Ragnotti, G., Bernelli-Zazzera, A., and Bassi, M. State and function of liver polysomes during recovery from ischemia. *Exp. Mol. Pathol.* **14** (1971), 392-403.
11. Tacchini, L., Schiaffonati, L., Pappalardo, C., Gatti, S., Bernelli-Zazzera, A. Expression of HSP 70, immediate-early response and heme oxygenase genes in ischemic-reperfused rat liver. *Lab. Invest.* **68** (1993), 465-471.
12. Cajone, F., Schiaffonati, L., and Bernelli-Zazzera, A. Protein synthesis in liver injury. Soluble factors of protein synthesis in the cytosol from ischemic rat liver. *Lab. Invest.* **34** (1976), 387-393.
13. Tacchini, L., Pogliaghi, G., Radice, L., Anzon, E., and Bernelli-Zazzera, A. Differential activation of heat-shock and oxidation-specific stress genes in chemically induced oxidative stress. *Biochem. J.* 309 (1995), 453-459.
14. Cairo, G., Schiaffonati, L., Rappocciolo, E., Tacchini, L., and Bernelli-Zazzera, A. Expression of different members of heat shock protein 70 gene family in liver and hepatomas. *Hepatology* **9** (1989), 740-746.
15. Tacchini, L., Schiaffonati, L., Rappocciolo, E., Cairo, G., and Bernelli-Zazzera, A. Expression pattern of the genes for different members of the heat shock protein 70 family, ornithine decarboxylase and c-Ha-ras during the early stages of hepatocarcinogenesis. *Mol. Carcinog.* **2** (1989), 233-236.
16. Morimoto, R.I. Cells in stress: transcriptional activation of heat shock genes. *Science* **259** (1993), 1409-1410.

Section II

PATHOPHYSIOLOGY OF BILE SECRETION

CHAPTER 15

CYTOTOXIC AND PROTECTIVE EFFECTS OF BILE SALTS *IN VITRO*

FRANCESCA CARUBBI, M. EUGENIA GUICCIARDI, MAURO CONCARI, MARA BOZZOLI, NICOLA CARULLI.

Dipartimento di Medicina Interna, Università di Modena, Italy

SUMMARY

Toxicity and cytoprotective effects of bile salts were studied in the human Hep G2 cell line, grown for 24 up to 72 hours with free and conjugated bile salts at increasing concentrations. Toxicity was observed with 300 μmol deoxycholate and chenodeoxycholate and was enhanced in a dose and time dependent manner. Cell viability inversely correlated with enzyme release, whereas a decrease in DNA synthesis occurred at lower doses. Free hydrophobic bile salts appeared to be more toxic than their conjugates. In delipidated media the toxic effect of bile salts was enhanced and became evident at lower doses. Addition of 50-100 μmol ursodeoxycholate significantly reduced the hepatotoxicity of deoxycholate 350 μmol. The protective effect was similar with cholate and with tauroursodeoxycholate. Higher doses of hydrophilic bile salts added to 350 μmol of deoxycholate resulted always less toxic than equimolar doses of deoxycholate alone. Cytotoxicity of bile salts is correlated to their physico-chemical properties and is enhanced by reduction of lipid availability in the media. Toxicity of deoxycholate is significantly reduced by addition of low doses of hydrophilic bile salts.

Physico-chemical properties of Bile Salts (BS) depend on their molecular structure; in particular, the capacity to solubilize cholesterol and phospholipids is highly different for each bile salt, due to the differences in their hydrophobic or hydrophilic properties. Both "detergency" and toxicity of bile salts were found to be directly correlated to their hydrophobicity (1-4). Biliary secretion of lipids as well as enzymatic proteins depends on the interaction of hydrophobic BS with the canalicular plasma membranes of the hepatocyte (5-9). *In vitro* studies have confirmed that BS at high doses have similar "detergent" properties on plasma membrane of many other cells, including erythrocytes

P. Gentilini and M. U. Dianzani. New Trends in Hepatology, 133-141

(10), intestinal epithelial cells (11) mast cells (12) and on isolated reconstituted membranes (13-17). Cholestasis causes an increase of total BS within the liver, which in turn may account for some of the liver injuries occurring in cholestatic disorders. The beneficial effects of therapy with Ursodeoxycholic acid (UDCA), the 7β epimer of chenodeoxycholic acid (CDCA) on various forms of chronic liver diseases (18-22) suggested that hydrophilic bile salts may protect against the harmful effects of "toxic" bile salts (BS) in cholestasis, as seen *in vivo* in rats (23). Several *in vitro* studies showed that UDCA may reduce damages induced by more hydrophobic BS on hepatocytes (24, 25), erythrocytes (24) and reconstituted liver membranes (26). This has stimulated great interest in the cellular mechanisms of BS toxicity and the hepatoprotective effect of UDCA.

Toxicity of Bile Salts *in vitro*

We have investigated the effect of low doses of BS on the human hepatoblastoma Hep G2 cell line, in relation to the time of exposure, the availability of lipids in the media and the BS conjugation (35), to study the toxic and protective properties of different bile salts.

The Hep G2 cell line is derived from a well differentiated human hepatoblastoma (27) and maintains several differentiated functions of human hepatocyte, such as membrane potential regulation (28), fatty acids transport (29), lipoprotein and bile acid metabolism (30, 31), sensitivity to sex hormones (32) and synthesis of apolipoprotein receptors (33). Advantages of liver cell line include the high reproducibility of the results, the possibility to control variables and to detail cellular processes, by excluding the enterohepatic circulation.

1. When Hep G2 cells were treated with several increasing concentrations of individual bile salts both as free and conjugated salts, transaminase AST release in the media of Hep G2 cells increased as a function of BS concentration for all BS (35). Toxicity greatly differed for individual BS depending on their hydrophobicity, being much higher for hydrophobic, Deoxycholate (DCA) and CDCA, than for hydrophilic BS, UDCA and Cholate (CA). All the BS resulted not toxic at concentrations 50-200 μmol. Hydrophobic BS at 300-600 μmol were toxic, whereas hydrophylic BS were not. All of these findings were enhanced prolonging the incubation time at 48-72 hours (35)· Free BS were significantly more toxic than their corresponding conjugates.

2. DNA synthesis (36) decreased even with very low concentrations of DCA; cell viability correlated with AST release, with increasing concentrations (35).

At low doses of DCA (200 μmol) the decrease in DNA synthesis preceded the increase of AST in the media.

3. Reducing the availability of lipids in the culture medium by incubating cells with serum free or delipidated media, the toxic effect of BS increased (35), for each incubation time.

4. Low doses of UDCA (50-200 μmol) plus 350 μM DCA reduced enzyme release as compared to what observed with DCA alone. The protective effect of UDCA was evident at 24 up to 72 hours, as well as with CA (35). 400 μmol UDCA resulted not protective, but the mixture of DCA plus UDCA was still less toxic than the equimolar concentration (750 μmol) of DCA alone.

Our data demonstrate that: a) liver cell injury is dependent on bile acid structure and concentration and is time related; b) hydrophobic bile acids cause hepatic cell injury at a concentration; c) hydrophilic bile acids (UDCA, CA) are not toxic and prevent injury caused by hydrophobic BS; c) cell DNA synthesis decreases even at low doses of hydrophobic BS, which do not cause enzyme release in the media; d) availability of lipids plays an important role in cell injury determined by hydrophobic BS; e) the hepatoprotective effect of UDCA and other hydrophilic BS is related to the reduced exposure of liver cells to hydrophobic BS (35).

BS at high concentrations may induce cholestasis and liver-cell injury (8, 37, 38). UDCA can prevent the hepatotoxic effect of other bile salts in experimental cholestasis (39, 40) and ameliorate liver function tests in cholestatic diseases (18, 21, 22, 41). Our data clearly demonstrate a direct relationship between liver cell injury and hydrophobicity of bile salts: DCA and CDCA, resulted more toxic than hydrophilic BS (UDCA, CA). Taurine or glycine conjugation of hydrophobic BS reduced their toxicity. DCA and CDCA caused enzyme release at concentrations as low as 300 μmol; DCA beyond 800 μmol determined total cell death. Hep G2 cells seems to be damaged by bile acids at lower concentrations as compared with rat hepatocytes (24, 25, 42).

One of the major criticisms about previous studies on BS toxicity *in vitro* (1, 10, 12-17, 24-26, 42) is the use of high, not physiological doses of bile acids, as it is not known whether such concentrations bear any relation to the elevated total BS concentrations actually found in vivo in hepatobiliary diseases. BS concentrations in rat portal blood are estimated to reach 40-50 μmol (43) and even in severe cholestasis, total BS concentration in portal venous blood hardly exceeds 400 μmol and 800 μmol within the hepatocytes, so that the basolateral membrane of hepatocytes could rarely be exposed to concentrations higher than

these (15, 44). In previous studies, the concentrations of BS used to investigate their toxic effects have been higher than the critical micellar concentration, thus exploring the detergent like effect of the steroid molecule. Recent studies have investigated the non detergent mechanisms of BS toxicity, suggesting that hydrophobic BS are toxic by acting as mitochondrial toxins and may induce apoptosis (45-47). Moreover, studies on isolated hepatocytes have never explored the effect of prolonged time of exposure of the cells to BS, due to the short limited life span of isolated hepatocytes. Our study (35) has shown that hydrophobic BS (DCA, CDCA) are toxic in a time and dose dependent fashion.
Another important issue raised by previous *in vitro* experimental studies in cell culture is the use of high concentrations of unbound bile acids, due to the absence of albumin in the culture media. BS are bound to plasma proteins, mainly albumin, even in cholestasis (15, 48); the unbound fraction of BS is presumably very toxic to cells (44). Hep G2 cells can synthesize and secrete albumin and many other human plasma proteins (27, 31) and albumin has also been added, so that the BS unbound fraction could not be elevated (35). A novel, interesting finding of our study is that DNA synthesis decreases at low doses of DCA which do not increase enzyme release in the media yet, thus suggesting a complex metabolic action of BS, impairing macromolecule synthesis at the nuclear level. Availability of lipids in the media was also shown to influence bile salt toxicity in our *in vitro* system: a marked increase of enzyme release occurred in the absence of lipids in the media (35). Cholesterol has a membrane stabilizing effect (49, 50). Lipid availability may allow the formation of a less toxic cholesterol-BS complex or allow the repair of membrane damage induced by detergent BS.
Hydrophobic BS like GCDCA, at low concentrations, can induce influx of extracellular calcium (Ca^{2+}) into the cell (45, 47), due to their Ca^{2+} ionophore effect, thus increasing cytosolic calcium (50, 51, 54). GCDCA can also increase the release of Ca^{2+} from the endoplasmic reticulum, thus activating intracellular hydrolases and proteases. In addition, toxic BS can increase membrane permeability, induce cell ATP depletion and mitochondrial membrane permeability transition (MMPT) by inhibiting several enzyme complexes of the mitochondrial respiratory chain (45-47), thus activating hydrolases, Ca^{2+} dependent proteolysis and cell injury (45, 47, 54). Failure of oxidative phosphorylation and increase of cytosolic ionized calcium can be a common event in cell injury determined by different cytotoxic factors and seem to be a final common pathway of lethal injury, casting doubt on a specific role of

individual BS on this mechanism. Moreover, also the non toxic BS, TUDCA, increases cytosolic calcium in isolated rat hepatocytes (52, 55), modulates Ca^{2+} signaling and glucose release, activating phosphorilase *a* (52), thus suggesting complex metabolic effects, yet to be elucidated.

Hepatoprotective effects of UDCA *in vitro*

The mechanism by which UDCA improves chronic liver diseases is still debated.

In our model (35), low doses of hydrophilic BS, either CA or UDCA (50-200 μ mol) added to 350 μmol DCA reduce enzyme release in the culture media, thus suggesting that protection is not a peculiar property of UDCA, but is rather related to the physico-chemical properties of hydrophilic BS (35). Our data suggest that the hepatoprotective effect of UDCA and other hydrophilic BS may depend also on changes induced on hepatocyte metabolic pathways besides the dilution of hydrophobic BS they bring about. Hydrophobic and hydrophilic BS could compete for the same BS transporter, allowing a lower amount of toxic BS to interact with hepatocytes. Alternatively, the addition of an hydrophilic BS to a more detergent one could expand the simple micellar phase, thus decreasing the mixed micellar solubilization of membrane lipids (26). This hypothesis is consistent with the increase of BS toxicity observed when BS are added in delipidated media (35): Heuman et al., by using membrane models entirely composed of egg lecithin and cholesterol (26), demonstrated that UDCA consistently reduced membrane disruption caused by hydrophobic BS via a physico-chemical mechanism: the cholesterol and phospholipid content in membranes was critical for the protective effect of UDCA (26). Guldutuna et al. have suggested that the sensitivity of membranes to toxic BS increases with decreasing membrane cholesterol content (51). Another possible protective mechanism of UDCA and conjugates is that they are bound to plasmamembranes and incorporated into the hydrophobic part of the membranes (51), thus stabilizing membranes and influencing membrane receptors. An effect of UDCA on intracellular disposal of calcium has also been suggested (52, 54). Recent studies suggest that UDCA can antagonize the GCDCA induced MMPT, thus preventing cell injury and apoptosis (47).

Whatever the precise mechanism leading to cell death, several experimental evidences (56) suggest that the initial event of both DCA-induced cell damage and hepatoprotection by UDCA are of physico-chemical nature, mainly dependent on the interaction of BS with hepatocyte membranes and mithochondria: our results are entirely in sound with *in vitro* findings in hepatocytes and erythrocytes (14, 24, 26).

Our study explores the effect of BS at the hepatocyte level, thus excluding the enterohepatic circulation: clearly, the observed hepatoprotective effect of hydrophilic BS cannot be related to changes induced by UDCA in the intestinal absorption of BS (57), which may still play an additional role *in vivo,* as well as on BS synthesis, which is also related to the hydrophobic hydrophilic properties of BS: CDCA and DCA are more potent innhibitors of *de novo* synthesis than UDCA and CA (56, 58). A choleretic property of UDCA has been reported *in vivo*, but the role of bicarbonate rich hypercholeresis in the hepatoprotective action of UDCA appears to be minor (56). Studies reporting a decreased expression of major histocompatibility complex class 1 molecules on hepatocytes (59) or of class 2 molecules on biliary epithelium under treatment with UDCA has focused interest on the direct effect of UDCA on the immune system. Lacaille and Paradis recently showed the immunosuppressive effect of UDCA by inhibition of mononuclear cells proliferation, suggesting that UDCA may decrease cytokine production (60).

In conclusion, toxicity of BS seems related to the hydrophobic-hydrophylic balance of the added BS mixture. UDCA and other hydrophilic BS exert hepatoprotective effects at the cell level, suggesting a direct effect of BS on liver cell membranes and metabolism.

References

1. Salvioli G, Lugli R, Pradelli JM. Effects of bile salts on membranes. In: Calandra S, Carulli N, Salvioli G, eds. *Liver and lipid metabolism.* New York: Elsevier Science Pub., 1984: 163-179.

2. Attili AF, Angelico M, Cantafora A, Alvaro D, Capocaccia L. Bile acid-induced liver toxicity: relation to the hydrophobic-hydrophilic balance of bile acids. Med Hypotheses 1986; 19: 57-69.

3. Carulli N, Loria P, Bertolotti M, Ponz de Leon M, Menozzi D, Medici G. Effect of acute changes of bile acid pool composition on biliary lipid secretion. J Clin Invest 1984; 74: 614-624.

4. Loria P, Carulli N, Medici G, Menozzi D, Salvioli GF, Bertolotti M, Montanari M. Effect of Ursocholic acid on bile lipid secretion and composition. Gastroenterology 1986; 90: 865-874.

5. Yousef IM, Barnwell S, Gratton F, Weber A, Roy CC. Liver cell membrane solubilisation may control maximum secretory rate of cholic acid in the rat. Am J Physiol 1987; 252:G84-G91.

6. Barnwell SG, Lowe PJ, Coleman R. Effect of taurochenodeoxycholate or tauroursodeoxycholate upon biliary output of phospholipids and plasma-membrane enzymes, and the extent of cell damage, in isolated perfused rat livers. Biochem J 1983; 216: 107-111.
7. Bilhartz LE, Dietschy JM. Bile salt hydrophobicity influences cholesterol recruitment from rat liver in vivo when cholesterol synthesis and lipoprotein uptake are constant. Gastroenterology 1988; 95: 771-779.
8. Hofmann AF. Bile acid hepatotoxicity and the rationale of UDCA therapy in chronic cholestatic liver diseases: some hypotheses. In: Paumgartner G, Stiehl A, Barbara L, Roda E; eds. *Strategies for the treatment of hepatobiliary diseases*. Dordrecht, The Netherlands: Kluwer Acad. Press, 1990: 13-33.
9. Schmucker DL, Otha M, Kitani S, Sato Y. Hepatic injury induced by bile salts: correlations between biochemical and morphological events. Hepatology 1990; 12: 1216-1222.
10. Salvioli G, Gaetti E, Panini R, Lugli R, Pradelli JM. Different resistance of mammalian red blood cells to hemolysis by bile salts. Lipids 1993; 11: 999-1003
11. Mekhjian HS, Phillips SF. Perfusion of canine colon with unconjugated bile acids: effect of water and electrolyte transport, morphology and bile acid absorption. Gastroenterology 1970; 59: 120-131.
12. Quist RG, Ton-nu TT, Lillienau J, Hofman AF, Barrett KE. Activation of mast cells by bile acids. Gastroenterology 1991; 101: 446-456.
13. Scholmerich J, Becher MS, Schmidt K, Schubert R, Kremer B, Feldhaus S, Gerok W. Influence of hydroxylation and conjugation of bile acids on their membrane-damaging properties: studies on isolated hepatocytes and membrane vesicles. Hepatology 1984; 4: 661-666.
14. Human DM, PandaK WM, Hylemon PB, Vlahcevic ZR. Conjugates of Ursodeoxycholate protect against cytotoxicity of more hydrophobic bile salts. Hepatology 1991; 14:, 1991: 920-926.
15. Ostrow JD. Metabolism of bile salts in cholestasis in humans. In: Tavoloni N, Berk PD, eds. *Hepatic transport and bile secretion*. New York: Raven Press 1993: 673-712.
16. Scharschmidt BF, Keeffe EB, Vessey DA, Blankenship NM, Ockner RK. *In vitro* effect of bile salts on rat liver plasma membrane, lipid fluidity, and ATPase activity. Hepatology 1981; 1: 137-145.
17. Billington D, Evans CE, Godfrey PP, Coleman R. Effects of bile salts on plasma membrane of isolated rat hepatocytes. Biochem J 1980; 88: 321-323.
18. Poupon RE, Balkan B, Eschwege E, Poupon R. A multicenter, controlled trial of ursodiol for the treatment of primary biliary cirrhosis. N Engl J Medicine 1991; 324: 1548-1554.
19. Chazouillères O, Poupon R, Capron J-P, Metman E-H, Dhumeaux D, Amouretti M, Couzigou P, et al. Ursodeoxycholic acid for primary sclerosing cholangitis. J Hepatol 1990; 11: 120-123.
20. Beuers U, Spengler U, Zwiebel FM, Pauletzki J, Fischer S, Paumgartner G. Effect of ursodeoxycholic acid on kinetics of the major hydrophobic bile acid in health and in chronic cholestatic liver disease. Hepatology 1992; 15: 603-608.
21. James OFW. Ursodeoxycholic acid treatment for chronic cholestatic liver disease. J Hepatol 1990; 11: 5-8.
22. Leuschner U, Fischer H, Kurtz W, Guldutuna S, Hubner K, Hellstern A, Gatzen M, Leuschner M. Ursodeoxycholic acid in primary biliary cirrhosis: results of a controlled double-blind trial. Gastroenterology 1989; 97: 1268-1274.

23. Heuman DM, Mills AS, McCall J, Hylemon PB, Pandak WM, Vlahcevic ZR. Conjugates of Ursodeoxycholate protect against cholestasis and hepatocellular necrosis caused by more hydrophobic bile salts: in vivo studies in the rat. Gastroenterology 1991; 100: 203-211.
24. Heuman DM, Pandak WM, Hylemon PB, Vlahcevic ZR. Conjugates of ursodeoxycholate protect against cytotoxicity of more hydrophobic bile salts: *in vitro* studies in rat hepatocytes and human erythrocytes. Hepatology 1991; 14: 920-926.
25. Galle PR, Theilmann L, Raedsch R, Otto G, Stiehl A. Ursodeoxycholate reduces hepatotoxicity of bile salts in primary human hepatocytes. Hepatology 1990; 12: 486-491.
26. Heuman DM, Bajaj R. Ursodeoxycholate conjugates protect against disruption of cholesterol-rich membranes by bile salts. Gastroenterology 1994; 106: 1333-1341.
27. Knowles BB, Howe CC, Aden DP. Human hepatocellular carcinoma cell lines secrete the major plasma proteins and hepatitis B surface antigen. Science 1980; 209: 497-499.
28. Motzkin SM, Feinstein J, Tiribelli C. Modulation of resting membrane potential of human and rat hepatocytes by sex steroids. Biochem Biophys Res Commun 1990; 172: 1163-1166.
29. Stremmel W, Diede HE. Fatty acid uptake by human hepatoma cell lines represents a carrier-mediated uptake process. Biochim Biophys Acta 1989; 1013: 218-222.
30. Javitt NB, Pfeffer R, Kok E, Burstein S, Cohen BI, Budai K. Bile acid synthesis in cell culture. J Biol Chem 1989; 264: 10384-10387.
31. Javitt NB. Hep G2 cells as a resource for metabolic studies: lipoprotein, cholesterol, and bile acids. FASEB J 1990; 4: 161-168.
32. Tam SP, Archer TK, Deeley RG. Biphasic effects of estrogen on apolipoprotein synthesis in human hepatoma cells: mechanism of antagonism by testosterone. Proc Natl Acad Sci USA 1986; 83: 3111-3115.
33. Krempler G, Kostner GM, Friedl W, Paulwebar B, Bauer H, Sandhofer F. Lipoprotein binding to cultured human hepatoma cells. J Clin Invest 1987; 80: 401-408.
34. Goldstein JL, Basu SK, Brown MS. Receptor-mediated endocytosis of low-density lipoprotein in cultured cells. In: Fleischer S, Fleischer B, eds. *Methods in enzymology*. New York: Academic Press, 1983; 98, part L: 241-260.
35.Carubbi F, Guicciardi ME, Concari M, Bozzoli M, Loria P, Tagliazucchi M, Carulli N. Cytotoxic and protective effects of bile salts are dependent on their physico-chemical properties in vitro. Hepatology 1996 (in press).
36. Goldspink DF, Goldberg AF. Problems in the use of (Me-^{3}H) thymidine for the measurement of DNA synthesis. Biochim Biophys Acta 1973; 299: 521-532.
37. Desmet VJ. Current problems in diagnosis of biliary disease and cholestasis. Semin Liver Dis 1986; 6: 233-248.
38. Raedsch R, Lauterburg GH, Hofmann AF. Altered bile acid metabolism in primary biliary cirrhosis. Dig Dis Sci 1981; 26: 394-400.
39. Kitani K, Ohata M, Kanai S. Tauroursodeoxycholate prevents biliary protein excretion induced by other bile salts. Am J Physiol 1985; 248: G 407-418.
40. Kitani K, Kanai S.Tauroursodeoxycholate prevents taurocholate induced cholestasis. Life Sci 1982; 30: 515-523.
41. Poupon RE, Poupon R. Ursodeoxycholic acid for the treatment of cholestatic diseases. In: Boyer JL, Ockner RK, eds. *Progress in liver diseases*. Vol 10. Philadelphia: WB Saunders, 1993: 219-238.

42. Ohiwa T, Katagiri K, Hoshino M, HayakawaT, Nakai T. Tauroursodeoxycholate and tauro-βmuricholate exert cytoprotection by reducing intrahepatocyte taurochenodeoxycholate content. Hepatology 1993; 17: 470-476.
43. Cronholm T, Sjovall J. Bile acids in portal blood of rats fed different diets and cholestyramine. Bile acids and steroids 189. Eur J Biochem 1967; 2: 375-383.
44. Ostrow JD. *In vitro* studies of bile salt toxicity. Hepatology 1994; 19: 1538-1539.
45. Spivey JR, Bronk SF, Gores GJ. Glycochenodeoxycholate-induced lethal hepatocellular injury in rat hepatocytes. J Clin Invest 1993; 92: 17-24.
46. Krahenbuhl S, Talos C, Fischer S, Reichen J. Toxicity of bile acids on the electron transport chain of isolated rat liver mitochondria. Hepatology 1994; 19: 471-479.
47. Rosser BG, Gores GJ. Liver cell necrosis: cellular mechanisms and clinical implications. Gastroenterology 1995; 108: 252-275.
48. Chitranukroh A, Billing BH. Changes in the binding of radioactive conjugated bile salts to serum proteins in cholestatic jaundice. Clin Sci 1983; 65: 77-84.
49. Schubert R, Schmidt KH. Structural changes in vesicle membranes and mixed micelles of various lipid compositions after binding of different bile salts. Biochemistry 1988; 27: 8787-8794.
50. Yeagle PL. Cholesterol and the cell membrane. Biochim Biophys Acta 1985; 822: 267-287.
51. Guldutuna S, Zimmer G, Imhof M, Bhatti S, You T, Leuschner U. Molecular aspects of membrane stabilization by ursodeoxycholate. Gastroenterology 1993; 104: 1736-1744.
52. Bouscarel B, Fromm H, Nussbaum R. Ursodeoxycholate mobilizes intracellular Ca^{2+} and activates phosphorilase *a* in isolated hepatocytes. Am J Physiol 1993; 264: G243-250.
53. Anwer MS, Engelking LR, Nolan K, Sullivan D, Zimniak P, Lester R. Hepatotoxic bile acids increase cytosolic Ca^{2+} activity of isolated rat hepatocytes. Hepatology 1988; 8: 887-891.
54. Combettes L, Dumont M, Berthon B, Erlinger S, Claret M. Release of calcium from the endoplasmic reticulum by bile acids in rat liver cells. J Biol Chem 1988; 263: 2299-2303.
55. Beuers U, Nathanson MH, Boyer JL. Effects of Tauroursodeoxycholic acid on cytosolic Ca^{2+} signals in isolated rat hepatocytes. Gastroenterology 1993; 104: 604-612.
56. Heuman DM. Hepatoprotective properties of Ursodeoxycholic acid. Gastroenterology 1993; 104: 1865-1870.
57. Stiehl A, Raedsch R, Rudolph G. Acute effect of ursodeoxycholic and chenodeoxycholic acid on the small intestinal absorption of bile acids. Gastroenterology 1990; 98: 424-428
58. Pandak WM, Vlahcevic ZR, Heuman DM, Redford KS, Chiang JYL, Hylemon PB. Effects of different bile salts on steady state mRNA levels and trascriptional activity of cholesterol 7α hydroxylase. Hepatology 1994; 19:941-947
59. Calmus Y, Gane P, Rouger P, Poupon R. Hepatic expression of class I and class II major histocompatibility complex molecules in primary biliary cirrhosis: effect of ursodeoxycholic acid. Hepatology 1990; 11:12-15
60. Lacaille F, Paradis K. The immunosoppressive effect of ursodeoxycholic acid: a comparative *in vitro* study on human peripheral blood mononuclear cells. Hepatology 1993; 18: 165-172.

CHAPTER 16

LAMELLAR BODIES IN HUMAN GALLBLADDER BILE

URSODEOXYCHOLIC ACID TREATMENT INCREASES THE AMOUNT OF CHOLESTEROL TRANSPORTED BY BILIARY LAMELLAE

S. GINANNI CORRADINI[1], M. ANGELICO[2], P. DELLA GUARDIA[1], L. BAIOCCHI[2], C. RIPANI[1], L. GIOVANNELLI[1], G. ARANCIA[3], A. CALCABRINI[3], AND L. CAPOCACCIA[1].
[1]Department of Clinical Medicine, Division of Gastroenterology La Sapienza University, [2]Department of Public Health, Tor Vergata University and [3]Department of Ultrastructure, Istituto Superiore di Sanità, Rome, Italy.

1. Summary

Two topics are covered in this chapter: a) current knowledge on cholesterol biliary lipid carriers, with particular emphasis on whether biliary lamellae are real structures existing in bile or methodological artifacts and, b) the effect that ursodeoxycholic acid treatment exerts on biliary lipid carriers. Lamellae are real lipid structures occurring in bile as they can be isolated and characterized with different techniques, including quasielastic light scattering, that cause little or no physical perturbation of bile. Ursodeoxycholic acid treatment increases the percentage of cholesterol carried by biliary lamellae.

2. Characterization of Cholesterol Carriers in Bile

Biliary PC and Ch are assembled in structures such that they may be secreted by hepatocytes and solubilized in bile. For practical reasons of sample availability, gallbladder bile is mostly used to study lipid carriers in human Ch supersaturated bile. To study biliary lipid carriers they must first of all be separated from other biliary components. Classic separation procedures of biliary lipid carriers are based on size (gel filtration) or density (density gradient ultracentrifugation). The isolated carriers are then further characterized, from a qualitative point of view, using methods that assess their size and/or shape (different type of microscopy, quasielastic light scattering, X-ray diffraction techniques, etc...).

A certain caution is required when interpretating qualitative, morphological data on the structure of biliary lipid carriers. The techniques used both for their separation and characterization could, in fact, induce the artifactual formation of non physiologically occurring structures. A good strategy to minimize these pitfalls is to use techniques that are relatively fast and induce the smallest possible physico-chemical perturbations of bile.

Mixed Ch, PC and bile salt micelles were the first biliary carriers described. They are about 2-6 nm in diameter, as inferred from data obtained by quasielastic light scattering (QLS) on both model and native bile (1). The exact shape of mixed micelles is still under discussion as they are too small to obtain reliable pictures by transmission microcopy. A disc- or rod-like structure is the most probable.

P. Gentilini and M. U. Dianzani. New Trends in Hepatology, 142-148

In the early 1980's the existence of another biliary lipid carrier, unilamellar vesicles, was demonstrated by laser light scattering (2,3), gel filtration (4,5) and negative staining (3) and freeze fracture (6) electron microscopy. These vesicles are spherical structures visible at electron microscopy and have been shown to vary in size from 10 up to 70 nm in diameter. They are composed of a closed Ch and PC membrane, delimiting an inner aqueous compartment. These vesicles are currently considered very unstable structures, the final source of Ch for crystal formation (7,8), and the initial event in the development of gallstones.

Moreover, negative staining electron microscopy has revealed multilamellar structures, of variable shape, in bile. These structures are not surrounded by a membrane and range from well defined elongated or cigar-shaped stacks to concentric stacked discs separated by regular interspaces. In the 1970's these were interpreted as being the artifactual appearance of micelles induced by the negative staining procedure prior to electron microscopy (9-11). This view was supported by the reproducible finding that, by means of low-resolution gel filtration using conventional matrixes and columns, only two lipid peaks were separable from bile - vesicles and putative mixed micelles. However, in 1990, for the first time, investigators from Israel (12), by using larger columns with the conventional matrix Sephacryl S-300 and hence increasing the resolution of the gel-chromatographic run, were able to resolve the putative micellar fraction in two peaks. At negative staining electron microscopy, only the first of the last two peaks contained the multilamellar structures described above and the lipid carrier eluting in this fraction was called lamellae. The second of these two lipid peaks did not show any microscopically distinguishible structures and was identified as micellar by its lipid composition.

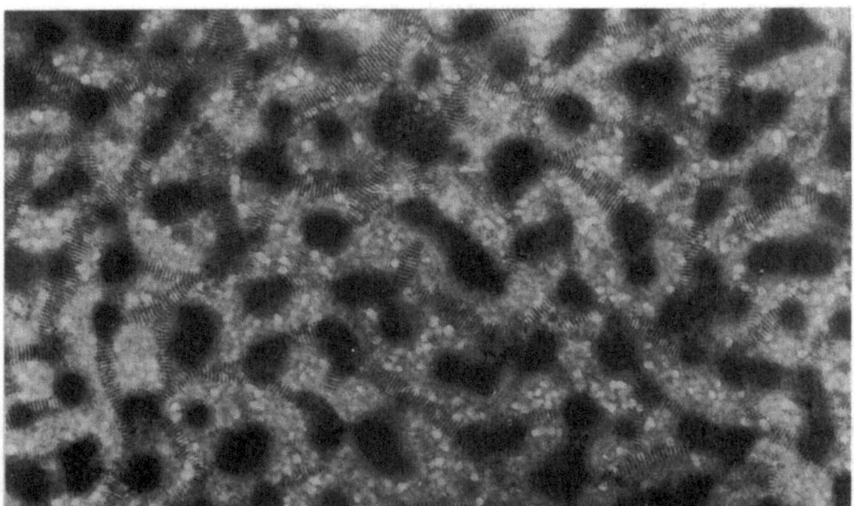

Figure 1 Negative staining electron micrograph (150,000x) of an isotropic (ultracentrifuged) sample of native gallbladder bile, obtained at surgery from an untreated cholesterol gallstone patient. Elongated lamellar stacks and cigar-shaped lamellae coexist with roundish vesicles.

The presence of lamellar stacking in bile, not fractionated by gel-chromatography, was further confirmed by the same authors using X-ray diffraction (13). In addition, another group from Japan was able to separate lamellae from micelles by gel-chromatography (14).

Despite these reports, and the common finding of lamellar bodies in many cells and body fluids (15), biliary lamellae continued to be considered methodological artifacts (16) caused by gel-chromatography or by negative staining electron microscopy.

2.1. BILIARY LAMELLAE ARE NOT ARTIFACTS

Theorethically, the gel-chromatographic conditions used by the Israeli group (12) to separate lamellae from micelles, could have artifactually created the lamellar peak. This could be due to the use of a gel-filtration media (Sephacryl S-300) with heterogeneous bead sizes, which requires relatively large columns (1.6 x 68 cm) and low eluant flow rates to reach high resolution, resulting in long running times (4 hours). Alterations in metastable lipid structures could occur during such a prolonged period. Chemical interactions between biliary lipids and the particular matrix used could also cause artifacts.

Prompted by this discussion, to establish whether lamellae are artifacts or not, we analyzed gallbladder bile obtained at cholecystectomy from Ch gallstone patients (17). As a first step, we submitted to negative staining electron microscopy the optically isotropic intermediate phase obtained after bile ultracentrifugation. Lamellar and small vesicular structures were found to coexist (Fig. 1). Lamellae were cigar-shaped or elongated stacks of variable length, usually with 5 nm interspaces and up to 30 nm in width, often overlapping to form a thick network. Less frequently lamellae appeared as multiple curved parallel sheets. Roundish vesicles, ranging from 7 to 20 nm in diameter, were observed within the lamellar network.

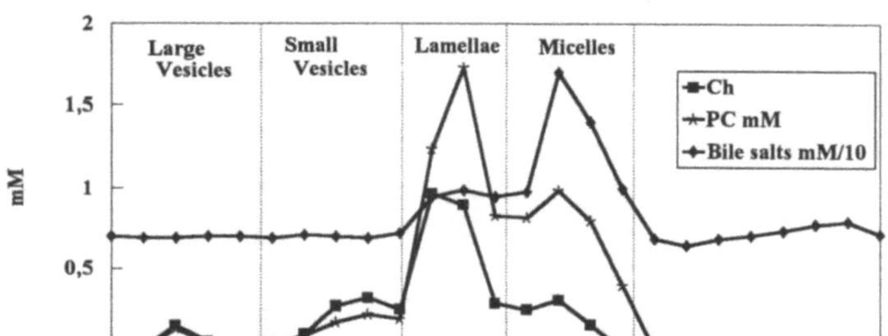

Figure 2 High-resolution gel chromatographic separation of biliary lipid carriers from whole (not ultracentrifuged) human gallbladder bile, obtained at surgery from an untreated patient with cholesterol gallstones. The bile sample is the same as in Fig. 1. Chromatographic conditions were as follows: column Superose 6 column (HR 10/30, Pharmacia); flow rate, 0.5 ml/min; buffer: 20 mM Tris/HCl (pH 7.8), 140 mM NaCl, 7.0 mM Na taurocholate, 3 mM Na azide. Collection was performed in 1 ml fractions. The elution pattern of cholesterol (Ch) and phosphatidylcholine (PC) is based on radiochemical determinations, that of total bile salts on enzymatic measurements.

Although the presence of lamellae in samples not submitted to gel-chromatography is, per se, proof that the latter technique does not artifactually create these structures, we were also able to isolate lamellae from the other biliary lipid carriers by a high resolution gel-chromatographic system different from that used by the Israeli group (12). The gel-chromatographic media we used (Superose 6), because of the more homogeneous bead sizes, permits faster running times (1 hour) in shorter columns (1 x 30 cm), achieving a very high resolution power. In such a short running time artifactual re-arrangement of lipid structures is less likely to occur. Vesicles and lamellae with the same appearance as those identified in isotropic unfractionated native bile were observed upon electron microscopic analysis of the selected lipid containing elution zones, obtained after gel-chromatography of the correspondent whole native bile. In particular, we were able to separate four distinct gel-chromatographic fractions (Fig. 2). The first fraction in elution order, in which small amounts of PC and Ch were eluted only in a few dilute samples, showed no distinct structures at electron microscopy. This region was not further characterized. The second fraction, at electron microscopy, contained exclusively small roundish vesicles, 7-20 nm in diameter (Fig. 3, left panel). The third fraction contained exclusively lamellae, with various morphologies, similar to those observed in the respective unfractionated biles (Fig. 3, right panel). The fourth fraction had no distinct structures at electron microscopic examination and was identified by chemical composition as micellar.

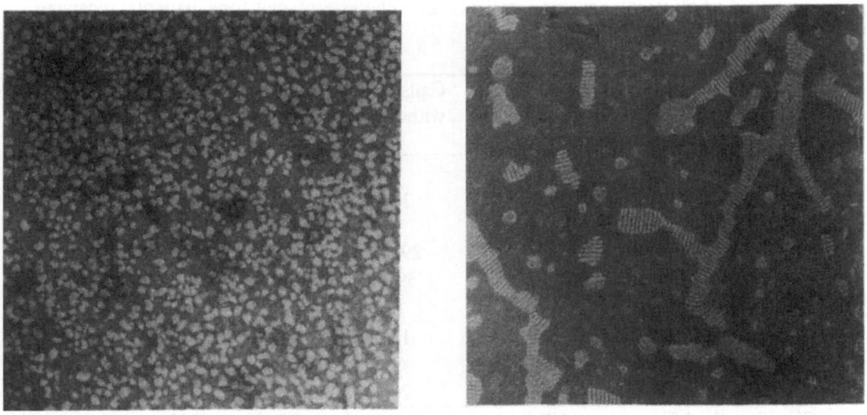

Figure 3 Negative staining electron micrograph (150,000x) of the gel chromatographic elution fractions of the chromatogram shown in Fig. 2, (i.e. native gallbladder bile of an untreated cholesterol gallstone patient).

Left panel: in the second peak in elution order, corresponding to the "vesicular" peak, only a great abundance of small vesicles, 7-20 nm in diameter, and no lamellar bodies were present.

Right panel: in the third peak in elution order, corresponding to the "lamellar" peak, only lamellar stacks were detected, without evidence of vesicles.

The main criticism of the occurrence of lamellae as physiological lipid carriers in bile and not as artifacts has been the failure to back-up the lamellar hypothesis using a less artifact-prone technique than electron microscopy, such as QLS (16). Because of this lack of confirmation lamellae continued to be considered as artifacts, possibly due to exposure of mixed micelles to heavy metal ions and subsequent dehydratation of the sample during negative staining preparation before electron microscopy. Our group recently obtained, for the first time, both by QLS and negative staining microscopy, simultaneous characterization of lamellae isolated from native bile (17). In our gel-chromatographic region, where only lamellae were detected at electron microscopy (third peak in elution order in Fig. 2), the QLS data showed a mean hydrodynamic radius ranging from 21.9 to 29.4 nm. These values are too large to be mixed micelles and are compatible with lamellar bodies. In addition, the high polydispersity found by QLS (range of percent variance 21-45%) is in keeping with the heterogeneity of lamellar sizes and shapes detected by electron microscopy.

As a second, independent demonstration that lamellae are not artifacts due to negative staining electron microscopy, some aliquots of the lamellar fractions, isolated by gel-chromatography, were immediately submitted to electron microscopy while the remaining were incubated under sterile conditions. When electron microscopy was repeated after a few days, lamellar forms were absent, having been substituted by vesicles, with the occasional finding of transitional structures (17).

TABLE 1. Total lipids, cholesterol crystal observation time and percent distribution of cholesterol and phosphatidylcholine among biliary lipid carriers, isolated by high-resolution gel-chromatography from gallbladder bile. A comparison between untreated cholesterol gallstone patients and cholesterol gallstone patients receiving UDCA (means±SD).

	Gallstone patients without treatment (n=9)	UDCA-treated gallstone patients (n=8)
Total lipids (g/dl)	8.4±4.1	9.1±4.2
Cholesterol crystal observation time (days)	3.1±4.1**	19.0±1.9
% Cholesterol in vesicles	29.1±12.4**	8.3±4.3
% Cholesterol in lamellae	59.1±6.2**	81.2±9.5
% Cholesterol in micelles	11.8±9.4	11.6±9.0
% Phosphatidylcholine in vesicles	13.3±7.8*	3.9±2.8
% Phosphatidylcholine in lamellae	66.3±6.6	73.4±15.7
% Phosphatidylcholine in micelles	20.4±11.7	22.7±14.4

Significantly different from UDCA treated patients: *=p<.05; **=p<.001.

3. The Effect of Ursodeoxycholic Acid Administration on Biliary Lamellae

Ursodeoxycholic acid (UDCA) treatment of Ch gallstone patients prolongs the crystal observation time of their gallbladder bile to values found in gallstone-free controls (20,21).

We have recently addressed the issue of the mechanism by which UDCA restores a normal metastability in bile of Ch gallstone patients. We measured Ch and PC concentrations in the isolated lipid carriers of gallbladder bile, comparing untreated versus UDCA-treated (600 mg/die for one week prior to cholecystectomy) Ch gallstone patients (17). In the same bile samples the crystal observation time, as an index of bile lithogenicity, was also measured.

In keeping with other studies, we found that UDCA treatment reduces the percentage of biliary Ch carried by vesicles (17,20,21). In fact, significantly more Ch (p<0.001) and PC (p<0.01) carried by vesicles in untreated than in UDCA- treated patients (Table 1) was present (17). Furthermore our data showed that UDCA-treated patients had more Ch carried by lamellae (p<0.001) than untreated patients. A significant inverse correlation was found between the Ch crystal observation time and the percent of Ch (r= 0.851, p< 0.001) and PC (r= 0.750, p< 0.001) carried by vesicles. On the other hand, the Ch crystal observation time was directly correlated with the percent of Ch (r= 0.858, p< 0.001) carried by lamellae. In untreated patients, Ch crystal observation time was also directly correlated (0.573, p<0.01) with the fraction of Ch carried by mixed micelles. These data, taken together, suggest that a) both lamellae and mixed micelles are metastable aggregates and b) that UDCA enhances bile metastability by increasing the fraction of cholesterol solubilized by lamellae.

4. Conclusions

We revised current knowledge on biliary lipid carriers, with particular emphasis on biliary lamellae. Evidence of the occurrence of lamellae, not as a methodological artifact, but, rather, as a major lipid carrier in gallbladder bile from cholesterol gallstone patients, has been provided. Further research is needed to ascertain the contribution of lamellae to cholesterol transport in bile of gallstone-free subjects.

Ursodeoxycholic acid treatment prevents cholesterol crystal precipitation in gallbladder bile by increasing the percentage of cholesterol carried by biliary lamellae. The knowledge that biliary vesicles are unstable structures, prone to cholesterol crystal formation, while lamellae and mixed micelles are more stable, is crucial for future studies on cholesterol gallstone pathogenesis and treatment.

References

1. Mazer NA, Schurtenberger P,Carey MC, Preisig R, Weigand K and Kanzig W. Quasi-elastic light-scattering studies of native hepatic bile from the dog: comparison with aggregative behavior of model biliary lipid systems. Biochemistry 1984;23:1994-2005.
2. Somjen GJ, Gilat T. A non micellar mode of cholesterol transport in human bile. FEBS Lett. 1983; 156: 265:265-268.
3. Cohen DE, Angelico M, Carey MC. Quasielastic light scattering evidence for vesicular secretion of biliary lipids. Amer J Physiol 1989; 257: G1-G8.
4. Ulloa N, Garrido J, Nervi F. Ultracentrifugal isolation of vesicular carriers of biliary cholesterol in native human bile. Hepatology 1987; 7: 235 244.
5. Somjen GJ, Gilat T. Contribution of vesicular and micellar carriers to cholesterol transport in human bile. J Lipid Res 1985; 26: 699-704.
6. Somjen GJ, Marikovski Y, Leike, Gilat T. Cholesterol phospholipid vesicles in human bile: an ultrastructural study. Biochim Biophys Acta 1986; 879: 14-21.
7. Kibe A, Dudley MA, Halpern Z, Lynn MP, Breuer AC, Holzbach RT. Factors affecting cholesterol monohydrate crystal nucleation time in model systems of supersaturated bile. J Lipid Res. 1985; 26: 1102-1111.
8. Harvey PR, Somjen G, Lichtenberg MS, Petrunka C, Gilat T, Strasberg SM. Nucleation of cholesterol from vesicles isolated from bile of patients with and without cholesterol gallstones. Biochim Biophys Acta 1987; 921: 198-204.

9. Howell JI, Lucy JA, Pirola RC, Bouchier AD. Macromolecular assemblies of lipid in bile. Biochim Biophys Acta 1970; 210:1-6.
10. Manzato E, Fellin R, Gaggio G, Walch S, Neubeck W, Seidel D. Formation of lipoprotein X: its relationship to bile components. J Clin Invest 1976; 57:1248-1260.
11. Holzbach RT, Corbusier C. Liquid crystals and cholesterol nucleation during equilibration in supersaturated bile analogs. Biochim Biophys Acta 1978; 528: 436-444.
12. Somjen GJ, Marikovsky Y, Wachtel E, Harvey PRC, Rosenberg R, Strasberg SM, Gilat T. Phospholipid lamellae are cholesterol carriers in human bile. Biochim Biophys Acta 1990; 1042:28 35.
13. Somjen GJ, Coleman R, Koch MHJ, Wachtel E, Billington D, Towns Andrews E, Gilat T. The induction of lamellar stacking by cholesterol in lecithin bile salt model systems and human bile studied by synchrotron X radiation. FEBS Lett 1991, 289: 163-166.
14. Mizuno S, Tazuma S, Kaijyma G. Stabilization of biliary lipid particles by ursodeoxycholic acid. Prolonged nucleation time in human gallbladder bile. Dig Dis Sci 1993; 38: 684-693.
15. Schmitz G, Muller G. Structure and function of lamellar bodies, lipid protein complexes involved in storage and secretion of cellular lipids. J Lipid Res 1991; 32:1539-1570.
16. Cohen DE, Kaler EW, Carey MC. Cholesterol carriers in human bile: are "lamellae" involved ? Hepatology 1993; 18: 1522-1532.
17. Ginanni Corradini S, Arancia G, Calcabrini A, Della Guardia P, Baiocchi L, Nistri A, Giacomelli L, Angelico M. Lamellar bodies coexist with vesicles and micelles in human gallbladder bile. Ursodeoxycholic acid prevents cholesterol crystal nucleation by increasing biliary lamellae. J Hepatol 1995;22: 642-657.
18. Somjen GJ, Koch MHJ, Wachtel E, Coleman R, Gilat T. Bile salt species determine lipid particle structure and cholesterol solubilizing capacity in gallbladder bile models. A synchroton small angle X-ray scattering study. XIII international Bile Acid Meeting, Falk Symposium no. 80, San Diego, CA, September 30-October 2, 1994, abstract 9.
19. Donovan JM, Jackson AA. Rapid determination by centrifugal ultrafiltration of inter-mixed micellar/vesicular (non lecithin associated) bile salt concentrations in model bile: influence of Donnan equilibrium effects. J Lipid Res 1993; 34:1121-1129.
20. Sahlin S, Thyberg P, Ahlberg J, Angelin B, Einarsson K. Distribution of cholesterol between vesicles and micelles in human gallbladder bile: influence of treatment with chenodeoxycholic acid and ursodeoxycholic acid. Hepatology 1991;13:104-110.
21. Hirota I, Chijiiwa K, Noshiro H, Nakayama F. Effect of chenodeoxycholate and ursodeoxycholate on nucleation time in human gallbladder bile. Gastroenterology 1992; 102:1668-1674.

Acknowledgement: Thanks to MJ Crowley for editing the text.
Address for correspondence: S. Ginanni Corradini MD, Via Asmara 9B, 00199, Rome, Italy

CHAPTER 17

HEPATOCYTE LIPID-METABOLIC INTERPLAYS AND THE CHOLESTEROL SECRETION PROCESS TO BILE: INSIGHTS FROM RAT STUDIES.

MASSIMINO CARRELLA

Cattedra di Gastroenterologia, Facoltà di Medicina e Chirurgia, Università degli Studi di Udine - Udine, Italy

Summary

Besides water, electrolyte and protein components, bile secretion is composed of a consistent lipid proportion mainly represented by cholesterol and phospholipid in close association with bile acids for reasons of solubilization and transport (1, 2). While bile acids are still considered the main drivers of bile lipid secretion, increasing interest has been addressed to the multiple hepatic metabolic functions in which cholesterol is involved, such as lipoprotein uptake and degradation and the rates of cholesterogenesis and VLDL secretion, with the purpose of understanding the mechanisms of increased cholesterol secretion in bile. In the present editorial these aspects will be examined, mainly focusing on data obtained in in vivo rat models.

The lipoprotein-biliary sterols relationship

About 2/3 of the sterols excreted in bile, mainly comprising cholesterol and bile acid, can be traced to deriving from plasma lipoproteins (3). However, a different contribution to this process might derive from the various lipoprotein classes in view of their different metabolic functions, lipid and apolipoprotein composition, and especially mechanisms of hepatic uptake and processing (4, 5). LDL and chylomicron remnants, responsible for most endogenous and exogenous cholesterol transport, are removed by the hepatocyte apoB, E receptor (4) or by apoE-LRP remnant receptor (6, 7) to undergo endocytosis and lysosomal degradation supplying cholesterol which can be esterified with fatty acids for temporary storage, re-secreted at the sinusoidal pole in newly assembled VLDL, or transported to bile as such or after conversion to bile acid (2, 5). The hepatic uptake of HDL is more complex and variable for the different HDL subclasses. Whereas apoE-rich HDL-1 and the HDL-1c follow the remnant pathway (5), a different mechanism of hepatic cholesterol delivery occurs for the apoE free-

P. Gentilini and M. U. Dianzani. New Trends in Hepatology, 149-157

HDL species by way of an apoAI-receptor-mediated uptake not leading to lysosomal degradation, or, a direct association and fusion with the outer leaflet of the sinusoidal plasma membrane (5, 8).

The relationships between lipoprotein cholesterol and biliary sterols have generally been studied in acute or chronic bile-fistula rat models by the i.v. administration of single lipoproteins labelled in their free or esterified cholesterol moiety, and by following the radioactivity of biliary cholesterol and bile acid. In these studies, a more consistent biliary elimination of either a free or cholesterol ester-label was shown for HDL at variance with other lipoproteins. Thus, the 24 h biliary elimination of a cholesteryl ester-label incorporated in HDL (9) and LDL (10) was found 28 % and 10 % of dose, the radioactivity appearing maximally associated to bile acid. Intriguingly, the upregulation of the apo B,E receptor obtained by ethinylestradiol administration led to an increased label elimination not only from LDL but also from HDL (23 and 35 % of dose/24 h) (9). With the injection of free cholesterol-labeled lipoproteins (11), the recovery in biliary radioactivity was relatively greater than that of cholesteryl ester-labeled lipoproteins, and a greater proportion of it associated to the cholesterol fraction rather than bile acid. Again, HDL seemed more active in the biliary sterol excretion process, 2.3 % and 0.2 % of administered dose being excreted in 3h bile by HDL or LDL, respectively. Furthermore, in the latter studies (11), 11.7 % of dose was excreted in bile after administration of HDL-2, a HDL subclass functioning as a scavenger of unesterified cholesterol and phospholipid during the lipolysis of chylomicrons and VLDL.

These studies would suggest a preferential function of HDL in feeding the biliary sterol excretion pathway, representing a useful homeostatic extension of the role attributed to this lipoprotein in the reverse cholesterol transport from the peripheral tissues to the liver. However, all trace-labeled lipoprotein studies may be affected by significant drawbacks, among which the exchange of labeled free cholesterol among plasma lipoproteins and the difficulty establishing any quantitative evaluation of experimental data without knowledge of the intrahepatic pool size of injected label. To partially avoid these drawbacks, the biliary sterol excretory pathway has been examined in relation to an acute *increase in plasma and liver cholesterol levels* induced by the administration of an unlabeled cholesterol mass contained in single lipoproteins. In these studies, small time-related changes in the mass of secreted biliary sterols were observed, compounding 24 h elimination of 15.6 % of LDL cholesterol dose while HDL was ineffective, a difference which appeared unrelated to hepatic uptake (12). In another study using the same experimental setup, a greater biliary sterol contribution from chylomicron remnants was found amounting to 37.3 % of cholesterol dose in 24 h (13). While in agreement with findings obtained under labeled remnant trace injection (14), these sterol changes were small on an hourly basis and partially quenched by physiological circadian secretory variations. Interestingly, when the injected remnant mass was simultaneously labeled in the cholesterol moiety, a definite biliary radioactivity peak was detected between 3 and 12 h with a maximum at 6 h from injection which was in striking contrast with the small hourly changes observed in the mass of excreted biliary sterols consistent with the existence of a small, poorly-expandable, intrahepatic cholesterol pool ultimately connected to biliary sterols, as from earlier suggestions (2).

The greater biliary elimination of free rather than esterified cholesterol of lipoproteins (10, 11) reproduces the more rapid elimination kinetics obtained in early studies with injection of free- as compared to esterified-cholesterol labeled liposomes (15). In this regard, it may be speculated that unesterified cholesterol may be able to enrich, in a more immediate way, the proposed cholesterol precursor pool at the canalicular plasma membrane of the hepatocyte, while lipoprotein cholesteryl esters may need both particle degradation and/or esters hydrolysis to generate free cholesterol to reach such a pool. In this context, the intrahepatic balance between cholesterol esterification by the acyl CoA:cholesterol acyltransferase (ACAT) enzyme and the hydrolysis of cholesteryl esters by cholesteryl esters hydrolase(s) appears to be of remarkable importance.. An increased *cholesterol esterification* rate, following the administration of dietary (16) or lipoprotein (17) cholesterol, or the inhibition of ACAT activity by progesterone (18), have been shown to decrease or increase the biliary cholesterol elimination rate, respectively. Also, the ACAT-mediated usual esterification of the cholesterol supplied through LDL or remnants degradation may set the basis for a preferential use of these cholesteryl esters in the process of VLDL assembly (19) and plasma secretion.

Overall, the available data suggest that HDL and chylomicron remnants might be better sources of biliary sterols as compared to LDL but this proposition needs validation, as discussed above. It is also to be stressed that both exogenous and endogenous cholesterol appear to ultimately reach bile, and that in no way does available knowledge support any mechanistic relationship between the increase in a single plasma lipoprotein class and the amount of sterols secreted into bile.

Impact of cholesterol synthesis and VLDL secretion

Cholesterol synthesis and VLDL secretion are two other different but related functions of the hepatocyte which may significantly influence the biliary sterols excretion pathway; the first by providing new cholesterol substrate addressed to plasma membrane and potentially to bile, the second by channeling intrahepatic cholesterol to the plasma compartment instead of to bile. A functional role has been assigned to neosynthetic cholesterol in complementing dietary cholesterol to provide the substrate needed to the VLDL packaging at the level of the endoplasmic reticulum (19). Indeed, cholesterol synthesis is turned down subsequent to the hepatic uptake of lipoprotein cholesterol of either exogenous or endogenous origin. In these situations, downregulation of cholesterogenesis and an increased cholesterol conversion to bile acid are the main mechanisms by which cholesterol overaccumulation is prevented in the rat species (2).

Cholesterol synthesis is a multistep biochemical pathway regulated at the level of the microsomal enzyme HMG CoA reductase acting in concert with lipoprotein uptake and catabolism to constantly provide cells with this essential structural and metabolic molecule. Neosynthetic cholesterol is also known to feed bile acid synthesis whose limiting enzyme cholesterol-7α hydroxylase undergoes concordant regulation with HMGCoA reductase in respect to several experimental conditions (20). By the use of triparanol, an inhibitor of the desmosterol to cholesterol conversion step, it has been estimated that up to 28 % of biliary cholesterol may derive from a synthetic source (3). As for bile acids, 25 % have been traced to neosynthetic cholesterol (3), and this proportion has more than doubled according to studies employing synthetic HMG CoA reductase inhibitors (21). In rat studies conducted under infusion of tritiated water precursor, the proportion of biliary labeled cholesterol was 16 % of total in controls, and 34 % and 3.5 % under cholestyramine or cholesterol feeding (22), situations associated to large increases or decreases of cholesterogenesis. Much to surprise, however, no mass change appeared to occur in any of these experimental groups in the biliary output of either cholesterol and bile acid, or phospholipid (16). In addition, no association with hepatic cholesteryl esters levels and no difference in the bile acid-induced secretion of biliary cholesterol was detected (16). These studies led to the conclusion that biliary cholesterol and bile acid preferentially derive from an, as yet unidentified, pool of preformed cholesterol. However, several observations have been made (2) following pregnenolone-16α-carbonitrile or β-sitosterol administration in the rat, or feeding an essential fatty acid deficient diet in the hamster, or in human obesity (23), showing an increase in both biliary cholesterol output and cholesterogenesis. Thus, it is possible that other metabolic factors, additional to the rate of cholesterogenesis, might concur in determining cholesterol availability for transport to bile.

One of such potential factors may be the *VLDL secretion rate*, a powerful mechanism by which the liver accomplishes its regulatory role in the lipid metabolism between intestinal and peripheral tissues. In this process, apoB peptide of various lengths and lipid affinity, determined by post-translational modifications, concur with lipids, mainly cholesteryl esters, triglycerides, and also phospholipids, in the assembly of a lipoprotein precursor at the level of the endoplasmic reticulum which may proceed to the Golgi apparatus for targeting glycosilations and then be secreted to plasma as VLDL. An increased hepatic lipid availability as fatty acid, triglyceride or cholesteryl ester is known to stimulate VLDL secretion (19). On the other hand, defects in either the apoB peptide maturation or the quantitative or qualitative lipid supply may lead to an impaired VLDL assembly/secretion, in some instances resulting in an increased level of hepatic lipids. Experimental models have described lipid-related alterations in the VLDL secretion occurring under n-3 fatty acid feeding or choline deficiency or the acute administration of competitive HMG CoA reductase inhibitors (21). In addition, the concomitant elevation in the biliary phospholipid and cholesterol secretions also raises interesting questions as to the transport mechanisms involved and the significance of this coupling. An inverse secretory relationship between biliary and plasma VLDL cholesterol was shown to occur during diosgenin, orotate, or fish-oil treatment (24, 25). In recent studies during prolonged feeding of pravastatin, a hydrophylic HMG CoA reductase inhibitor, we found increased biliary secretion of cholesterol and phospholipid, but not of bile acid, in the presence of reduced VLDL secretion (26). Furthermore, these changes were accompanied by stimulated rates of cholesterol and fatty acid synthesis consequent to an adaptive bypass of the biochemical drug's block, and increased hepatic levels of cholesteryl esters and especially triglycerides (27). While in line with the suggested inverse relationship between biliary and VLDL cholesterol secretion, our data also suggest a role for stimulated cholesterol biosynthesis, a change also found with diosgenin or orotate feeding (25, 28). Altogether the data propose an interesting relationship between multiple synergistic defects, which are necessary to turn on the biliary sterols secretion pathway. In addition, the concomitant rise in biliary phospholipid secretion also poses questions concerning the mechanisms involved in these transports and their significance.

Conclusions

The data reviewed support the contention that physiological cholesterol and bile acid secretion into bile is subserved by a small and hardly expandable hepatic free cholesterol pool which is fed both by a neosynthetic source and lipoprotein degradation. However, due to the modulatory responses interrelating these two metabolic processes and the characteristics of the precursor pool, no change is observed in the biliary sterol output following any of their stimulation, even though large. On the other hand, neosynthetic and catabolic cholesterol also concur to VLDL assembly and plasma secretion, a rapid and effective response to balance the cell cholesterol excess. There are several experimental drug-related observations in which increased biliary cholesterol secretion is found in association with an increased cholesterol synthesis and an impaired VLDL secretion. A double synergistic metabolic defect, consisting of lipid increased cell inflow and decreased plasma export, which may force the hepatocyte to expand the biliary lipid secretion pathway, may be proposed as a working hypothesis. What mechanisms may mediate the selection of such homeostatic response, and also what really defines the hepatic cholesterol precursor pool for biliary sterols will be the next challenging question.

Acknowledgements

Funding for the mentioned studies was provided by the italian MURST National Project "Cirrosi Epatica ed Epatite Virale" led by Professor Paolo Gentilini. The expert typing assistance by Mrs. Sandra Cescutti is gratefully acknowledged. The author also wishes to express profound gratitude to Professors Fabrizio Bresadola and Marzio Strassoldo for any academic support to his research endeavors.

References

1 Coleman R, Rahman K, Bellringer ME, Carrella M. Biliary lipid secretion and its control. In: Northfield T, Jazrawi R, Zentler-Munro P, eds. Bile Acids in Health and Disease. Dordrecht: Kluwer Academic Publishers, 1988:43-60.

2 Turley SD, Dietschy JM. Cholesterol metabolism and excretion. In: Arias IM, Popper H, Jackoby WM, Schachter D, Shafritz DA, eds. The Liver:Biology and Pathobiology.New York: Raven Press, 1988;617-641.

3 Long TTL, Jakoi R, Stevens R, Quarfordt S. The sources of rat biliary cholesterol and bile acids. J Lipid Res 1978;19:872-878.

4 Brown MS, Kovanen PT, Goldstein JL. Regulation of plasma cholesterol by lipoprotein receptors. Science 1981;212:628-635.

5 Havel RJ, Hamilton RL. Hepatocytic lipoprotein receptors and intracellular lipoprotein catabolism. Hepatology 1988;8:1689-1704.

6 Carrella M, Cooper AD. High affinity binding of chylomicron remnants to rat liver plasma membranes. Proc Natl Acad Sci USA 1979;76:338-342.

7 Kowal RC, Herz J, Goldstein JL, Esser V, Brown MS. Low-density lipoprotein receptor-related protein mediates uptake of cholesteryl esters derived from apoprotein E-enriched lipoproteins. Proc Natl Acad Sci USA 1989;86:5810-5814.

8 Knecht TP, Pittman RC. A plasma membrane pool of cholesteryl esters that may mediate the selective uptake of cholesteryl esters from high-density lipoproteins. Biochim Biophys Acta 1989;1002:365-375.

9 Pieters MN, Schouten D, Bakkeren HJF, Esbach B, Brouwer A, Knook DL, van Berkel TJC. Selective uptake of cholesteryl esters from apolipoprotein-E-free high density lipoproteins by rat parenchymal cells in vivo is efficiently coupled to bile acid synthesis. Biochem J 1991;280:359-365.

10 Nagelkerke JF, Bakkeren HF, Kuipers F, Vonk RJ, van Berkel TJC. Hepatic processing of the cholesteryl ester from low density lipoprotein in the rat. J Biol Chem 1986;261:8908-8913.

11 Bravo E, Cantafora A, Argiolas L. Hepatic uptake and metabolism of free cholesterol from different lipoprotein classes: an in vivo study in the rat. Biochim Biophys Acta 1989;1003:315-320.

12 Carrella M, Del Piano C. Effects on the secretion of biliary lipids and bile acids from the pool expansion of different plasma lipoproteins. In: Gentilini P, Dianzani MU, eds. Experimental and Clinical Hepatology. Amsterdam, The Netherlands: Elsevier Science Publishers, 1991:119-131.

13 Carrella M, Csillaghy A, De Mercato R, D'Arienzo A. Biliary excretion of chylomicron remnant cholesterol: responses to the expansion of their plasma pool and promoting role of stimulated bile-acid synthesis. Clin Sci 1995;89:121-128.

14 Smit MJ, Kujpers F, Vonk RJ, Temmerman AM, Jackle S, Windler EET. Effects of dietary cholesterol on bile formation and hepatic processing of chylomicron remnants cholesterol in the rat. Hepatology1993;17:445-454.

15 Ogura M, Shiga J, Yamasaki K. Studies on the cholesterol pool as the precursor of bile acids in the rat. J Biochem 1971;70:967-972.

16 Turley SD, Dietschy JM. Regulation of biliary cholesterol output in the rat: dissociation from the rate of cholesterol synthesis, the size of hepatic cholesteryl-ester pool, and the hepatic uptake of chylomicron cholesterol. J Lipid Res 1979;20:923-934.

17 Nervi F, Bronfman M, Allalon W, Depiereux E, Del Pozo E. Regulation of biliary cholesterol secretion in the rat. Role of hepatic cholesterol esterification. J Clin Invest 1984;74:2226-2237.

18 Stone BG, Erickson SK, Craig WY, Cooper AD. Regulation of rat biliary cholesterol secretion by agents that alter intrahepatic cholesterol metabolism: evidence for a distinct biliary precursor pool. J Clin Invest 1985;76:1773-1781.

19 Fungwe TV, Cagen LM, Wilcox HG, Heimberg M. Regulation of hepatic secretion of very low density lipoprotein by dietary cholesterol. J Lipid Res 1992; 33:179-191.

20 Myant NB, Mitropoulos KA. Cholesterol 7α-hydroxylase. J Lipid Res 1977;18:135-153.

21 Pandak WM, Heuman DM, Hylemon PB, Vlahcevic ZR. Regulation of bile acid synthesis.IV. Interrelationships between cholesterol and bile acid biosynthesis pathways. J Lipid Res 1990;31:79-90.

22 Turley SD, Dietschy JM. The contribution of newly synthesized cholesterol to biliary cholesterol in the rat. J Biol Chem 1981;256:2438-2446.

23 Bennion LJ, Grundy SM. Effects of obesity and caloric intake on biliary lipid metabolism in man. J Clin Invest 1976;57:473-477.

24 Nervi F, Marinovic I, Rigotti A, Ulloa N. Regulation of biliary cholesterol secretion. Functional relationship between the canalicular and sinusoidal cholesterol secretion pathways in the rat. J Clin Invest 1988;82:1818-1825.

25 Stone BG, Evans CD. Evidence for a common biliary cholesterol and VLDL cholesterol precursor pool in the rat liver. J Lipid Res 1992;33:1665-1675.

26 Carrella M. Decrease in plasma triglycerides as a reflection of an altered VLDL metabolism in pravastatin-fed rats. Ital J Gastroenterol 1994;26:38.

27 Carrella, M., and A. Colombatti. 1995. Increased output of biliary lipids during a long-term pravastatin administration may relate to an enhanced hepatic synthesis of cholesterol and fatty acids. Ital J Gastroenterol 1995;27:206.

28 Cayen MN, Dvornik D. Effect of diosgenin on lipid metabolism in rats. J Lipid Res 1979;20:162-174.

Section III

INSIGHTS IN HEPATIC CARCINOGENESIS

CHAPTER 18

LIPID PEROXIDATION AND HEPATOCARCINOGENESIS: γ-GLUTAMYL TRANSPEPTIDASE-DEPENDENT OXIDANT STRESS IN HEPATIC PRENEOPLASTIC LESIONS AND HEPG2 HUMAN HEPATOMA CELLS

A. POMPELLA, A. PAOLICCHI (°), P. TONARELLI (°), R. TONGIANI (°), S. DOMINICI & M. COMPORTI

Istituto di Patologia Generale, Università di Siena and, (°) Dipartimento di Biomedicina Sperimentale, Università di Pisa

Summary

The role(s) possibly played by oxidant stress and lipid peroxidation in the carcinogenic process are multifold and complex. Recent studies have shown that γ-glutamyl transpeptidase (γ-GT) - an activity normally involved in the metabolism of extracellular glutathione - can favour, in the presence of iron, the ignition of free radical processes and lipid peroxidation. Our studies indicate that γ-GT-dependent lipid peroxidation can involve the lipids of cell membranes, including those of intact living cells. Moreover, the lipid peroxidation stimulated by γ-GT expressed at the surface of hepatoma cells can be propagated to extracellular lipid substrates. These oxidative processes might be operative *in vivo* in chemically-induced experimental hepatic preneoplastic lesions expressing high levels of γ-GT, as well as in other γ-GT-rich neoplastic tissues, such as e.g. several hepatoma cell lines, and could play a role in tumor progression.

The problem of lipid peroxidation (LPO) and related oxidative phenomena in neoplastic and pre-neoplastic tissue has been debated for a long time by many authors, and a number of studies have appeared in the literature in the past two decades. Lipid peroxidation products have been shown in fact to be potentially able to intefere with the carcinogenic process at many levels, due to their well-established antiproliferative (1,2), as well as mutagenic (3,4) and tumor-promoting effects (5,6). However, it has long been known that tumor cells, like other rapidly dividing cells, show low rates of LPO compared to corresponding normal tissues (reviewed in 7); this aspect was also clearly shown by histochemical means, in chemically-induced preneoplastic lesions of rat liver (8). The phenomenon of lower LPO inducibility in neoplastic and preneoplastic tissue has been mostly attributed to de-differentiation of trasformed cells causing a decrease of the enzymes involved in the initiation of NADPH-dependent LPO (9), as well as to the lower content of oxidizable substrate (unsaturated fatty acids) usually present in tumor cell membranes (10).

P. Gentilini and M. U. Dianzani. New Trends in Hepatology, 161-168

Against this background, recent experimental evidence obtained in liver preneoplastic lesions and in other neoplastic cells expressing high levels of γ-glutamyl transpeptidase, allows now to obtain novel insights into the possible roles played by oxidative phenomena during the carcinogenic process.

γ-Glutamyl transpeptidase (γ-GT) activity and oxidant stress. In several models of experimental hepatocarcinogenesis, a precocious marker of cell transformation is the overexpression of γ–GT activity (11, 12). γ–GT (EC 2.3.2.2.) is a membrane-bound enzyme, with its active site oriented towards the outer surface of the cell, capable of affecting the hydrolysis of extracellular glutathione (GSH), thus allowing the cellular uptake of precursor aminoacids for the intracellular re-synthesis of GSH (13).

On this basis, the marked increase in γ–GT activity during chemical hepatocarcinogenesis has been interpreted as one aspect of the new phenotype of transformed cells, which generally results in a higher resistance towards chemical insults. It has in fact been documented that increased γ–GT levels result in an increased resistance of several cell types against injury caused by hyperoxia, menadione, other quinones. γ–GT Re-expression is also observed in human neoplasia - notably colon carcinoma and ovarian cancer; in the latter, it is thought to play a role in tumor resistance against chemotherapeutic agents (14, 15).

Recent studies however have shown that the γ–GT-mediated hydrolysis of GSH can favour - in the presence of chelated iron ions - the ignition of free radical processes. The dipeptide cysteinyl-glycine, resulting from GSH cleavage, is in fact more reactive than the parent compound and - by interacting with chelated iron (III) - can start its redox-cycling with oxygen; altogether, these reactions have been shown to be able to initiate a process of lipid peroxidation (LPO) (16), with the mechanism suggested in Figure 1.

Prooxidant effects of γ-GT in chemically-induced hepatic preneoplastic lesions. In preneoplastic foci of rat liver induced by the administration of N-nitroso-diethylamine and 2-acetylaminofluorene, followed by partial hepatectomy (17), we have tested the possibility that the overexpression of γ–GT may result in a selective induction of LPO. On fresh, serial liver cryostat sections, histochemical procedures were performed for evaluation of γ–GT activity, protein thiols and susceptibility to LPO. The latter was revealed by means of the NAH-FBB procedure (18). The results indicate that GGT-positive tissue is indeed susceptible to undergoing a selective γ–GT-mediated LPO, when exposed in vitro to low concentrations of GSH and chelated iron (19).

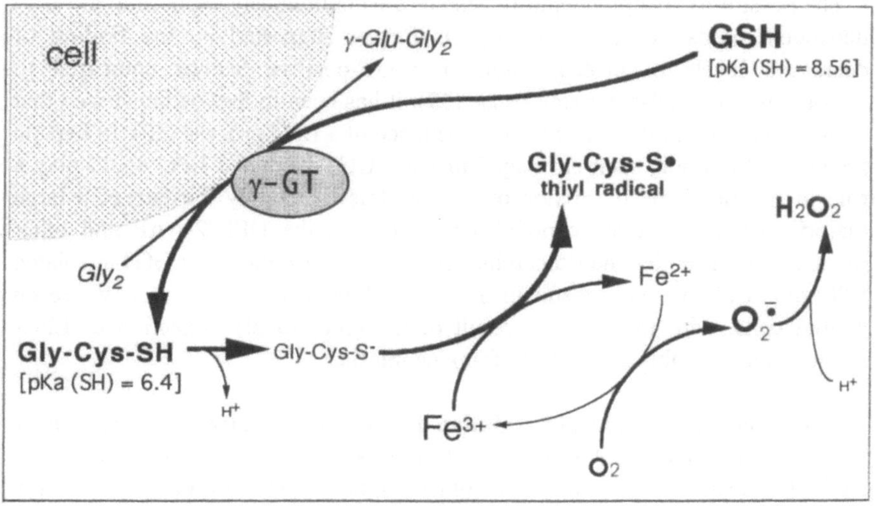

Figure 1. Proposed mechanism for the generation of thiyl radicals and reactive oxygen species during γ-GT-mediated metabolism of extracellular GSH. *After Stark et al. (16).*

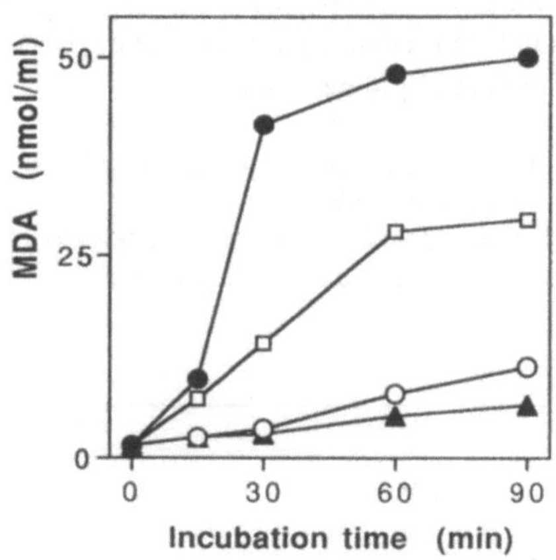

Figure 2. γ-GT-dependence of iron-stimulated lipid peroxidation (production of malonaldehyde, MDA) in rat liver microsomes. Incubations were carried out in Hank's buffer, and had the following composition: (❑) 2 mM GSH, 1.5-0.15 mM ADP-Fe^{3+}, 200 mU/ml γ-GT; (●) as above, plus 20 mM glycyl-glycine; (O) 2 mM GSH, 1.5-0.15 mM ADP-Fe^{3+}, 20 mM glycyl-glycine (no added γ-GT); (▲) like ●, plus 0.2 mM BHT. A typical experiment of five is shown. *(Pompella, Paolicchi, Tongiani and Comporti: unpublished results).*

The possibility that preneoplastic lesions are continuously exposed to a γ–GT-dependent oxidative stress *in vivo* is further suggested by the finding of decreased levels of protein thiols in γ–GT-positive lesions compared to surrounding normal-appearing tissue (19); it has been in fact demonstrated that a loss of protein thiols can be the consequence of a LPO process (20). In hepatic preneoplastic tissue, such envisaged *in vivo* GGT-mediated LPO could play a role in favour of the regression of lesions; this is actually the fate of a large majority of the hepatocyte nodules produced in the DEN/2-AAF and other models of rat chemical hepatocarcinogenesis (12). A continuing GGT-mediated LPO might alternatively result in the establishment of a selective pressure on altered cells, with the possible result of the (occasional) selection of LPO-resistant clones liable to evolve to frank neoplasia.

γ-GT-Dependent lipid peroxidation in liver microsomes. The possibility that γ–GT activity might stimulate a LPO process in cellular membranes was studied in detail with rat liver microsomes (Figure 2). Microsomes exposed only to GSH and ADP-chelated ferric iron exhibited increasing levels of lipid peroxidation. However, the addition of γ–GT to the incubation mixture greatly stimulated the process, and even higher lipid peroxidation levels were attained when the incubation included glycyl-glycine, acting as γ-glutamyl acceptor and therefore as a stimulant for γ–GT activity (21). The addition of the lipid soluble, chain-breaking antioxidant butylated hydroxytoluene (BHT) resulted in the suppression of γ–GT-stimulated lipid peroxidation.

Table 1. GSH-dependent lipid peroxidation (production of TBA-reactive substances, TBARs) in γ–GT-rich Hep-G2 hepatoma cells[a].
(Data from: Pompella, Paolicchi, Tongiani and Comporti, manuscript in preparation).

Incubation system[b]	TBARs, nmol/mg protein[c]
HepG2 (control)	0.71 ± 0.05
HepG2 + ADP-Fe	3.30 ± 0.02
HepG2 + ADP-Fe + GSH	4.29 ± 0.05
HepG2 + ADP-Fe + GSH + glycyl-glycine	5.11 ± 0.18
HepG2 + ADP-Fe + GSH + glycyl-glycine + acivicin	2.54 ± 0.11

[a] Incubations were carried out at 37°C for 60 min. [b] Concentration of reagents was as follows: GSH, 2 mM; glycyl-glycine, 20 mM; ADP-Fe, 1.5 mM-150 μM; acivicin, 1 mM. [c] Data are means ± S.E.M. of three experiments.

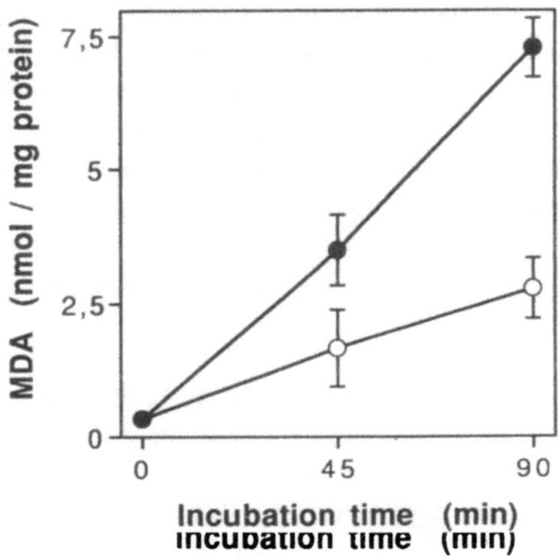

Figure 3. Prooxidant effect of γ-GT in isolated rat hepatocytes exposed to glutathione, glycyl-glycine and ADP-iron. Incubations were carried out in Hank's buffer containing 2 mM GSH, 1.5-0.15 mM ADP-Fe^{3+} and 20 mM glycyl-glycine, in the presence (●), or absence (○) of γ-GT (200 mU/ml). *(Data from: Pompella, Paolicchi, Tongiani and Comporti, manuscript in preparation).*

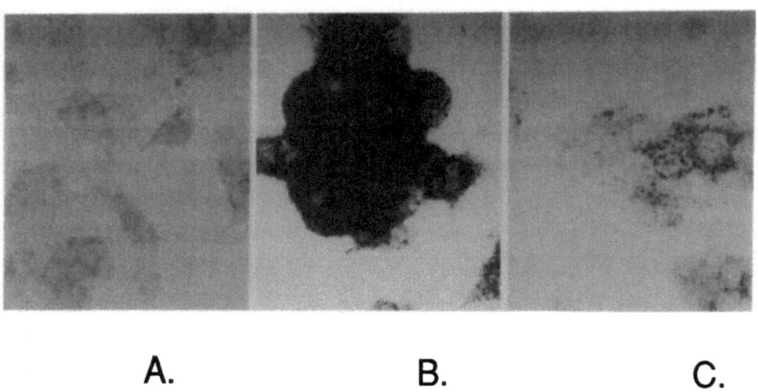

Figure 4. Production of superoxide anion (reduction of Nitro Blue Tetrazolium, NBT) by HepG2 cells following activation of intrinsic γ-GT. Cells were cultured in chamber-slides, to which O_2-bubbled Krebs-Ringer buffer was added containing 1.25 mg/ml NBT. The medium also contained: (**A**) 20 mM glycyl-glycine and 1.5-0.15 mM ADP-Fe^{3+}, (**B**) as (A) plus 2 mM GSH, (**C**) as (B) plus 1 mM acivicin, an inhibitor of GGT. Slides were then incubated for 45 min at 37°C, gently washed and mounted.

γ-GT-Dependent lipid peroxidation in cultured rat hepatocytes. The possibility was then verified, that the described γ–GT-stimulated lipid peroxidation might involve the membranes of intact, living cells (Figure 3). Primary cultures of isolated rat hepatocytes were studied. As in the case of liver microsomes, lipid peroxidation developed in cultured rat hepatocytes in the presence of GSH, glycyl-glycine and ADP-iron; the addition of γ–GT to the incubation mixture was however able to cause a marked stimulation of the process. Up to the latest time of incubation studied (90 min), hepatocyte viability - as assessed by LDH leakage - was not affected by γ–GT-simulated lipid peroxidation.

Prooxidant effect of cell-bound γ–GT activity in HepG2 hepatoma cells. Studies were then dedicated to the possible prooxidant effects of *intrinsic* γ–GT, i.e. the γ–GT expressed on the surface of living cells. In human HepG2 hepatoma cells - expressing high levels of γ–GT - the exposure to GSH and chelated iron results in γ–GT-dependent extracellular production of superoxide anion, as evidenced by the NBT reduction test and by determination of ferricytochrome c reduction (Figure 4). At the same time, the functioning of γ–GT is accompanied by the induction in HepG2 cells of (non-lethal) lipid peroxidation, which is preventable by adding the γ–GT inhibitor, acivicin (Table 1). When rat liver microsomes were included (as a target system) with HepG2 cells in the incubation mixture, the propagation of γ–GT-dependent LPO to microsomes was also observed; again, the phenomenon was preventable by inhibiting γ–GT by a specific inhibitor, the serine-boric acid complex (Table 2).

Table 2. Lipid peroxidation in rat liver microsomes exposed to γ–GT-rich HepG2 hepatoma cells, in the presence of γ–GT substrates[a].
(Data from: Pompella, Paolicchi, Tongiani and Comporti, manuscript in preparation).

Incubation system[a]	TBARs, nmol/mg protein[b]
microsomes + GSH + glycyl-glycine + ADP-Fe	14.8 ± 1.38
+ HepG2 cells	26.0 ± 2.24
+ HepG2 cells + serine borate	12.6 ± 1.59
HepG2 + GSH + glycyl-glycine + ADP-Fe	2.9 ± 0.24

[a] Incubations were carried out at 37°C for 60 min. Concentration of reagents was as follows: GSH, 2 mM; glycyl-glycine, 20 mM; ADP-Fe, 1.5 mM-150 μM; microsomes, 1 mg protein/ml; serine 10 mM-boric acid 20 mM. [b] Data are means ± S.E.M. of three experiments.

The data reported indicate that both rodent and human membranes are susceptible to undergoing a pro-oxidant effect induced by the γ–GT-mediated metabolism of GSH. GSH metabolites appear able - prior to their absorption by the cell - to participate in metal-catalyzed redox reactions, leading to the production of radical oxygen species and to lipid peroxidation. The enzyme catalytic site, its substrates and the potential targets of the pro-oxidant reactions are extracellular, thus out of reach for the cellular antioxidant systems. γ–GT-rich tumor cells could induce such reactions in vivo in their vicinity, thus exposing themselves and the surrounding cells to a pro-oxidant environment. Due to the complex effects that oxidative reactions are known to exert on the mechanisms of cell proliferation at many levels (22), these findings appear of potentially considerable significance.

References

1. Esterbauer H, Schaur RJ, Zollner H (1991) Chemistry and biochemistry of 4-hydroxynonenal, malonaldehyde and related aldehydes. Free Rad Biol Med 11: 81-128.

2. Gonzalez MJ, Schemmel RA, Gray JI, Dugan L Jr, Sheffield LG, Welsch CW (1991) Effect of dietary fat on growth of MCF-7 and MDA-MB231 human breast carcinomas in athymic nude mice: relationship between carcinoma growth and lipid peroxidation product levels. Carcinogenesis 12: 1231-1235.

3. Esterbauer H, Eckl P, Ortner A (1990) Possible mutagens derived from lipids and lipid precursors. Mutat Res 238: 223-233.

4. Zhang J-R, Sevanian A (1993) The genotoxic effects of arachidonic acid in V79 cells are mediated by peroxidation products. Toxicol Appl Pharmacol 121: 193-202.

5. Bartoli GM, Bartoli S, Galeotti T, Bertoli E (1980) Superoxide dismutase content and microsomal lipid composition of tumors with different growth rates. Biochim Biophys Acta 620: 205-211.

6. Greenley TL, Davies MJ (1994) Direct detection of radical generation in rat liver nuclei on treatment with tumor-promoting hydroperoxides and related compounds. Biochim Biophys Acta 1226: 56-64.

7. Dianzani MU (1993) Lipid peroxidation and cancer. Crit Rev Oncol Hematol 15: 125-147.

8. Benedetti A, Malvaldi G, Fulceri R, Comporti M (1984) Loss of lipid peroxidation as a histochemical marker for preneoplastic hepatocellular foci of rats. Cancer Res 44: 5712-5717.

9. Minotti G, Borrello S, Palombini G, Galeotti T (1986) Cytochrome P-450 deficiency and resistance to t-butyl hydroperoxide of hepatoma microsomal lipid peroxidation. Biochim Biophys Acta 876: 220-225.

10. Masotti L, Casali E, Galeotti T (1988) Lipid peroxidation in tumor cells. Free Rad Biol Med 4: 377-386.

11. Kalengayi MM, Ronchi G, Desmet VJ (1975) Gamma-glutamyltranspeptidase in rat liver during aflatoxin B1 induced carcinogenesis. J Natl Cancer Inst 55: 579-588.

12. Enomoto K, Farber E (1982) Kinetics of phenotypic maturation of remodeling of hyperplastic nodules during liver carcinogenesis. Cancer Res 42: 2330-2335.

13. Tate SS, Meister A (1985) γ–Glutamyl transpeptidase from kidney. Meth. Enzymol. 113: 400-419.

14. Hanigan MH, Frierson HF jr, Brown JE, Lovell MA, Taylor PT (1994) Human ovarian tumors express γ–glutamyl transpeptidase. Cancer Res. 54: 286-290.
15. Paolicchi A, Pompella A, Tonarelli P, Gadducci A, Genazzani AR, Zunino F, Tongiani R (1996) γ–Glutamyl transpeptidase activity in primary and metastatic human ovarian tumors. Anticancer Res. *(manuscript submitted).*
16. Stark A-A, Zeiger E, Pagano DA (1993) Glutathione metabolism by γ–glutamyl transpeptidase leads to lipid peroxidation: characterization of the system and relevance to hepatocarcinogenesis. Carcinogenesis 14: 183-189.
17. Solt D, Farber E (1976) New principle for the analysis of chemical carcinogenesis. Nature 263: 701-706.
18. Pompella A, Comporti M (1991) The use of 3-hydroxy-2-naphthoic acid hydrazide and Fast Blue B for the histochemical detection of lipid peroxidation in animal tissues - a microphotometric study. Histochemistry 95: 255-262.
19. Pompella A, Paolicchi A, Dominici S, Comporti M, Tongiani R (1996) Selective colocalization of lipid peroxidation and protein thiol loss in chemically induced hepatic preneoplastic lesions: the role of γ–glutamyltranspeptidase activity. Histochemistry Cell Biol. *(in press).*
20. Pompella A, Romani A, Benedetti A, Comporti M (1991) Loss of membrane protein thiols and lipid peroxidation in allyl alcohol hepatotoxicity. Biochem Pharmacol 41: 1255-1259.
21. Huseby NE, Strömme JH (1974) Practical points regarding routine determination of γ–glutamyl transferase (γ–GT) in serum with a kinetic method at 37°C. Scand.J.Clin. Lab.Invest. 34: 357-361.
22. Sun Y (1990) Free radicals, antioxidant enzymes and carcinogenesis. Free Rad.Biol. Med 8: 583-599.

CHAPTER 19

ANTIOXIDANT SYSTEM IN HEPATOCELLULAR CARCINOMA

ANNA GRATTAGLIANO, GIAN LUDOVICO RAPACCINI, ANTONIO GASBARRINI, PATRIZIA MARINO AND GIOVANNI GASBARRINI.

Department of Internal Medicine, Catholic University, Roma, Italy.

Summary

Oxygen radicals play an important role in the course of experimental and human carcinogenesis. Antioxidant enzymes have been shown to protect cells against oxidative damage and, thus, to inhibit both initiation and promotion of carcinogenesis. The antioxidant enzyme superoxide dismutase catalyses the dismutation of superoxide anion, a very toxic radical, into hydrogen peroxide and exists as two types: one containing manganese and found in the mitochondria matrix and one containing copper-zinc and found in the cytosol. The superoxide dismutase activity has been shown to be impaired in some human neoplasm and in rat hepatocarcinoma. We found, in a recent study, a progressive reduction of superoxide dismutase activity progressing from chronic liver diseases to hepatocellular carcinoma; this finding seems consistent with current knowledge on the natural history of hepatocellular carcinoma.

INTRODUCTION

Oxidative damage is involved in the pathogenesis of different imflammatory, ischaemic, and degenerative diseases. Oxygen free radicals have been shown to play an important role both in the experimental promotion of tumors and in spontaneous mutagenesis and have been assumed to be implicated in human neoplasms. Antioxidant enzymes have been demonstrated to inhibit both initiation and promotion in carcinogenesis and to counteract in vitro cell immortalization and transformation. The main antioxidant enzymes are glutathione peroxidase (GSH-PX), catalase (CAT) and superoxide dismutase

P. Gentilini and M. U. Dianzani. New Trends in Hepatology, 169-173

(SOD). In vivo and in vitro studies have shown a reduction of these enzymes during carcinogenesis and in tumors (1).

Liver cirrhosis could be considered an interesting human model. In this disease, in fact, regenerant hepatocytes are present and hepatocellular carcinoma (HCC) frequently appears in its natural history. HCC, moreover, almost always arises from cirrhotic liver and epidemiological studies and those on the natural history have led to the hypothesis that cirrhosis is a preneoplastic condition independent from its etiology (2-4). In fact, liver regeneration can favor, due to the large number of mitoses, the development of mutations.

Continuous improvement in imaging techniques has allowed certain hyperplastic-regenerative nodular lesions to be identified in liver cirrhosis with increasing frequency; however, the clinical and prognostic value of these lesions is not clear. Thus, since the transformation from normal cell to neoplastic cell can include a dysplastic phase, the identification of this stage appears to be very important in the early diagnosis of HCC (5-6).

HEPATOCELLULAR CARCINOMA AND ANTIOXIDANT ENZYMES

Corrocher et al. showed a reduction in GSH-Px and CAT activity in HCCs submitted to surgical resection. However, this study considered patients selected for surgery, thus the hepatocarcinoma was associated with cirrhosis in only 5 of the 24 cases and only 8 patients were positive for hepatitis B surface antigen (7).

The role of SOD in primary liver neoplasms has been examined: in animal models, such as rat HCC, a reduction in both the activity and quantity of SOD and its mRNA have been shown to be directly proportional to tumor growth rate (8); furthermore, in human hepatoma cell lines (Hep 3B) with B virus genoma, low levels of SOD (either MnSOD or CuZnSOD) and CAT and the absence of GSH-Px was found (9). The absence of the MnSOD protein and the reduction of theCuZnSOD protein in HCC have been reported by immunohistochemical assay (10). Nevertheless, there is no data in literature on the enzymatic activity of SOD in human hepatocarcinomas or displastic nodules, possibly due to past difficulties in obtaining tissue from these lesions in that the underlying cirrhosis almost always prevents patients from undergoing surgical resection. The introduction of ultrasonography in clinical practice has permitted the follow up of cirrhotic patients and the consequent discovery of neoplastic and preneoplastic lesions in the preclinic phase. It has also provided the possibility of guiding percutaneous biopsies into the lesions, with high diagnostic accuracy for both cytologic and histologic samples (11).

Our recent studies (12-13), performed on bioptic specimens, show a reduction in both types of SOD, cytoplasmic and mitochondrial, which is progressively greater in chronic hepatitis (CH), cirrhosis, Dysplastic Nodules (DN) and HCC in cirrhotic liver (Tab.1). Furthermore, this finding seems to be consistent with current knowledge on the natural history of HCC. We evaluated HCC stemming from liver cirrhosis, mainly of viral aetiology. It would also be interesting to evaluate SOD activity also in rare, primary tumors stemming from normal liver.
It must be stressed that in CH and cirrhosis the ratio of MnSOD to CuZnSOD is similar to that normal liver, whereas in DNs and HCCs this ratio abruptly decreases. Moreover, there is not only a statistically significant difference between the activity of the HCCs and the normal liver, but also of CHs and cirrhoses. Our results suggest that in viral liver diseases a correlation exists between carcinogenesis and CuZnSOD depletion. It could be inferred that chronic liver diseases are a predisposing condition to neoplasms, both because the liver has already come into contact with a hypothetical initiator (virus ?) and because liver regeneration behaves like a promoting agent.
The levels of SOD activity in the DNs are not very different from those of HCCs. This suggests that DNs, when correctly identified (6), have the same biological properties of HCCs and thus the same therapeutic approach is proposable. Two of the four DNs in our study showed an increase in size with subsequent histological diagnosis of HCC within one year from the first biopsy. Nevertheless, in order to confirm the above hypothesis it would be necessary to perform further assays of SOD activity on more DNs with adequate follow-up time.

CONCLUSION

Our study, in agreement with previous reports, shows a reduction in SOD enzymatic activity in chronic hepatitis and primary neoplastic liver lesions. The mechanism leading to changes in the levels of antioxidant enzymes still needs to be identified. Furthermore, whether these modifications are a consequence of a transformation in the liver or, rather, an early event of carcinogenesis which favors the transformation itself must also be determined . In vivo and in vitro evidence of pretranscriptional control of SOD genomic expression (8), inducibility of SOD from cytokines (14), and repression by Transforming Growth Factor (15) need to be confirmed on human tissue and placed in the context of the natural history of chronic liver diseaeses.

TABLE 1

	Mn-SOD µg/mg prot	CuZn-SOD µg/mg prot
Normal liver	6.4 ± 0.8	6.0 ± 0.4
CH	4.5 ± 0.5°	3.4 ± 0.4*
Cirrhosis	3.6 ± 0.4°	3.4 ± 0.5*
DN	3.1 ± 0.6°	2.1 ± 0.2*
HCC	3.6 ± 0.6°	1.3 ± 0.5*

Mean value ± standard error of superoxide dismutase activity in liver specimens evaluated. CH: chronic hepatitis. DN: dysplastic nodules. HCC: hepatocellular carcinoma.

* $p < 0.001$, ° $p < 0.05$ vs normal livers

REFERENCES

1) Sun Y. Free radicals, antioxidant enzymes, and carcinogenesis. Free Rad Biol Med. 1990; 8: 583-599.

2) Johnson PJ, Williams R. Cirrhosis and the aetiology of hepatocellular carcinoma. J Hepatol. 1987; 5: 140-147.

3) Zaman SN, Johnson PJ, Williams R. Silent cirrhosis in patients with hepatocellular carcinoma. Cancer. 1990; 65: 1607-1610.

4) Simonetti RG, Cammà C, Fiorello F, Pagliaro L. Hepatocellular carcinoma: a worldwide problem. The maijor risk factors. Dig Dis Sci. 1991; 36: 962-972.

5) Rapaccini GL, Pompili M, Caturelli E, Anti M, Cedrone A, Amadei E, Grattagliano A, et al. Focal ultrasound lesions in liver cirrhosis diagnosed as regenerating nodules by fine-needle biopsy. Follow-up of 12 cases. Dig Dis Sci. 1990; 35: 422-427.

6) Pompili M, Rapaccini GL, Gambassi G. Review of adenomatos hyperplastic nodules in liver cirrhosis: pathological features, imaging diagnosis and prognostic significance. Gastroenterol Int. 1991; 4: 120-124.

7) Corrocher R, Casaril M, Bellisola G, Gabrielli GB, Nicoli N, Guidi GC, De Sandre G. Severe impairement of antioxidant system in human hepatoma. Cancer. 1986; 58: 1658-1662.

8) Borrello S, De Leo ME, Galeotti T. Defective gene expression of MnSOD in cancer cells. Molec Aspect Med. 1993; 14: 253-258.

9) Bannister WH, Federici G, Heath JK, Bannister JV. Antioxidant systems in tumour cells: the level of antioxidant enzymes, ferritin and total iron in a human hepatoma cell line. Free Radic Res Commun. 1986; 1: 361-367.

10) Inagaki T, Katoch K, Takiya S, Ikuta K, Kobayashi S, Suzichi M, Fukuzawa Y, et al. Relationship between superoxide dismutase (SOD) and viral liver disease. Gastroenterol Jpn .1992; 27: 382-389.

11) Rapaccini GL, Pompili M, Caturelli E, Fusilli F, Trombino C, Gomes S, Squillante MM, M.M.,Castelvetere M,Aliotta A,Grattagliano A, et al. Ultrasound-guided fine-needle biopsy of hepatocellular carcinoma: comparison between smear cytology and microhistology. Am J Gastroenterol. 1994; 89: 898-902.

12) Grattagliano A, Rapaccini GL, De Leo ME, Marino P, Borrello S, Pompili M, Galeotti T, Gasbarrini G. Human hepatocarcinogenesis: assay of Superoxide Dismutase activity. Hepatology. 1994; 20: 352A, 1022,.

13) Grattagliano A, Rapaccini GL, De Leo ME, Marino P, Borrello S, Pompili M, Galeotti T, Gasbarrini G. Superoxide dismutase activity in human cirrhosis and in hepatocellular carcinoma. Gut. 1994; 35, suppl.4: 1018.

14) Ono M, Kohda H, Kawagushi T, Ohhira M, Sekiya C, Namiki M, Takeyasu A, et al. Induction of Mn-superoxide dismutase by tumor necrosis factor, interleukin-1 and interleukin-6 in human hepatoma cells. Biochem Biophys Res Commun. 1992; 182: 1100-1107.

15) Kayanoki Y, Fuji J, Suzuki K, Kawata S, Matsuzawa Y, Taniguchi N. Suppression of antioxidative enzyme expression by transforming growth-factor β1 in rat hepatocytes. J Biol Chem. 1994; 269: 15488-15492.

CHAPTER 20

LOSS OF HETEROZYGOSITY OF THE LONG ARM OF CHROMOSOME 16 IN HEPATOCELLULAR CARCINOMA ON LIVER CIRRHOSIS.

LAURA GRAMANTIERI, ANNA CASALI, STEFANO GAIANI, FABIO PISCAGLIA, BARBARA STECCA, ALIGHIERO MAZZIOTTI, ANTONINO CAVALLARI, LUIGI BOLONDI.

Dipartimento di Medicina Interna e Gastroenterologia, Clinica Chirurgica II, Università di Bologna

SUMMARY

The analysis of loss of heterozygosity in human neoplasms, has shown that several genomic regions are frequently lost, suggesting their involvement in the pathogenesis of cancer as putative sites for tumor suppressor genes. The long arm of chromosome 16 has been implicated in breast, prostate and hepatocellular carcinomas. Previous studies made on large, advanced cases of HCC, revealed large areas of deletion on 16q. A recent report from a Japanese series of large HCC delimitated a common area of deletion at 16q22-23. We tested 16 small (<3 cm) HCC for loss of somatic heterozygosity using a set of 8 polymorphic microsatellite markers spanning 16q22-24. Three out of 10 informative cases showed loss of heterozygosity at 16q24.3, defining a commonly deleted region, possible site for a tumor suppressor gene.

GENETIC ALTERATIONS IN HCC

Several factors (hepatitis virus infections, alcohol, chronic hepatitis and liver cirrhosis, exposure to mycotoxins and some chemical carcinogens) have been found to be associated with the development of primary liver cancer, but the pathways of hepatocarcinogenesis are still unknown. So far our knowledge of genes playing a key role in the development and the progressive growth of HCC is limited (1). Similarly to other malignant tumors, hepatocarcinogenesis is regarded as a long term, multistep process where cumulative mutations in oncogenes, tumor suppressor genes and overexpression of growth factors are required for transformation of a normal cell to a malignant one.

P. Gentilini and M. U. Dianzani. New Trends in Hepatology, 174-182

Several genetic mechanisms have been analyzed: point mutations, translocations, insertional mutagenesis of a viral genome, gene amplifications, loss or gain of whole chromosomes or part of a chromosome can activate oncogenes or inactivate tumor suppressor genes.

It is unlikely that a single genetic alteration will account for all HCC, given their etiological, biochemical, histological and clinical heterogeneity (2). As for most other tumor types, experimental evidences suggest that the malignant phenotype results from the cumulative effect of multiple genetic alterations, similarly to what has been found for colo-rectal cancer (3) but, so far, not confirmed for other tumor types.

Hepatits B virus has been proposed as a major cause of HCC (4) and experimental evidences supporting its causal role are based on the finding of integration of HBV-DNA in the hepatocellular genome of a large percentage of HCC (5), independently from the presence of serum markers indicative for HBV infection (6). Even if some studies have identified a region commonly deleted in HBV-related hepatocellular carcinoma on chromosome 17 near to the p53 gene (7), evidence of a precise genomic locus of integration of HBV-DNA, similarly to woodchuck HBV in the development of woodchuck HCC (8), is still lacking. An important role in HBV-related carcinogenesis seems to be played by transcriptional transactivators and particularly by HBX (9) and the preS2/S genes products of HBV (10). The X gene of HBV, which was also demonstrated to interact with the wild type p53, thus inhibiting its sequence-specific DNA binding and transcriptional activity, has been found integrated in the hepatocyte genome in a very high percentage of cases (2).

The clinical experience however shows other conditions closely linked to the development of HCC: HCV infection, mycotoxin exposure, metabolic disorders (hemocromatosis, Wilson' s disease), autoimmune diseases (primary biliary cirrhosis), so that different mechanisms have been hypothesized for hepatocarcinogenesis. Activated oncogenes have in fact been found in spontaneous and experimentally-induced HCC, but, as yet, no single oncogene has been shown to be preferentially or always activated in human HCC (1).

TUMOR SUPPRESSOR GENES AND HCC

Another possible genetic alteration is the inactivation of one or more tumor suppressor genes (TSG). The existence of TSG was first indirectly suggested by studies with Restriction Fragment Length Polymorphism

(RFLP) that indicated a loss of specific chromosomal regions in tumor DNA when compared to somatic DNA from the same patients.

Mutation of a tumor suppressor gene and subsequent loss of the corresponding normal allele is widely considered a pathway common to many types of neoplasms. Retinoblastoma (RB) gene, localized on chromosome 13q14 is the first characterized TSG. It was recognized in the region commonly deleted in retinoblastoma, breast cancer, osteosarcoma and lung cancer.

Several other TSG such as p53, Wilms' tumor gene, the DCC (deleted in colorectal carcinomas) gene, APC (adenomatous polyposis coli) gene, neurofibromatosis type 1 gene, have been subsequently cloned.

p53 and RB gene are the two best known TSG and they have been extensively studied in HCC. Mutation of the p53 gene have been frequently found in advanced HCC, particularly from areas with high dietary exposure to aflatoxin B1 such as China, Senegal, Mozambique and South Africa (11). The role of p53 mutation however, has not been confirmed for HCC in aflatoxin's low exposure areas (12).

Concerning the retinoblastoma (RB) gene, Nishida et al (13) reported allelic losses on 13q in 47% of advanced HCC, suggesting that RB gene is involved in development or progression at least of a subset of human HCC. These findings however were not confirmed by Seki and coworkers (14) who analyzed an HCC cell line (OCUH-16) and 11 biopsy specimens from patients with HCC and reported that the RB gene is preserved and expressed at reasonable level in OCUH-16 cells and detected the RB protein by immunostaining in biopsy specimens of early and advanced HCC.

Several studies on different neoplasms including HCC, detected allelic losses in tumor DNA at precise genomic loci. These frequent genetic losses, occurring in a significant number of tumors suggest the existence of several other tumor suppressor genes, different from RB and p53, which may participate in the development and/or progression of cancer (15). The first evidence that some chromosomal regions were involved more frequently in deletions or translocations derived from analysis of karyotype. Then more sensitive examinations could be conducted by means of molecular biology techniques like RFLP analysis of genomic DNA.

This technique consists of digestion of high molecular weight DNA with appropriate restriction enzymes, electrophoretical fractioning on 0.8%

agarose gel, transfer to nylon membrane and hybridization with specific labeled DNA probes. Tumor and constitutional DNA obtained from normal tissue (blood lymphocytes or non tumor tissue) from the same patients are compared to detect any allelic imbalance at the tested loci.
Recently the detection of loss of heterozygosity (LOH) has been performed by microsatellite PCR analysis: specific genomic loci are amplified by PCR performed on very little amounts of genomic DNA extracted from tumor and control tissue from the same patient. The amplification products are separated on a 6% polyacrylamide gel and revealed by means of autoradiography or other staining procedures. This technique can be utilized for LOH detection in large series of cases and it employs little amounts of DNA, so that more chromosome's loci can be examined.
Several genomic regions have been studied in different neoplasms, including HCC, and some of them have been found to be deleted in high percentages of cases and in different types of tumors (non random deletions).

LOSS OF HETEROZYGOSITY ON CHROMOSOME 16
As regard HCC, previous cytogenetical and RFLP studies showed LOH at chromosomes 1p, 4q, 5q, 10q, 11p 13q, 16q, 17p (13). RFLP studies, made on human HCC, breast and prostate cancer reported high incidence of LOH on 16q but, as regard HCC, advanced cases were mostly considered.
Tsuda and coworkers (16) analyzed 70 surgically resected tumors by RFLP and reported large percentage (52%) of loss regarding chromosome 16 (both 16p and 16q were analyzed). These authors included in their study a large majority of advanced HCC, since 31 out of 69 cases had neoplastic thrombosis of the portal vein or intrahepatic metastasis and only 6 out of 69 cases could be considered early lesions. Among the 36 tumors which showed LOH on 16q, 21 lost the whole chromosome 16 and in 30 cases all informative loci on 16q showed LOH, suggesting loss of the entire long arm of chromosome 16. The losses were more frequently detected in poorly differentiated HCC, of large size and with metastasis. These findings don't allow the identification of a limited chromosomal region of loss of heterozygosity. The 6 early cases of HCC did not show any loss and the advanced cases, where probably late genetic events have occurred during tumor progression also in aspecific way, showed large areas of deletion. In the HCC series analyzed by Tsuda et al. (16) the most

common region of loss was located between HP (16q22.1) and CTRB loci (16q22.3-q23.2).

Sakai et al. (17) in a RFLP study made on 68 samples of paired tumor and non tumor tissue, analyzed 3 sites on chromosome 16: HBA on 16p 13.3, MT2 on 16q21-22.1 and HP on 16q22.1-q22.2, which were found deleted respectively in 22%, 15% and 39%. In this study the most telomeric regions of chromosome 16q were not analyzed. These authors could not confirm the correlation found by Tsuda et al. between 16q losses and advanced stage of HCC but they underlined the limited number of well differentiated HCC analyzed in both (16, 17) these studies.

Nishida and coworkers (13) analyzed one locus (D16S7) on chromosome 16q, and found loss of heterozygosity in 40% of cases, being these chromosomal losses more frequent in large, poorly differentiated HCCs, with intrahepatic metastasis or portal vein thrombosis. The analysis of only one locus does not allow the identification of a deletion map of the chromosome, since LOH at one locus can also be detected when the entire chromosome arm or the whole chromosome is lost, especially in advanced neoplasms, where aspecific genomic alterations can be frequently found. In this study, the authors consider also the accumulation of allelic loss on three different chromosomes (13q, 16q and 17p) and confirm that more progressive and poorly differentiated tumors show deletion of multiple chromosome's arms and they can't exclude their random nature. Nevertheless the frequent finding of LOH on chromosome 16q is confirmed to be important, at least in a subset of HCC.

A recent study by Yeh and coworkers (18) reports a 70% frequency of loss of heterozygosity on 16q in large hepatocellular carcinomas (>5 cm). These authors defined the commonly affected region at 16q22-23.

PERSONAL EXPERIENCE

To analyze the allelotype in HCC and to identify candidate sites for tumor-suppressor genes in the development of HCC, we have examined by means of PCR analysis of LOH 16 small (<3 cm) HCC, resected at surgery, using a set of 8 highly polymorphic markers spanning a region on 16q which was found frequently deleted in advanced HCC from eastern countries. The following microsatellite markers were used for PCR analysis of LOH: D16S522 (16q22.1), HSD17β2 (16q24.1), D16S422 (16q24.1), D16S402, D16S393, D16S520 (16q24.2), D16S305, D16S413 (16q24.3) (fig.1). PCR reaction was performed with 50 ng of DNA in a 25

Fig. 1.

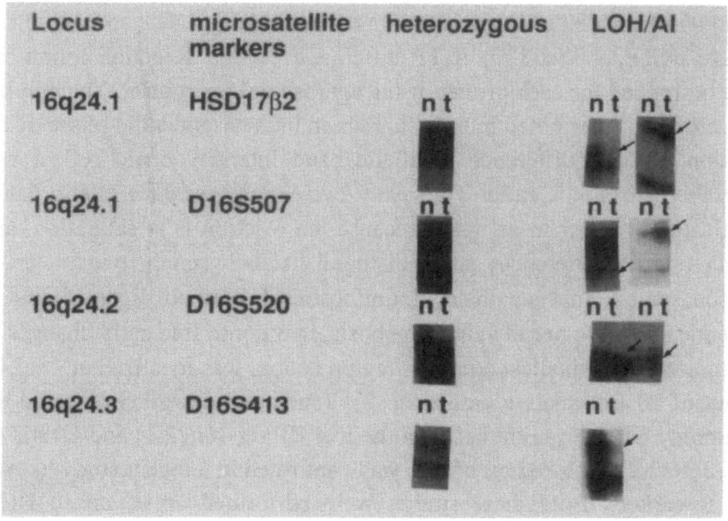

Examples of LOH at chromosome 16q in representative hepatocellular carcinomas. Analysis of normal (n) and tumor tissue (t) DNA. Arrows: alleles showing LOH or allelic imbalance.

Fig. 2

	1	2	3	4	5	6	7	8	9	10	11	12	13	14	15	16
D16S522	H	H	H	H	H	H	O	H	H	H	LOH	H	O	O	H	H
HSD17b2	H	O	AI	H	H	H	O	O	H	H	LOH	AI	O	AI	H	O
D16S422	O	H	O	H	H	H	H	H	H	H	LOH	AI	H	AI	H	O
D16S402	H	H	H	H	H	H	H	H	H	H	LOH	H	H	H	H	O
D16S393	O	H	H	H	H	H	H	H	H	H	LOH	H	H	H	H	H
D16S520	O	H	H	H	H	H	H	H	H	H	LOH	O	H	H	H	H
D16S305	O	H	H	H	O	H	O	H	O	H	LOH	H	H	H	H	H
D16S413	O	H	H	O	O	H	O	O	O	H	LOH	LOH	H	LOH	H	H

Summary of the of genetic alterations at 8 loci on chromosome 16q in 16 HCC samples, detected by microsatellite polymorphism analysis. Microsatellite markers used are indicated in the left column. H: heterozygous; O: omozygous; LOH: loss of heterozygosity.; AI: allelic imbalance.

μl volume, using 0.5 Unit Taq DNA-polymerase (from Boehringer-Mannheim) with 50 μM concentration each of dATP, dGTP and dTTP and 2,5 μM dCTP, and (α-32P) dCTP at 0.5 μCi/reaction. Reaction conditions were optimized for each primer, using agarose gel for control. The number of cycles was determined in order to remain in the esponential phase of the reaction, so that difference in allelic band intensity could reflect real differences in allelic ratio. Too many cycles may produce allelic bands which do not differ in intensity because the reaction is at saturation, and no quantitative differences can be distinguished between the two alleles.

We focused our analysis on small, unifocal HCC, without signs of local or systemic spread or portal vein thrombosis, in order to find early changes.

In our series the smallest common region of loss was localized at 16q24.3 (3 out of 10 informative cases, fig. 2). Tsuda and coworkers located the commonly deleted region between the loci HP (at 16q22.1) and CTRB (at 16q22.3-23.2). This region of loss was confirmed in a recent study by Yeh and coworkers. Both these studies were performed on advanced HCC, from eastern countries (respectively Tokio and Taiwan). The common region of deletion in our patients series was different from the one described by these two studies. This can be possibly due to different risk factors that can act through different molecular pathways, as already documented for p53 tumor-suppressor gene. A recent report by Cleton-Jansen and coworkers (19) detected LOH on 63% of 79 cases of sporadic breast carcinomas and restricted the area of loss at two distinct regions on 16q: the first one between APRT and D16S303 (16q24.3) deleted in 52% of cases, the second one between D16S398 and D16S301 (16q22.1) involved in 47% of cases. These authors, in agreement with previous studies (20, 21) made on breast cancer, suggest that these two distinct regions emerge as likely sites for tumor suppressor genes. Furthermore they underline that loss of chromosome arm 16q is probably an early event in carcinogenesis since, as concerns breast cancer, it has been observed in tumors with few or even no other cytogenetic abnormalities.

Further studies on HCC at a different stage will indicate if LOH on chromosome 16q can be considered a key genetic alteration in the development of this neoplasms.

References

1) Okuda K. hepatocellular carcinoma: recent progress (1992). Hepatology 15: 948-963

2) Unsal H, Yakicier C, Marcais C, Kew M, Volkmann M, Zentgraf H, Isselbacher KJ, Ozturk M (1994). Genetic heterogeneity of hepatocellular carcinoma. Proc. Natl Acad Sci USA 91: 822-826

3) Fearon ER, and Vogelstein B (1990). A genetic model for colorectal tumorigenesis. Cell, 61: 759-767

4) Beasley RP. Hepatitis B virus as the etiologic agent in hepatocellular carcinoma-epidemiologic considerations (1982). Hepatology 2: 21-26

5) Shafritz DA, Shouval D, Sherman HI, Hadziyannis SJ, Kew MC (1981). Integration of hepatitis B virus DNA into the genome of liver cells in chronic liver disease and hepatocellular carcinoma. N Engl J Med 305: 1067-1073

6) Paterlini P, Gerken G, Nakajima E, Terre S, D'Errico A, Grigioni W, Nalpas B, Franco D, Wands J, Kew M, Pisi E, Tiollais P, Brechot C (1990). Polymerase chain reaction to detect hepatitis B virus DNA and RNA sequences in primary liver cancers from patients negative for hepatitis B surface antigen. N Engl J Med 323: 80-85)

7) Slagle BL, Zhou YZ, and Butel JS (1991). Hepatitis B virus insertion event in human chromosome 17 near the p53 gene identifies the region of the chromosome commonly deleted in virus positive hepatocellular carcinoma. Cancer Res, 51: 49-54

8) Hsu TY, Moroy T, Etiemble J, Louise A, trepo C, Tiollais P, buèndia MA (1988). Activation of c-myc by woodchuck hepatitis virus infection in hepatocellular carcinoma. Cell 55: 627-635

9) Wollersheim M, Deveika Y, Hofschneider PH (1988). A transactivating function encoded in the hepatitis B virus X gene is conserved in the integrated state. Oncogene 3: 545-552

10) Kekulè AS, Lauer UM, Meyer M, caselmann WH, Hofschneicer PH, Koshy R (1990). The preS2/S region of integrated hepatitis B virus DNA encodes a transcriptional transactivator. Nature 343: 457-461

11) Ozturk M (1991). p53 mutations in hepatocellular carcinoma after aflatoxin exposure. Lancet 338: 1356-9

12) Kubicka S, Trautwein C, Schrem H, Tillmann H, Manns M (1995). Low incidence of p53 mutations in european hepatocellular carcinomas with heterogeneous mutation as a rare event. J Hepatol 23: 412-419

13) Nishida N, Fukuda Y, Kokuryu H, Sadamoto T, Isowa G, Honda K, Yamaoka Y, Ikenaga M, Imura H, Ishizaki K (1992). Accumulation of allelic loss on arms of chromosomes 13q, 16q, and 17p in the advanced stages of human hepatocellular carcinoma. Int J Cancer 51, 862-868

14) Seki S, Kawakita N, Yanai A, Kitada T, Sakai Y, Nakatani K, Yamada T, Sakaguchi H, Kuroki T (1995). Expression of the retinoblastoma gene product in human hepatocellular carcinoma. Hum Pathol 26: 366-374

15) Lasko D, Cavenee W, Nordenskjold M (1991). Loss of constitutional heterozygosity in human cancer. Annu. Rev. genet. 25: 281-314

16) Tsuda H, Zhang W, ShimosatoY, Yokota J, Terada M, Sugimura T, Miyamura T, Hirohashi S (1990). Allele loss on chromosome 16 associated with progression of human hepatocellular carcinoma. Proc. Natl. Acad. Sci. USA, 87: 6791-6794

17) Sakai K, Nagahara H, Abe K, Obata M (1992). Loss of heterozygosity on chromosome 16 in hepatocellular carcinoma. J Gastroenterol Hepatol 7: 288-292
18) Yeh SH, Chen PJ, Lai MY, Chen DS (1996). Allelic loss on chromosomes 4q and 16q in hepatocellular carcinoma: association with elevated α-fetoprotein production. Gastroenterology 110: 184-192
19) Cleton-Jansen AM, Moerland EW, Kuipers-Dijkshoorn NJ, Callen DF, Sutherland GR, Hansen B, Devilee P, Cornelisse CJ (1994). At least two different regions are involved in allelic imbalance on chromosome 16q in breast cancer. Genes Chrom Cancer 9: 101-107
20) Sato T, Akiyama F, Sakamoto G, Kasumi F, Nakamura Y (1991). Accumulation of genetic alterations and progression of primary breast cancer. Cancer Res 51: 5794-5799
21) Callen DF, Hildebrand CE, Reeders S (1992). Report of the second international workshop on human chromosome 16 mapping. Cytogenet Cell Genet 60: 158-167

CHAPTER 21

POTENTIAL MOLECULAR MECHANISMS OF VIRAL LIVER CARCINOGENESIS

M.S. DE MITRI, P. BACCARINI, C. BONAZZI, P. PATERLINI, E. PISI
Istituto di Clinica Medica Generale e Terapia Medica, Università di Bologna, Italy

Summary
Hepatocellular carcinoma is one of the most common malignant tumors worldwide. The geographic prevalence of HCC is largely variable and this reflects the different distribution of possible etiological factors. Liver cirrhosis is the major determinant of neoplastic transformation (1). The strong association between chronic HBV and HCV infection and developement of HCC is widely demonstrated by epidemiological studies (2,3) but the exact mechanism by which malignant trasformation occurs remains still unclear. HBV might exert a direct role in liver carcinogenesis by a combination of different non exclusive effects as DNA integration (4) and transactivating activity of HBX and truncated pre-S2/S proteins (5,6). Concerning HCV related liver oncogenesis, it is still obscure whether HCV might exert, in addition to inducing cirrhosis, a direct effect in malignant transformation. The evidence that HCV persists and replicate in HCC developing in absence of cirrhosis (7) may be a basis for further molecular studies on the potential oncogenic effect of HCV.

Hepatitis B virus and hepatocellular carcinoma

Structure and organization of viral genome

The human hepatitis B virus, a member of the hepadnavirus family, is the smallest DNA virus known, having only 3200 nucleotides in its genome. The genome exhibits an unusual and characteristic structure, a partially double-stranded circular DNA molecule. The "minus" strand (L-) is almost a complete circle of a fixed length and contains four overlapping open reading frames (ORFs), termed S, C, P and X, which encode for structural proteins (surface and core) and replicative proteins (polymerase and X). In contrast, the "plus" strand (S+) is short, variable in length and does not contain any ORFs. The S region codes for the protein of the viral envelope (HBsAg) and is divided into the S gene, pre-S1 and pre-S2 regions. HBV

P. Gentilini and M. U. Dianzani. New Trends in Hepatology, 183-196

envelope proteins display morphogenetic and regulatory functions: whereas all the information required to produce HBsAg particles is contained in the S region, the protein encoded by the pre-S1 domain plays a key role for the outcome of a viral infection and in virion assembly. The C gene with a pre-C region encodes the principal structural protein of the viral nucleocapsid (HBcAg) and a cleavage product, e antigen (HBeAg), respectively (8). HBeAg has significant clinical importance because its persistence in infected patients is probably associated with active viral replication, high infectivity and potential cronicity. A mutation in the pre-C region abolishes the synthesis of HBeAg, and these cases are associated with more severe liver disease and a high rate of progression to cirrhosis (9). The enzymatic activities required for the initiation of reverse transcription, central step in the viral replication cycle, the synthesis of DNA minus- and plus-strand and removal of the RNA template are encoded in the P region which produces the DNA polymerase, a single multidomain protein. About the X gene, so-called because the function of gene product was unknown when the gene was identified, its molecular functions are still unclear. The X protein appears to have potent transactivating effect that might be responsible for activation of cellular oncogenesis (10).

Molecular mechanisms of HBV carcinogenesis

Extensive epidemiological studies have shown a strong association between HBV chronic infection and HCC development (1,2). However, despite the important knowledges acquired in the last years, the mechanism involved in liver carcinogenesis remains still enigmatic. The HBV carcinogenic potential has been linked to the combination of different non exclusive effects: the capacity to induce liver cirrhosis, the possibility to integrate into the hepatocyte genome and the transactivating and possible transforming activity of HBX protein. Liver cirrhosis is strongly associated to HCC and this link suggests that chronic hepatic injury and successive regeneration may promote the induction or selection of malignant clones (11). In these cases the developement of liver cancer is a complication of cirrhosis rather than a consequence of potential direct viral mechanisms of carcinogenesis as integration and transactivation. Although there is general agreement on the importance of cirrhosis in the carcinogenic process, the existence of a direct effect of HBV in liver cell trasformation is still controversial.

HBV sequences are frequently found integrated into the genome of HCC cells and this feature leads to an unknown cascade of events that ultimately trasform normal hepatocytes in malignant cells, possibly through activation of genes or oncogenes associated with cell proliferation or, more likely, inactivation of tumor-suppressor genes (12). The consequences of viral DNA integration might be chromosomal rearrangements, insertional mutagenesis and synthesis of truncated X and pre-S2/S proteins.

In woodchucks liver cancer, infected by woodchuck hepatitis virus, viral DNA has been frequently found integrated into *c-myc* or N-*myc* oncogenes (13). In contrast, in human HCC viral DNA integration in a cellular gene has been shown in single cases. In one HCC, the pre-S1 region was found integrated in the retinoic acid receptor ß gene which has a well established important role in cell differentiation and proliferation (14). In an early small cancer developed on a non-cirrhotic liver, HBV DNA integration was found in the second intron of cyclin A gene on chromosome 4 (4q27) (15), in the proximity of a chromosomal locus (4q32) which is frequently rearranged in HCC (16). Cyclin A plays a key role in the control of cell division and several studies indicate that it acts, in combination with $p34^{cdc2}$ and $p33^{cdk2}$ kinase, in both the G2/M and S transitions. The $p34^{cdc2}$-cyclin A complex is a constituent of the maturation-promoting factor (17). A potential mechanism for the role of cyclin A in liver carcinogenesis might be the loss of cyclin A function through allelic loss at its locus. To determine if a cyclin A allelic loss occurs frequently in liver cancer, we studied tumorous and non-tumorous tissue from 50 patients with HCC to search for allelic loss in the cyclin A gene. We based the study on TaqI polymorphism previously described on the 7th intron of cyclin A gene (18), and on the polymerase chain reaction (PCR) tecnique. We found that the allelic loss in the cyclin A gene is a rare event in liver cancer (5%) (19). In a recent work, we investigated whether cyclin A gene structure and expression are frequenly dysregulated in liver cancer by Southern blot analysis and whether cyclin A expression, known to take place after cell commitment to DNA synthesis up to mitosis, correlates with the HCC cell proliferation rate (cells in S and G2/M phases assessed by flow cytometry). Also this study showed that rearrangements and allelic losses are rare events in HCC but the findings indicated that the level of cyclin A RNA is generally low and proportional to the percentage of cycling cells, indicating that cyclin A has potential as a new index of tumor cell proliferation in liver cancer (20). Recently, further observations of viral DNA integration in cellular genes involved in cell proliferation, as the gene encoding human mevalonate kinase and an epidermal growth factor gene, have been described in single cases (21,22). While these results argue for a role of HBV insertion in liver cell transformation through the identification of critical genes encoding proteins involved in cell proliferation and differentiation, these findings have remained isolated.

In addition to the effect of HBV integration into the cellular genome, viral proteins X, synthesized from both free and integrated HBV sequences, and C terminally truncated PreS2/S protein (MHBst) encoded by integrated viral genomes, might be involved in liver carcinogenesis (23,24).

The HBX protein appears to have potent transactivating properties that might be responsible for transactivation of both viral and cellular genes through transcriptional regulatory factors such as AP-1, AP-2, NF-*k*B, etc, including proto-oncogenes as c-*myc* and c-*fos*. It has recently been reported that X protein has serine/threonine kinase-activity and the mechanism for transactivation may be related to the phosphorylation and consequently alteration of cellular proteins (25).

Several studies have investigated the expression of HBV transcripts in HCC by means of PCR and Northern blot techniques. With the aim to evaluate the presence and cellular localization of HBV RNAs in histological sections of HCC, we analyzed the expression of HBV RNAs (C; PreS2-S and X) in tumour and non tumour liver tissues of 19 HCC HBsAg-positive by means of a non-isotopic *in situ* hybridization method. The results demonstrated a low level of viral replication with different patterns of expression of the four main HBV transcripts (3.5 Kb, 2.4 Kb, 2.1 Kb and 0.8 Kb). Moreover, with the sense cDNA probe corresponding to the X gene, the presence of "antisense" X-specific transcripts was identified in two cases (Table 1). This study represents the first *in situ* demonstration of "antisense" transcripts of the X gene in human HCC, confirming the postulated bi-directional transcription of HBX gene. However, the role of these HBV transcripts, in particular of the "antisense" transcripts, in the pathogenesis of HCC needs to be further investigated.

TABLE 1. HBV replication in HCC from patients HBsAg positive, with different patterns of expression of the four main HBV transcripts.

	Gene specific cRNA probes for HBV RNA			
	C	preS2/S	X	X-antisense
1	+	+	+	+
2	+	+	+	-
3	+	-	+	-
4	+/-	-	+	-
5	-	-	+/-	+
6-19	-	-	-	-

HBV DNA in HBsAg-negative HCCs

Several works have suggested that HBV might be involved in the developement of HCC in patients negative for serum HBsAg. Indeed, the HBV sequences persist in a high proportion of HBsAg negative patients with or without antibodies (anti-HBs and anti-HBc), which indicate past exposure to the virus and resolved infection (26). Since in these patients the number of viral copies per cell is much lower than those found in HBsAg positive patients, it is not known if the viral oncogenic mechanism is different from that observed in HBsAg carriers. The prevalence of HBsAg negative and HBV DNA positive HCC cases has been debated but now it is known that the different results were due to distinct epidemiological factors and to different specifity and sensibility of the techniques used (27).

In our studies, using PCR assay and distinct sets of primers specific for S, pre/S, C and X coding regions, we have demonstrated a high rate of persistence of HBV DNA in the liver of HBsAg negative patients with HCC. The combination of the four specific primers showed, in several patients, positive results with all primers covering the different HBV regions; in other cases the DNA resulted positive only with some of the sets of primers. These findings are consistent, in the first observation, with the absence of large deletions in viral genome, in the second result with the presence of defective HBV genomes (28).

We confirmed these results in a recent study in which we looked for the persistence of HBV genome in a selected group of HBsAg negative patients with HCC, developed in the absence of cirrhosis (Table 2). Seven of 19 patients were HBV DNA positive in the tumorous and non tumorous tissue and 5 of them were anti-HBc positive. In three cases HBV DNA were expressed as complete viral genome, resulting positive for all the viral regions tested (S, Pre-S, C, X), whereas the remaining four cases showed the presence of defective HBV genomes (Table 3)(7).

Hepatitis C virus and hepatocellular carcinoma

Structure, organization and variability of viral genome

The hepatitis C virus was discovered recently using a recombinant complementary DNA (cDNA) assay (29). The viral genome consists of a small positive single-stranded RNA molecule comprising approximately

TABLE 2. Clinical and histological features of patients HBsAg negative with HCC developed on non cirrhotic liver

	Sex	Age	α-FP	HCC grade°	Ks* NT liver
1	M	22	3	III	2
2	M	64	nd	III	10
3	M	71	6	II	10
4	F	76	4	III	6
5	M	69	4	II	1
6	M	72	7	III	1
7	F	35	2	II	1
8	M	59	2	II	6
9	M	25	nd	IV	1
10	F	28	9	Fib.^	2
11	M	64	2	II	2
12	F	70	460	III	6
13	M	58	9000	III	13
14	M	57	2	III	9
15	F	66	11	IV	6
16	M	59	5	II	10
17	M	43	290	II	1
18	M	74	150	III	8
19	M	65	15	II	6

°Edmonson's grade; *Knodell's score; ^fibrolamellar type;
nd= not determined.

TABLE 3. HBV DNA; HCV RNA, HCV genotype in patients HBsAg negative with HCC developed on non cirrhotic liver

	HBV DNA		Anti-HCV	HCV RNA		Genotype		
	T	NT		T	NT	T	NT	S
1	-	-	-	+	+	2a	2a	
2	-	-	-	+	+	1b	1b	
3	-	-	+	+	+	1b	1b	
4*	-	-	nd	+	+	1b	1b	
5*	-	-	nd	+	+	1b	1b	
6	-	-	-	+	+	1b	1b	
7*	+	+	-	-	-	/	/	
8	+	+	-	-	-	/	/	
9	-	-	-	-	-	/	/	
10	-	-	-	-	-	/	/	
11*	+	+	-	-	-	/	/	
12	-	-	+	+	+	1b	1b	1b
13	-	-	+	+	+	2a	2a	2a
14*	+	+	+	+	+	1b	1b	1b
15*	-	-	-	-	-	/	/	/
16	-	-	+	+	+	1b	1b	1b
17	+	+	+	+	+	1b	1b	1b
18*	+	+	+	+	+	1b	1b	1b
19*	+	+	+	+	+	1b	1b	1b

*anti-HBc positive; T= tumour tissue; NT= non-tumour tissue; S= serum; /= not evaluable.

9,400 nucleotides, with a single continous traslational open-reading frame (ORF) which could encode a large viral polypeptide. At the 5' end there is a terminal region (non-coding region, NCR) of approximately 340 bases which is highly conserved among different HCV isolates analyzed, which contains small ORFs. There is no evidence and it is unlikely that these ORFs encode viral specific proteins. Its highly conserved character suggests that it may play a very important regulatory role during viral replication, probably at level of traslation of the HCV genome, and renders it suitable for diagnostic detection of viral RNA with PCR assay. In the organization of HCV genome, at 5' end are located the genes core and envelope (C and E1, E2/NS1) encoding for the structural viral proteins, while the four genes (NS2, NS3, NS3, NS4) encoding for the non-structural proteins are clustered at the 3' end of the genome. The C gene product is assumed to be the core protein of HCV (p22). The other viral structural proteins are the putative virion envelope glycoproteins (gp35 and gp70), encoded by E1 and E2/NS1 regions, that may be targets for neutralising antibodies. The non-structural regions have a role in virus replication and encode for protease (NS2, NS3), helicase (NS3), and an RNA-dependent RNA polymerase that replicates the RNA genome (NS5). The NS4 region encodes a hydrophobic protein with unknown function but it seems to be synthesized during the HCV replication. The genetic and polypeptide HCV organization is distantly related to human flavivirus and animal pestivirus and for this reason, it is considered a member of *Flaviviridae* family (30).

The 5' non-coding and nucleocapside regions of the genome are relatively conserved whereas the regions (N-terminus of the E1, E2/NS1) encoding the putative envelope proteins are highly variable. Rapid mutations in the envelope region suggests an ability of the virus to evade host immune response. The presence of hypervariable region in the HCV genome and the immune selection of viral escape mutants could explain the mechanism of HCV persistence and the difficulties in the vaccine developement (31).

The diversity in virus sequence has lead to its classification into six "genotypes" that differ substantially in nucleotide sequence and show varied geographic and epidemiological distribution (32).

Finally, like a wide variety of RNA virus, HCV exist in infected patients as quasispecies populations, composed of closely related genomes that contain one master sequence and a large spectrum of variants (33). The presence of different HCV quasispecies are related to several important biological properties and clinical aspects as evasion of host immunity, resistance to anti-viral agents and a more advanced liver disease (34).

Molecular mechanisms of HCV carcinogenesis

In spite of the accumulation of the epidemiological data which suggest the close relationship of HCV infection and the developement of HCC, the mechanism to explain the role of HCV in liver carcinogenesis remains unknown (3,35,36). At present, there is no evidence that HCV sequences can lead to DNA intermediates or become integrated within the genome of hepatocytes as occurs with HBV infection. Similarly, there is no evidence that viral product have any directly oncogenic activity or that it activates any oncogens or deactivates any tumor suppressor genes.

The more obvious mechanism by which HCV infection results in HCC is related to the presence of cirrhosis. HCV-related HCC generally develop on cirrhosis, mostly within regenerative nodules; which can be considered as a "preneoplastic" condition. HCV sequences have been found in liver cancer cells as HCV RNA negative strands representing replicative intermediate (37).

When discussing the role of HCV in liver cancer, a major issue is whether it is involved only in causing cirrhosis or might, in addition, have a direct oncogenic effect (38). In this context, the search for HCV RNA sequences in the rare group of HCCs developing without the intermediate step of cirrhosis should be highly informative, since only a few isolated cases have been reported so far and information on HCV genomes was not available (39). We looked for the persistence of HCV genomes in livers of patients with HCC developed in absence of cirrhosis and without recognized non viral risk factors, as a clue for the possible direct oncogenic role of HCV. Tumorous and non tumorous liver tissue, and serum of nineteen selected HBsAg negative patients were analyzed by PCR for the presence of HCV genome, HCV replication, HCV genotyping and HBV genome. Our findings show the persistence and replication of HCV genomes in 13 of 19 patients with HCC without cirrhosis (Table 3). The genotype 1b was predominant (11/13) (7). Several lines of evidence have suggested that the genotype variability of HCV has clinical implication. HCV type 1b has been shown to be more prevalent in older patients, in those with a long duration of viral infection, and it has been considered an independent risk factor for low response to alpha-interferon therapy (40). Moreover in a recent work on reinfection by HCV in liver transplant, the genotype 1b was more cytopathogenic than other types (41). We also observed the same high prevalence of HCV 1b infection in patients with cirrhosis who eventually developed HCC.

Finally, detection of both HBV DNA and HCV RNA sequences in liver tissue of HBsAg negative patients with HCC, with or without cirrhosis (2/7 and 4/19, respectively), underlines the important role of hepatitis viruses in liver carcinogenesis. The coinfection HBV and HCV may suppress HBV replication, thus contributing to the low level of HBV DNA in serum, which is only detectable by a highly sensitive method such as PCR (42). Moreover, clinical reports suggest a reciprocal inverse relation between HBV and HCV replication (43). Further studies are needed to establish whether the HCV genome is able to potentiate the oncogenic role of HBV.

References

1. Kew MC, Popper H. Relationship between hepatocellular carcinoma and cirrhosis. Sem Liver Dis 1984;2:136-46.

2. Beasley RP. Hepatitis B virus the major etiology of hepatocellular carcinoma. Cancer 1988;61:1942-56.

3. Colombo M, Choo QL, Del Ninno, et al. Prevalence of antibodies to hepatitis C virus in italian patients with hepatocellular carcinoma. Lancet 1989;ii:1006-8.

4. Bréchot C, Poucell C, Louise A, et al. Presence of integrated hepatitis B virus DNA sequences in cellular DNA of human hepatocellular carcinoma. Nature 1980;286:533-5.

5. Twu JS, Schloemer RH. Transcriptional trans-activating function of hepatitis. J Virol 1987; 62:3448-53.

6. Caselmann WH, Meyer M, Kékulé AS, et al. A trans-activator function is generated by integration of hepatitis B virus preS/S sequences in human hepatocellular carcinoma DNA. Proc Natl Acad Sci USA 1990;87:2970-4.

7. De Mitri MS, Poussin K, Baccarini P, et al. HCV-associated liver cancer without cirrhosis. Lancet 1995;345:413-5.

8. Tiollais P, Pourcell C, Dejean A. The hepatitis B virus. Nature 1985;317:489-95.

9. Brunetto MR, Stemler M, Bonino F, et al. A new hepatitis B virus strain in patients with severe anti- HBe positive chronic hepatitis B. J Hepatol 1990;10:258-61.

10. Coldrove R, Simon G, Ganem D. Transcriptional activation of homologous and heterologous genes by hepatitis B virus gene product in cells permissive for viral replication. J Virol 1989;63:4019-26.

11. Schirmacher P, Rogler CE, Dienes HP. Current pathogenetic and molecular concepts in viral liver carcinogenesis. Virchows Archiv B Cell Pathol 1993;63:71-89.

12. Edman JC, Gray P, Valenzuela P, et al. Integration of hepatitis B virus sequences and their expression in human hepatoma cell. Nature 1980;286:535-8

13. Hsu T, Möroy T, Etiemble J, et al. Activation of c-*myc* by woodchuck hepatitis virus insertion in hepatocellular carcinoma. Cell 1988;55:627-35.

14. Dejean A, Bougueleret L, Grzeschik KH, et al. Hepatitis B virus DNA integration in a sequence homologous to v-erbA and steroid receptor genes in a hepatocellular carcinoma. Nature 1986;322:70-2.

15. Wang J, Chenivesse X, Henglein B, et al. Hepatitis B virus integration in the cyclin A gene in a hepatocellular carcinoma. Nature 1990;343:555-7.

16. Pasquinelli C, Garreau F, Bougueleret L, et al. Rearrangement of a common cellular DNA domain on chromosome 4 in human primary liver tumors. J Virol 1988;62:629-32.

17. Henglein B, Chenivesse X, Wang J, et al. Structure and cell cycle regulated transcription of the human cyclin A gene. Proc Natl Acad Sci USA 1994;91:5490-4.

18. Paterlini P, De Mitri MS, Martin C, et al. A Taq I polymorphosm in the human cyclin A gene. Nucleic Acid Research 1991;19:2516.

19. De Mitri MS, Pisi E, Bréchot C, et al. Low frequency of allelic loss in the cyclin A gene in human hepatocellular carcinomas: a study in PCR. Liver 1993;13:259-61.

20. Paterlini P, Flejou JF, De Mitri MS, et al. Structure and expression of the cyclin A gene in human primary liver cancer. Correlation with flow cytometric parameters. J Hepatol 1995;23:47-52.

21. Graef E, Caselmann W, Wells J, et al. Insertional activation of mevalonate kinase by hepatitis B virus DNA in human hepatoma cell line. Oncogene 1994;9:81-7.

22. Zhang X-K, Egan JO, Huang D-P, et al. Hepatitis B virus DNA integration and expression of an Erb B-like gene in human hepatocellular carcinoma. Biochem Biophys Res Commun 1992;188:344-51.

23. Twu JS, Robinson WS. Hepatitis B virus X gene can transactivate heterologous viral sequences. Proc Natl Acad Sci USA 1989;86:1046-50.

24. Kékulé AS, Lauer U, Meyer M, et al. The preS2/S region of integrated hepatitis B virus DNA encodes a transcriptional transactivator. Nature 1990;343:457-61.

25. Wu JY, Zhou Z-Y, Judd A, et al. The hepatitis B virus-encoded transcriptional trans-activator hbx appears to be a novel protein serine/threonine kinase. Cell 1990;63:687-95.

26. Bréchot C, Degos F, Lugassy C, et al. Hepatitis B virus DNA in patients with chronic liver disease and negative tests for hepatitis B surface antigen. N Engl J Med 1985;312:270-6.

27. Bréchot C. Hepatitis B virus (HBV) and hepatocellular carcinoma: HBV DNA status and its implications. J Hepatol 1987;4:269-79.

28. Paterlini P, Gerken G, Nakajima E, et al. Polymerase chain reaction to detect hepatitis B virus DNA and RNA sequences in primary liver cancers from patients negative for hepatitis B surface antigen. N Engl J Med 1990;323:80-5.

29. Choo Q-L, Kuo G, Weiner AJ, et al. Isolation of a cDNA clone derived from a blood-borne non-A, non-B viral hepatitis genome. Science 1989;244:359-61

30. Houghton M, Weiner AJ, Han J, et al. Molecular biology of the hepatitis C viruses: implication for diagnosis, developement and control of viral disease. Hepatology 1991;14:382-8.

31. Weiner AJ, Geysen HM, Christopherson C, et al. Evidence for immune selection of hepatitis C virus (HCV) putative envelope glycoprotein variants: potential role in chronic HCV infection. Proc Natl Acad Sci USA 1992;89:3468-72.

32. Simmonds P, Alberti A, Alter HJ, et al. A proposed system for the nomenclature of hepatitis C genemes. Hepatology 1994;19:1321-4.

33. Martell M, Esteban JI, Quer J, et al. Hepatitis C (HCV) circulates as a population of different but closely related genomes: quasispecies nature of HCV genome distribution. J Virol 1992;66:3225-9.

34. Koizumi K, Enomoto N, Kurosaki M, et al. Diversity of quasispecies in various disease stages of chronic hepatitis C virus infection and its significance in interferon treatment. Hepatology 1995;22:30-5.

35. Saito I, Miyamura T, Ohbayashi A, et al. Hepatitis C virus infection is associated with the developement of hepatocellular carcinoma. Proc Natl Acad Sci USA 1990;87:6547-9.

36. Di Bisceglie AM, Simpson LH, Lotze MT, et al. Developement of hepatocellular carcinoma among patients with chronic liver disease due to hepatitis C viral infection. J Clin Gastroenterol 1994;19:222-6.

37. Paterlini P, Driss F, Pisi E, et al. Persistence of hepatitis B and C viral genomes in primary liver cancers from HBsAg negative patients: a study of a low endemic area. Hepatology 1993;17:20-9.

38. Blum HE. Comments to: does hepatitis C virus cause hepatocellular carcinoma? Hepatology 1994;19-251-5.

39. Herr W, Gerken G, Poralla T, et al. Hepatitis C virus associated primary hepatocellular carcinoma in a noncirrhotic liver. Clin Invest 1993;71:49-53.

40. Pontisso P, Ruvoletto MG, Nicoletti M, et al. Distribution of three major hepatitis C virus genotypes in Italy. A multicentre study of 495 patients with chronic hepatitis C. J Vir Hep 1995;2:33-8.
41. Feray C, Gigou M, Samuel D, et al. Influence of the genotypes of hepatitis C virus on the severity of recurrent liver disease after liver transpantation. Gastroenterology (in press).
42. Shih CM, Lo SJ, Miyamura SY, et al. Suppression of hepatitis B virus expression and replication by hepatitis C virus core protein in HuH7 cells. J Virol 1993;67:5823-32.
43. Pontisso P, Ruvoletto MG, Fattovich G, et al. Clinical and virological profiles in patients with multiple hepatitis virus infections. Gastroenterology 1993;105:1529-33.

CHAPTER 22

PREVALENCE OF WILD-TYPE AND VARIANT TRANSCRIPTS OF LIVER ESTROGEN RECEPTORS IN CHRONIC LIVER DISEASE

E. VILLA, A. DUGANI, L. CAMMELLINI, P. BUTTAFUOCO, A. GROTTOLA, I. FERRETTI, A. FERRARI, F. MANENTI

Chair of Gastroenterology, Department of Internal Medicine, University of Modena, Italy.

SUMMARY

Variant estrogen receptor transcripts (lacking exon 5 of the hormone binding domain) investigated by Reverse transcription/Polymerase chain reaction in a series of patients with chronic active hepatitis, cirrhosis, cirrhosis with dysplasia and with hepatocellular carcinoma, increased progressively from CAH to HCC. Patients with liver cell dysplasia showed the same alterations as patients with HCC. As the variant ER transcripts when translated could give rise to truncated receptors still able to constitutively activate transcription, overexpression of these ER transcripts could be a key factor in liver carcinogenesis.

1. Introduction

Hepatocellular carcinoma (HCC) is one of the leading causes of death both in western and eastern countries; a common characteristic in the different geographical areas is the striking male prevalence; the male/female ratio varies in fact from 4:1 to 7:1 in the different series reported (1).

These data have suggested that sexual hormone (and especially estrogens) could be involved in liver carcinogenesis. It is well known that estrogens influence growth, differentiation and functioning of many target tissues. Both male and female human liver have been shown to contain estrogen receptors (ERs) (2-3). In the liver, estrogens influence liver metabolism and the production of plasma proteins. In males which have high alcohol intake, ERs reach very high levels and hepatic metabolism becomes feminized (4). During the progression of chronic liver disease, especially when hepatocellular carcinoma develops, ER levels in males increase (5, 6); not all studies, however are concordant on this finding (7, 8). These data have given the rationale basis for the attempt of using antiestrogen, namely tamoxifen, for

P. Gentilini and M. U. Dianzani. New Trends in Hepatology, 197-203

palliative treatment of unresectable HCC. Tamoxifen acts by binding to the estrogen receptor in a manner which is competitive with estrogen. Although tamoxifen-bound ER binds to estrogen responsive elements, the complex is however unable to activate gene transcription, therefore the growth of cells is inhibited. The results, however, of the four controlled trials with this drug published up to now have been disappointing (9-12), although at least two of these studies showed a regression of tumor mass, decrease of alpha-fetoprotein and improved survival in some of the treated cases (9, 10). These findings have suggested that, in analogy with other hormone-dependent tumors, tamoxifen might lose its capacity of blocking estrogen receptor. In breast cancer (a tumor which is often dependent on estrogen for growth), the progression from hormone-dependence to hormone independence and the contemporary development of a more aggressive phenotype has been associated with the onset of variant liver estrogen receptors (13-17). Of special interest is one of these variants which appears to be missing the hormone-binding domain of the receptor but which maintains a constitutive transcriptional activity (18).

The hypothesis that a similar mutational event could also occur during hepatocarcinogenesis calls for the investigation of ER transcription in individual primary hepatocelluair carcinomas, especially looking for ER variants in the hormone binding domain.

2. Liver estrogen receptors transcripts in normal liver and in hepatocellular carcinoma

No data were available on the characteristics of ER transcripts in the liver, either normal or diseased, especially regarding the transcripts derived from the exons coding for the hormone binding domain (i.e. exons 4-6). Using reverse transcription and polymerase chain reaction (RT/PCR) with primers localized in the above named exons, we started investigating normal liver and found that it expressed almost exclusively the 438-base pair band: only one patient out of 5 displayed also the 298-base pair band, corresponding to the variant ER transcript. In this unique patient, however, the variant form was a minor component (Table 1).

In HCC patients, the finding was different in non-tumor and in tumor tissue. In non-tumor tissue, the 438-base pair band was the predominant in all cases studied, irrespectively of the sex of the patient studied. The variant form was present in all 7 males but only in 1 out of 7 females; its level of expression was about half of that of the wild-type. In tumor tissue the marked difference between males and females was maintained, the variant form being unique in 6 out of 7 male patients while in females it was weakly represented in 3 cases only; the wild-type form was always conserved in females while in males the wild-type transcript was present in only 1 patient ($p < 0.01$) (Table 1) (19).

TABLE 1. Distribution of wild-type (438 bp) and variant (298 bp) ER transcripts in 14 patients with HCC and 5 controls.

<u>HCC</u>

		Peri-tumoral tissue		Tumor tissue	
	Sex	438 bp	296 bp	438 bp	296 bp
1.-4.	F	+	-	+	-
5.-6.	F	++	-	+	±
7.	F	+	±	+	±
8.-12.	M	+	±	-	+
13.	M	±	+	-	+
14.	M	+	+	±	+

<u>Normal liver</u>

1.	M	+	±
2.-5.	M	+	-

*Northern analysis in these patients revealed smaller sized mRNA (3.8 kb) together with the normal 6.5 kb mRNA.

The presence of wild-type ER related positively with the measured levels of ER by ligand binding assay both in the normal liver and in the cirrhotic, non-tumorous liver tissue. ER levels ranged between 13 ± 4 fmol/mg cytosol protein (normal male liver), 15 ± 5 fmol/mg cytosol protein (non-tumor liver tissue from HCC patients) and 37 ± 9 fmol/mg cytosol protein (tumor liver tissue from female HCC). No specific binding was obtained in male HCC liver tissue.

3. Liver estrogen receptors mutagenesis during progression of chronic liver disease

The results obtained in HCC, although quite clear in indicating that the modification of ERs are a frequent occurrence in HCC, nevertheless do not clarify whether these events are associated only with the full-blown neoplastic transformation or are early events which occur when HCC is not yet present and which can somewhat favor the progression of cirrhosis to HCC. To investigate this aspect, we have addressed our attention to a series of patients with chronic but benign liver disease like chronic active hepatitis (CAH) or cirrhosis and in patients with cirrhosis but with a preneoplastic condition like liver cell dysplasia, in whom a liver biopsy had to be performed for diagnostic purposes.

3.1. PATIENTS WITH CAH AND CIRRHOSIS

Twenty-eight patients (20 males, 8 females) with a diagnosis of chronic active hepatitis were studied. In all patients the wild-type ER transcript was present and highly expressed while the 296 bp variant was present as a minor component in 15 patients, all males but 2. The difference between males and females is statistically significant ($p < 0.05$).

Twenty-five patients (15 males, 10 females) had liver cirrhosis and in all, independently from sex, the wild-type ER transcript was present. The variant transcript was present in 11 out of 16 males (68.7%) and in 5 out of 9 females (55.5%).

Variant ER transcript was significantly more often present in HBsAg-positive than in antiHCV-positive males with CAH; this difference was not present in cirrhotic subjects while it became again evident in patients with HCC, when the variant transcript was unique.

3.2. PATIENTS WITH LIVER CELL DYSPLASIA.

The result which can be most useful in evaluating the overall meaning of variant ERs in liver carcinogenesis has been obtained in 5 additional patients with cirrhosis (3 males, 2 females), in whom a histological diagnosis of liver cell dysplasia was obtained at biopsy of ultrasound-guided focal lesion. In these patients, like in HCC patients, the wild-type transcript was present in the cirrhotic tissue while the variant transcript was coexpressed in four; the level of expression being roughly the same for the two transcripts.

Again, like in tumor tissue of HCC patients, in the dysplastic tissue, the wild-type transcript was unique in 1 male patient; it was only weakly expressed in the 2 female patients and was totally absent in the other 2 male patients. In the latter four patients, the variant form was strongly expressed.

4. Conclusions

The variant ER transcript which we have demonstrated in the liver of patients with primary hepatocellular carcinoma appears to have the same characteristics as that reported in breast cancer. Although not all authors agree on their possible significance, their presence may be considered a relevant event in the natural history of breast cancer.In the first instance, the presence of the variant transcript in a substantial proportion of HCC patients, may clarify the discordant results obtained with antiestrogen therapy with tamoxifen.

The presence of a receptor altered in the hormone binding domain would in fact render ineffective a drug , like tamoxifen, which acts by competing with the hormone for the occupation of the receptor. The complex tamoxifen-receptor, furthermore, is unable to activate transcription.

The finding of the variant receptor in a substantial number of patients with benign conditions like CAH but even more with preneoplastic conditions like cirrhosis and liver cell dysplasia suggest that the appearance of the variant ER in HCC patients is an early event during the carcinogenetic process. Furthermore, it should be noted that in liver cell dysplasia there is an overexpression of the variant receptor which can lead to a gradual replacement of normal cells by cell overexpression of the variant ER, which can confer a growth advantage to these cells. It has been hypothesized for breast cancer that the presence of ERs in neoplastic cells, apart from being a marker of differentiation, would confer a survival advantage to the neoplastic cell (20). This would be even more so for these ERs altered in the hormone binding domain, as the normal dependence from hormonal control would be totally lost therefore offering a potential mechanism for tumor escape from hormone control (14). In human HCC, this mechanism would be mainly working in males since female tumors retain, in most instances, the wild-type ER, therefore remaining under normal hormonal constraint.

References

1. Villa, E., Baldini, G.M., Pasquinelli, C., Melegari, M., Cariani, E., Di Chirico, G., Manenti, F. Risk factors for hepatocellular carcinoma in Italy. Male sex, Hepatitis B virus, Non-A, Non-B infection, Alcohol. Cancer 1988; 62:611-615.

2. Porter, L.E., Elm, M.S., Van Thiel, D.H., Dugas, M.C., Eagon, P.K. Characterization and quantitation of human hepatic estrogen receptors. Gastroenterology 1983; 84:704-712.

3. Rossini, G.P., Baldini, G.M., Villa, E., Manenti, F. Characterization of estrogen receptors from human liver. Gastroenterology 1989; 96:1102-1109.

4. Villa, E., Baldini, M.G., Rossini, G.P., Pasquinelli, C., Melegari, M., Cariani, E., Tata, C., Bellentani, S., Ferrari, A., Manenti, F. Ethanol-induced increase in cytosolic estrogen receptors in human male liver: a possible explanation for biochemical feminization in chronic liver disease due to alcohol. Hepatology 1989; 8:1610-1614.

5. Nagasue, N., Ito, A., Yukaya, H., Ogawa,Y. Estrogen receptors in hepatocellular carcinoma. Cancer 1986; 57: 87-91.

6. Ohnishi, S., Murakami, T., Moriyama, T., Mitamura, K., Imawari, M. Androgen and estrogen receptors in hepatocellular carcinoma and in the surrounding non-cancerous liver tissue. Hepatology 1986; 6 440-443.

7. Eagon PK, Francavilla A, DiLeo A, Elm MS et al. Quantitation of estrogen and androgen receptors in hepatocellular carcinoma and adjacent liver tissue. Dig Dis Sci 1991; 36: 1303-1308.

8. Ikbal MJ, Wilkinson ML, Johnson PJ, Williams R. Sex steroid receptors proteins in foetal, adult and malignant human liver tissue. Br J Cancer 1983; 48: 791-796.

9. Farinati F, Salvagnini M, De Maria N, Fornasiero A, Chiaramonte M, Rossaro R, Naccarato R. Unresectable hepatocellular carcinoma. A prospective controlled trial with tamoxifen. J Hepat 1990; 11:297-301.

10. Martin-Cereso FJ, Tomas A, Enrichez J, Donoso L, Balanzo J, Guarner C. Tamoxifen improve survival in patients with advancedhepatocellular carcinoma. J Hepat. 1994; 20: 702-706.

11. Elba S, Giannuzzi V,Misciagna G, Manghisi OG. Randomized controlled trial of tamoxifen versus placebo in inoperable hepatocellular carcinoma. It. J. Gastroenterol. 1994; 26:66-68.

12. Castells A, Bruix J, Bru C, Ayuso C, Roca M, Boix L, Vilana R, Rodes J. Treatment of hepatocellular carcinoma with tamoxifen: a double-blind trial in 120 patients. Gastroenterology 1995; 109: 917-922.

13. Raam, S., Robert, N., Pappas, C.A., Tamura, H. Defective estrogen receptors in human mammary cancers: their significance in defining hormone dependance. J.Natl.Canc.Inst. 1988; 80: 756-761.

14. Graham, M.L. II, Krett, N.L., Miller, L.A., Leslie, K.K., Gordon, D.F., Wood, W.M., Wei, L.L.,and Horwitz, K.B. T4DCO cells, genetically unstable and containing estrogen receptors mutations, are a model for the progression of breast cancers to hormone resistance. Cancer Res. 1990; 50:6208-6217.

15. McGuire, W.L., Chamness, G.C., and Fuqua, S.A. Estrogen receptors variants on clinical breast cancer. Mol.Endocrinol. 1991; 5: 1571-1577.

16. Scott, G.K., Kushner, P., Vigne, J.L. and Benz, C.C. Truncated forms of DNA-binding estrogen receptors in human breast cancer. J.Clin.Invest 1991; 88:700-706.

17. Fuqua, S.A.W., Fitzgerald, S.D., Alred, D.C., Elledge, R.M., Nawaz, Z., McDonell, D.P., O'Malley, B.W., Gree, G.L., and McGuire, W.L. Inhibition of estrogen receptors action by naturally occurring variant in human breast tumors. Cancer Res.1992; 52: 483-486.

18. Fuqua, S.A.W., Fitzgerald, S.D., Chamness, G.C., Tandon, A.K., McDonnell, D.P., Nawaz, Z., O'Malley, B.W., McGuire, W.L. Variant human breast tumor estrogen receptor with constitutive transcriptional activity. Canc.Res 1991; 51: 105-109.

19. Villa E, Camellini, Dugani A , Zucchi F, Losi L, Buttafoco P, Grottola A, Merighi A, Manenti F.Variant estrogen receptors mRNA species detected in human primary hepatocellular carcinoma. Cancer Res 1995; 55:498-500.

20. Villa E, Camellini L, Dugani A, Grottola A, Buttafoco P, De Hemptinne B, Manenti F. Variant liver estrogen receptors transcripts occur in cirrhotic with liver cell dysplasia. Manuscript in preparation.

21. Israel, L., Band, P. Hormones as cancer growth factors. Lancet 1984; 2: 843-844.

Section IV

PATHOGENETIC ASPECTS OF HEPATITIS C VIRUS (HCV) INFECTION

CHAPTER 23

MOLECULAR BIOLOGY OF HCV: IMPLICATIONS IN EPIDEMIOLOGY AND DIAGNOSIS OF INFECTION

M. RAPICETTA, C. ARGENTINI, S. DETTORI, E. SPADA

Laboratory of Virology, Istituto Superiore di Sanità,

Viale Regina Elena n. 299 Rome, Italy

SUMMARY

The progress achieved in the molecular biology of HCV and the definition of viral variability have been crucial for developing more sensitive and specific diagnostic assays and for understanding the significance of relevant markers during the natural history of infection. Extensive phylogenetic studies have provided evidence of at least 11 major genotypes and several subtypes.

A wide spectrum of subtypes has been demonstrated for genotypes 2 and 4 in several African countries. In particular, we demonstrated, by a seroepidemiological study, the presence of 4 additional subtypes (namely: 2g, 2h, 2i, 2l) simultaneously circulating in the west central African country of Guinea Conakry.

The presence of HCV genotype 4 variants has been found in Tanzania in sera with an undetermined antibody pattern.

Specific epidemiological characteristics may have an impact on the wide variability of HCV in African countries.

P. Gentilini and M. U. Dianzani. New Trends in Hepatology, 207-216

Hepatitis C virus (HCV) a distant relative of Pestiviruses and Flaviviruses is the major ethiological agent of Non-A, Non-B hepatitis. The viral characterization is rather recent and the definition of the genome sequence was obtained in 1991 by means of a strategy of successive cloning and sequencing of partially overlapping genes, after the identification of the first specifically immunoreactive fragment (1).

From the deduced genome structure, structural (one Core and two envelope) and non structural proteins have been identified, however, the native particle has not been isolated nor visualized by electro microscopy and the viral characterization is still rather limited, because of the lack of suitable tissue culture systems and animal models (scimpanzè is the only available at present). In particular, several issues still remain undefined, such as: the exact replication mechanisms, the nature of viral receptor, the morphology of native particle and the functions of NS4 and NS5b proteins. Consequently, data on the interaction with host immune system are scarce.

In the last years, progresses have been achieved by expression studies in prokaryotic systems such as Escherichia Coli, or eucariotic systems such as HeLa cells transfected by recombinant vaccinia virus, baculovirus system and Hamster ovary cells (CHO). Important data on the expression of viral proteins, cleavage sites and involved enzymes have been obtained (2) that can be used for diagnostic and possible therapeutic purposes. In particular the cleavage sites by a cellular signal peptidase that gives rise to the structural proteins of Core and envelope (E1 and E2) and by the viral serineprotease, codified by NS3, that produces the non-structural proteins NS2, NS3, NS4, NS5 have been identified (3).

The analysis of sequence alignments of several viral isolates has enabled to identify the main immunoreactive sites for B and T cells. One of this corresponds to protein 5.1.1, that was first identified as specifically immunoreactive and used in the first generation diagnostic assay. Furthermore several epitopes, that have been shown to be experimentally immunoreactive, are present in the Core region. An extensive application of the first generation assay has enabled to define the global distribution of the infection, characterized by the presence of variable prevalence rates likewise the other hepatitis viruses.

One aspect of HCV research that has been crucial for further defining more sensitive and specific diagnostic assays and significance of relevant markers, has been represented by the definition of viral variability, even if other aspects, such as the definition of time appearance and persistence of the different markers during the natural history of infection in individuals, were important.

HCV viral population exhibit a "quasispecies" distribution in the single infected individual. Extensive phylogenetic studies of genome coding regions, such as E1 and NS5b, have provided evidence for the existence of at least 11 major HCV genotypes (4). Some of these are widely distributed around the world (genotypes 1, 2, 3) while others have been found in particular geographical regions. Genotypes 4 and 5 are regarded as African genotypes, while genotypes 6 to 11 seem to be mostly present in Eastern and Asian countries.

For genotype characterization various methods are at present in use with different degree of accuracy. The most accurate are based on sequence analysis. Simpler and more rapid methods are based on PCR with various sets of primers (Okamoto) (5) and on specific probes from 5'NCR (Innolipa) (6).

Differences, have been found, among HCV strains, in geographical distribution (7), antigenicity (8), level of viremia and severity of disease (9). A possible correlation with different routes of transmission has also been postulated (10).

Furthermore, the sequence differences between HCV types might be significant for screening HCV infection, given the present high degree of dependence on serological methods.

A different degree of variability in genome sequence and corresponding aminoacid sequences is present for the various structural and non structural proteins. The lowest level of structural conservation is found in E2 and El proteins, in NS4 protein (c100) and in the central part of NS5. This finding has important implications for the implementation of diagnostic assays. A different antibody response against the antigens relative to NS4, NS3 and Core has been observed in infections from viruses classified in different genotypes and, in particular, a higher variability in percentages of reactivity is found against the c100 protein that was used as antigen in the first generation assays (8). Higher homogeneity is found for the reactivity against the NS3 and Core antigens.

The viral variability also impacts on the HCV-RNA detection by means of PCR. The use of primers from 5' non coding region (NCR), which is the most conserved region, enables the highest level of sensitivity for the detection of HCV infection. The high sensitivity and specificity of this method is also due to the application of a double amplification with "nested" primers which are internal to the first amplified fragment. This assay is thus recommended in particular cases such as: for an early detection of acute infection, for the resolution of RIBA indeterminate cases, for the diagnosis of infection in immunocomprised patients and for the monitoring of therapies.

Further studies are needed to define the characteristics of HCV epidemiology and its relationship to the distribution of HCV genotypes, particularly in developing countries where the data are scarce.

Several studies are in course, in our research group, concerning the presence of HCV variants in Africa.

One study was carried out in an urban area of the West central African region of Guinea Conakry (11) with the aim of defining the prevalence of HCV infection in this region and to investigate the genetic relatedness and classification of HCV isolates. From this study an overall anti-HCV prevalence of 6.7%, with an increasing trend by age, was found in the town of Conakry, by the analysis (ELISA, Ortho) of sera from 1421 subjects belonging to the categories of blood donors, pregnant women and out- and in-patients (for non hepatic pathologies).

7 HCV isolates (DO12, MED007, MED011, MED017, PH33, PH48 and PH52), from a subsample of 73 sera of this population, collected for virological studies, were studied for genetic characterization and classification. The 5'NCR was analyzed by the Line Probe Assay. This method assigned the 7 isolates to the genotype 2. However, the analysis of the 5'NC Region sequences could not contribute to a more accurate assignment. The comparisons of sequences from the NS5b region (nt 7575-8196), both along the Guinea isolates and with the databank consensus sequences of isolates classified as genotype 2, showed, for five of these isolates, evolutionary distances in the 0.15-0.26 range (see Fig. 1A). Thus from this study a wide distribution of subtypes of genotype 2 was demonstrated, in sera collected in the same survey, with a supposed classification of the isolates into proposed 2g, 2h, 2i and 2l subtypes.

In another cooperative study on HCV infection, that we performed in Egypt (12), it has been shown that genotype 4 is present in 80% of chronic carriers, but also genotype 1 is present. The phylogenetic analysis has provided the evidence of a wide divergence for some isolates (EGS44; EGS193) (see Fig. 1B) that were classified, by Innolipa assay, as type 4. This finding is in accordance with

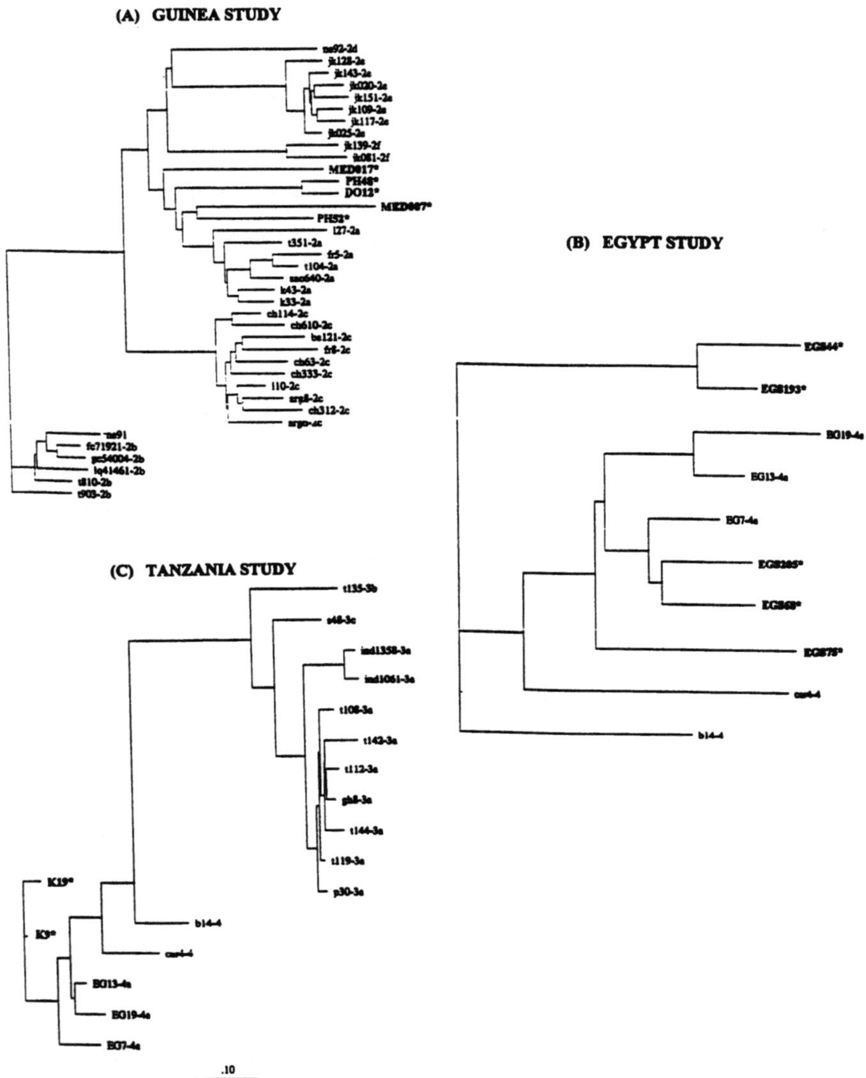

Figure 1. Phylogenetic analysis, performed on NS5b sequences) (nt 7575-8196) for HCV isolates from Guinea Conakry (MED017, PH48, DO12, MED007, PH52), from Egypt (EGS44, EGS193, EGS205, EGS68, EGS75) and from Tanzania (K19, K9).

* *Sequences of new isolates from our studies (bold character) and from databank.*

the data from other authors, that demonstrated high heterogeneity among genotype 4 isolates by the analysis of E1 region sequences (13).

A possible influence of peculiar transmission mechanisms can be postulated in relation to such wide spectrum of subtypes in several African Countries.

The studies, which we have carried out in Tanzania, on 1004 pregnant women and out-patients have shown that, in 41 sera that were above the cut-off level in the ELISA assay (Ortho Diagnostics), the antibody pattern was undeterminate or negative with the application of third generation supplemental assay RIBA (Ortho) (see Tab. 1). Nevertheless HCV-RNA was present in several cases. A preliminary characterization has shown the possible classification in the frame of genotype 4 in one case, genotype 1 in two cases, genotype 3 in two cases. Two further cases were not characterized. The presence of viral variants can be postulated. Preliminary data from phylogenetic analysis of NS5 genomic region (see Fig. 1C) have shown that a possible variant more related to genotype 4 could be present. More detailed analysis also from other genomic regions are however needed.

On the basis of all these findings we could conclude that non characterized HCV variants are present in Africa and that incomplete RIBA antibody patterns may occur as a consequence of the genotype variability. Higher sensitivity in diagnostic assays could be achieved by including peptides from genotypes other than the HCV-1 prototype, (which is at present used), toward the implementation of IV generation assays for general use. In fact, account should be taken of the possibility that different genotypes may change their distribution, due to the large population movements in the modern age.

ACKNOWLEDGEMENTS

We thank Cinzia Bisegna for editorial assistance.

Table 1. Antibody pattern in sera corresponding to HCV isolates from Tanzania

Sera	Values ELISA O.D.	IIIrd GENERATION RIBA				GENOTYPE (by Innolipa)
		C100	C33c	C22	NS5	
K19	***	-	±	-	±	4*
D31	***	±	±	±	±	1a
D776	***	-	±	-	+2	1a
K9	1.922	±	±	+2	-	3a
D714	1.889	±	±	-	-	NT
D70	0.623	-	±	-	-	1b-3a
D61	0.671	+2	±	-	-	3a

* *by 5' sequence analysis*

REFERENCES

1. Choo, Q.-L. Richman, K.H. Han, J.H. Berger, K. Lee, C. Dong, C. Gallegos, C. Coit, D. Medina-Selby, R. Barr, P.J. Weiner, A.J. Bradley, D.W. Kuo, G. and Houghton, M. (1991). Genetic organization and diversity of the hepatitis C virus. *Proceedings of the National Academy of Sciences USA* **88,** 2451-2455.
2. Ralston, R. Thudium, K. Berger, K. Kuo, C. Gervase, B. Hall, J. Selby, M. Kuo, G. Houghton, M. and Choo, Q.-L. (1993). Characterization of hepatitis C virus envelope glycoprotein complexes expressed by recombinant vaccinia viruses. *Journal of Virology*, **67,** 6753-6761.
3. Grakoui, A. Wychowski, C. Lin, C. Feinstone, S.M. and Rice, C. M. (1993). Expression and identification of hepatitis C virus polyprotein cleavage products. *Virology*, **67,** 1385-1395.
4. Tokita, H. Okamoto, H. Iizuka, H. Kishimoto, J. Tsuda, F. Lesmana, L.A. Miakawa, Y. and Mayumi, M. (1996). Hepatitis C virus variants from Jakarta, Indonesia classifiable into novel genotypes in the second (2e and 2f), tenth, (10a) and eleventh (11a) genetic groups. *Journal of General Virology* **77,** 293-301.
5. Okamoto, H. Sugiyama, Y. Okada, S. Kurai, K. Akahane, Y. Sugai, Y. Tanaka, T. Sato, K. Tsuda, F. Miyakawa, Y. and Mayumi, M. (1992). Typing hepatitis C virus by polymerase chain reaction with type-specific primers: application to clinical surveys and tracing infectious sources. *Journal of General Virology* **73,** 673-679.
6. Stuyver, L. Rossau, R. Wyseur, A. Duhamel, M. Vanderborght, B. Van Heuverswyn, H. and Maertens, G. (1993). Typing of hepatitis C virus isolates and characterization of new subtypes using a line probe assay. *Journal of General Virology* **74,** 1093-1102.
7. McOmish, F. Yap., P.L. Dow, B.C. Follett, E.A.C Seed, C. Keller, A.J. Cobain, T.J. Krusius, T. Kolho, E. Naukkarinen, R. Lin, C. Lai, C. Leong, S. Medgyesi, G.A. Hejjas, M. Kiyokawa, H. Fukada, K. Cuypers, T. Saeed, A.A. Alrasheed, A.M. Lin, M. and Simmonds, P. (1994). Geographical distribution of hepatitis C virus genotypes in blood donors-an international collaborative survey. *Journal of Clinical Microbiology* **32,** 884-892.
8. McOmish, F. Chan, S.-W. Dow, B.C. Gillon, J. Frame, W.D. Crawford, R.J. Yap, P.L. Follett, E.A.C. and Simmonds, P. (1993). Detection of three types of hepatitis C virus in blood donors: investigation of type-specific differences in serological reactivity and rate of alanine aminotransferase abnormalities. *Transfusion* **33,** 7-13.

9. Tanaka, S. (1994). Type C hepatitis and hepatocellular carcinoma in Japan. In *Viral Hepatitis and Liver Disease*, pp. 713-715. Edited by K. Nishioka, H. Suzuki, S. Mishiro & T. Oda. Springer-Verlag, Tokyo.
10. Pawlotsky, J.-M. Tsakiris, L. Roudot-Thoraval, F. Pellet, C. Stuyver, L. Duval, J. and Dhumeaux, D. (1995). Relationship between hepatitis C virus genotypes and sources of infection in patients with chronic hepatitis C. *The Journal of Infectious Diseases* **171**, 1607-1610.
11. Ruggieri, A. Argentini, C. Kouruma, F. Chionne, P. D'Ugo, E. Spada, E. Dettori, S. Sabbatani, S. and Rapicetta, M. (In press). Prevalence of HCV genotype 2 variants in West Central Africa (Guinea Conakry): identification of 4 additional subtypes. *Journal of General Virology.*
12. Angelico, M. Renganathan, E. Fathy, M. Gandin, C. Profili, M.C. Refai, W. De Santis, A. Capocaccia, L. Callea, F. Rapicetta, M. Badr, G. and Rocchi, G. for the Italian-Egyptian Schistosomiasis and Hepatitis C Study Group (1995). The nature of chronic liver disease in Alexandria, Egypt, an hyper-endemic area for schistosoma mansoni and hepatitis C infection. *(Inviato per la pubblicazione)*.
13. Bukh, J. Purcell, R.H. and Miller, R.H. (1993). At least 12 genotypes of hepatitis C virus predicted by sequence analysis of the putative E1 gene of isolates collected worldwide. *Proceedings of the National Academy of Sciences USA* **90**, 8234-8238.

CHAPTER 24

CELL-MEDIATED IMMUNE RESPONSE IN HEPATITIS C VIRUS (HCV) INFECTION: ARE DIFFERENT STRATEGIES ADOPTED BY HCV AND HEPATITIS B VIRUS TO PERSIST?

F. FIACCADORI, G. MISSALE, V. LAMONACA, R. BERTONI, A. VALLI, A. BERTOLETTI, C. BONI, A. CAVALLI, A. PENNA, C. FERRARI

Cattedra Malattie Infettive, Università di Parma

Via Gramsci 14, 43100 Parma

Summary

Immune-mediated mechanisms play an important role in the pathogenesis of liver cell injury and viral persistence in both HCV and hepatitis B virus (HBV) infections. However, the different vigor of HLA class I and class II restricted, anti-viral T cell responses in chronic hepatitis C and B and the different cytokine profiles within HCV and HBV infected livers suggest that these hepatotropic viruses have evolved different strategies to persist within their hosts and that different pathogenetic mechanisms are operative during HCV and HBV infections.

P. Gentilini and M. U. Dianzani. New Trends in Hepatology, 217-226

Introduction

The mechanisms responsible for viral clearance and liver cell injury in HCV infection are very poorly defined at present. Available data, however, suggest that the host's immune response almost certainly plays an important, perhaps central, role in these events (1).

In particular, HLA class I restricted CD8+ T cells are believed to be essential for elimination of intracellular virus by virtue of their cytolytic potential and their production of anti-viral cytokines, which may be responsible for suppression of viral gene expression within infected cells (2). On the other hand, optimal activation of HCV-specific cytotoxic T and B cells generally depends upon the helper function of HLA class II restricted CD4+ T lymphocytes which may also directly contribute to viral clearance by their cytokine production at the site of infection.

The CD4+ T cell response to HCV

Because of the high rate of chronic evolution, acute HCV infection represents an ideal model to study the peculiar features of the T cell response which are specifically associated with recovery or chronic viral persistence and to characterize the immune events which precede and perhaps determine the final outcome of the disease. In contrast, this type of analysis is almost completely impossible in hepatitis B because clinically overt acute HBV infections are generally self-limited and chronic evolution more commonly follows anycteric, subclinic infections.

Taking advantage of this natural model of chronic viral persistence, a group of 21 patients with acute HCV infection was studied for the proliferative T cell response to structural and non-structural HCV proteins sequentially from clinical presentation to the later stages of clinical recovery or chronic evolution . While T cell responses to structural (core and E2) as well as non-structural (NS3, NS4 and NS5) HCV antigens are readily detectable in the peripheral blood of patients who normalize the transaminase levels, the same responses are significantly weaker and less frequently measurable in patients with chronic evolution of hepatitis (3,4).

These results are compatible with the concept that an efficient and vigorous T cell response at the early stages of infection may be critical to limit the spread of the virus within the infected host and to keep viral replication under control. This implies that infection can probably be controlled only if the immune system has the capacity to avoid spread of the virus above a critical threshold beyond which infection would become irreversible.

Using recombinant HCV proteins to stimulate peripheral blood HCV specific T cells, HLA class II restricted responses in patients with long lasting chronic HCV infection (5-7) appear to be stronger than in acutely infected patients with persistent liver damage. This suggests that T cell responsiveness to HCV proteins in the peripheral blood compartment may progressively increase as a function of the time of infection. This may be due either to progressive induction of responses to subdominant epitopes as a result of continuous presentation of viral antigens (8) or to a different compartmentalization of T cells in different stages of infection or to recovery of the T cell function after an early stage of T cell hyporesponsiveness. $CD4^+$ T cells from chronically infected patients are characteristically polyclonal and multispecific for more than one viral antigen. A clear hierarchy of T cell responsiveness to HCV proteins has been defined in these patients. Specifically, core and NS4 are recognized by most patients whereas the putative envelope proteins (El and E2/NS1) and NS5 are immunogenic for a minor proportion of patients.

The high immunogenicity of NS4 at the T cell level has been confirmed by the isolation of NS4-specific T cells from the liver of chronic HCV patients (9). Remarkably, CD4 T cells sequestered within the inflamed liver are functionally and clonotypically different from NS4-specific T cells present in the peripheral blood suggesting a specific compartmentalization of some T cells at the site of infection. The presence of a vigorous HLA class II restricted T cell response in chronic HCV patients despite persistence of the virus, represents an important difference in the pathobiology of chronic HCV and HBV infections since this response is generally weak or undetectable in chronic hepatitis B (2). This probably reflects different pathogenetic mechanisms operative during infection by these hepatotropic viruses.

The $CD8^+$ T cell response to HCV.

While this response has not so far been investigated in acute HCV infection, HLA class I restricted HCV-specific CD8+ cytotoxic T lymphocytes (CTL) are detectable in the peripheral blood and the lymphocytic infiltrate in patients with chronic hepatitis C (10-15). A similar CTL response has been demonstrated in the liver of acutely infected chimpanzees, and the response has been shown to

persist indefinitely after infection, indicating that the virus can persist in the presence of these CTL (16).
The CTL identified thus far in infected patients are able to recognize both conserved and variable regions of the HCV core, E1, E2, NS2, NS4 and NS5 antigens in the context of several different HLA molecules (10-12,15,17). Moreover, the response is often polyclonal and multispecific in individual chronically infected patients. CTL clones have been isolated from the intrahepatic compartment using only antigen nonspecific stimuli, implying that these cells must be present at high frequency within the intrahepatic infiltrate (11,12). In contrast, it is necessary to expand the peripheral blood CTL precursor population with HCV derived peptides in order to demonstrate a CTL response to HCV. Nonetheless, the HCV-specific CTL response is probably stronger than the response to HBV because it can be relatively easily detected in the periphery during chronic infection, while the response to HBV cannot, and because virus specific lesional T cells seem to be more highly represented in HCV-infected than in HBV-infected livers.
This difference further supports the hypothesis that distinct mechanisms are likely to be involved in the immunopathogenesis of viral hepatitis due to HCV and HBV.

Cytokine production by intrahepatic T cells in chronic hepatitis B and C

In line with the possibility that HCV and HBV use different strategies to persist within the infected host are also the different cytokine patterns secreted by intrahepatic T cells in chronic HBV and HCV infections.
T helper 1 (Th1)-type cytokines, such as interleukin-2 (IL-2), interferon-γ (IFN-γ) and tumor necrosis factor-β, are principally involved in cell-mediated immune responses and play a crucial role in protection from intracellular pathogens, including viruses. Th2-type cytokines, such as IL4 and IL5, mostly regulate humoral immune responses; their effects can be beneficial against extracellular infectious agents but can be associated with progressive disease by intracellular pathogens (18,19).
At the beginning of a viral infection, the specific immune response is essential to focus immune reactions onto infected cells and to start the series of events that ultimately lead to massive non-specific recruitment of immune cells within the infected organ (20). Indeed, non-specific T cells generally represent the dominant population in the inflammatory infiltrates at the site of infection and the main

source of cytokines that in turn can cause T cell activation by antigen-independent mechanisms and amplification of the immune response (21). For this reason, the final commitment of intrahepatic virus non-specific T cells towards preferential Th1 or Th2 phenotypes is believed to exert a critical influence on the inflammatory environment and the final outcome of infection.

To understand whether a cytokine imbalance oriented towards preferential production of Th2 cytokines may be involved in the pathogenesis of viral persistence in HBV and HCV infections, the ability to secrete IFN-γ, IL4 and IL5 by wide series of T cell clones derived from the liver of patients with chronic active hepatitis B and chronic active hepatitis C was assessed (22). In order to avoid selective expansion in vitro of minor subsets of T cells, intrahepatic T cells were cloned immediately after isolation from liver tissue avoiding preliminary steps of antigen exposure in vitro, using cloning strategies able to expand with equal efficiency all T cell subsets (23).

Results indicate that T cell clones with a Th1-like pattern of cytokine production, able to secrete high amounts of IFN-γ, are enriched within the liver of patients with chronic HCV infection. A reciprocal pattern is observed in chronic hepatitis B, where the majority of liver infiltrating T lymphocytes are Th0 cells able to produce both Th2 cytokines and lower levels of IFN-γ. In line with these data, direct analysis of cytokine mRNA in liver tissue from patients with CAH-C showed high expression of IFN-γ (24).

Therefore, the liver environment in chronic hepatitis C appears to be dominated by anti-viral Th1 cytokines and should be favorable to viral clearance. Instead, HCV persists in the infected host with high efficiency. In contrast, the liver cytokine environment in chronic hepatitis B is more strongly influenced by Th2 cytokines that could create conditions more favorable to viral persistence.

Conclusions

Chronic active hepatitis caused by HBV and HCV is characterized by cellular infiltrates of the liver mostly represented by activated T cells, including variable proportions of $CD8^+$ T cells that have generally been regarded as the major determinant of liver cell damage (2). In both infections, $CD4^+$ and $CD8^+$ T cells specific for different viral antigens have been demonstrated within the liver (9,11,12,25,26). However, in most stages of chronic HBV infection, T cells are hyporesponsive to HBV antigens (27-29), whereas in most patients with chronic HCV infection the T cell reponse seems to be efficient despite its inability to

clear the virus (5,6,10-13). Moreover, suppressive Th2 cytokines seem to be more strongly represented in HBV than in HCV infected livers (22).
The two viruses have totally different biological features. HBV is a DNA virus apparently unable to cause a direct cytopathic effect. Chronic infection is generally characterized by high antigen concentrations in the serum and a wide spread of the virus within the liver (2). HCV is a RNA virus that probably induces hepatocellular damage by both cytopathic and immune-mediated mechanisms. In contrast to HBV, it does not generally cause high viremia (30).
Therefore, it is tempting to speculate that a critical factor that probably influences the pathogenetic mechanisms operative in HCV and HBV infections is the relative antigen load, which is very high in HBV infection and very low for HCV. While high antigen load may be responsible for T cell hyporesponsiveness as a possible result of T cell exhaustion (31,32) and preferential expansion of T cells able to produce suppressive Th2 cytokines (33), this pathway probably does not contribute to HCV persistence where more active viral escape mechanisms may play a more important role in view of the extremely high mutation rate of this virus.

Acknowledgments

Part of the studies described in this paper were supported by the Italian Ministry of the University and Scientific and Technological Research (project on Liver Cirrhosis and Viral Hepatitis) and by the National Institutes of Health, USA, Grant AI-26626.

References

1. Rice, C. M. and Walker, C. M. (1995) Hepatitis C virus-specific T lymphocyte responses. *Curr. Op. Immunol.* **7**,532-538.

2. Chisari, F. V. and Ferrari, C. (1995) Hepatitis B virus immunopathogenesis. *Annu. Rev. Immunol.* **13**,29-60.

3. Missale, G., Bertoni, R., Lamonaca, V., Valli, A., Massari, M., Mori, C., Rumi, M. G., Houghton, M., Fiaccadori, F., and Ferrari, C. (1996) Different clinical behaviors of acute hepatitis C virus infection are associated with different vigor of the anti-viral cell-mediated immune response. *Submitted.*

4. Diepolder, H. M., Zachoval, R., Hoffman, R. M., Wierenga, E. A., Santantonio, T., Jung, M. -C., Eichenlaub, D., and Pape, G. R. (1995) Possible mechanism involving T-lymphocyte response to non-structural protein 3 in viral clearance in acute hepatitis C virus infection. *Lancet* **346**,1006-1007.

5. Botarelli, P., Brunetto, M. R., Minutello, M. A., Calvo, P., Unutmaz, D., Weiner, A. J., Choo, Q. -L., Shuster, J. R., Kuo, G., Bonino, F., Houghton, M., and Abrignani, S. (1993) T-lymphocyte response to hepatitis C virus in different clinical courses of infection. *Gastroenterology* **104**,580-587.

6. Ferrari, C., Valli, A., Galati, L., Penna, A., Scaccaglia, P., Guiberti, T., Schianchi, C., Missale, G., Marin, M. G., and Fiaccadori, F. (1994) T-cell response to structural and nonstructural hepatitis C virus antigens in persistent and self-limited hepatitis C virus infections. *Hepatology* **19**,286-295.

7. Schupper, H., Hayashi, P., Scheffel, J., Aceituno, S., Paglieroni, T., Holland, P. V., and Zeldis, J. B. (1993) Peripheral blood mononuclear cell responses to recombinant hepatitis C virus antigens in patients with chronic hepatitis C. *Hepatology* **18**,1055-1060.

8. Lehmann, P. V., Forsthuber, T., Miller, A., and Sercarz, E. E. (1992) Spreading of autoimmunity to cryptic determinants of an autoantigen. *Nature* **358**,155-157.

9. Minutello, M. A., Pileri, P., Unutmaz, D., and et al, (1993) Compartmentalization of T-lymphocyte to the site of disease: Intrahepatic $CD4^+$ T-cells specific for the protein NS4 of hepatitis C virus in patient with chronic hepatitis. *J. Exp. Med.* **178**,17-26.

10. Cerny, A., McHutchison, J. G., Pasquinelli, C., Brown, M. E., Brothers, M. A., Grabscheid, B., Fowler, P., Houghton, M., and Chisari, F. V. (1995) Cytotoxic T lymphocyte response to hepatitis C virus-derived peptides containing the HLA-A2.1 binding motif. *J. Clin. Invest.* **95**,521-530.

11. Koziel, M. J., Dudley, D., Wong, J. T., Dienstag, J., Houghton, M., Ralston, R., and Walker, B. D. (1992) Intrahepatic cytotoxic T lymphocyte specific for hepatitis C virus in persons with chronic hepatitis. *J. Immunol.* **149**,3339-3344.

12. Koziel, M. J., Dudley, D., Afdhal, N., Choo, W-L., Houghton, M., Ralston, R., and Walker, B. D. (1993) Hepatitis C virus specific cytoxic T lymphocytes recognize epitopes in the core and envelope proteins of HCV. *J. Virol.* **67**,7522-7532.

13. Battegay, M., Fikes, J., Di Bisceglie, A. M., Wentworth, P. A., Sette, A., Celis, E., Ching, W., Grakoui, A., Rice, C. M., Kurokohchi, K., and et al., (1995) Patients with chronic hepatitis C virus-encoded peptides binding to HLA-A2.1 molecules. *J. Virol.* **69**,2462-2470.

14. Shirai, M., Okada, H., Nishioka, M., Akatsuka, T., Wychowski, C., Houghten, R., Pendleton, C. D., Feinstone, S., and Berzofsky, J. A. (1994) An epitope in hepatitis C core region recognize by cytotoxic T cells in mice and humans. *J. Virol.* **68**,3334-3342.

15. Kita, H., Moriyama, T., Kaneko, T., and et al, (1993) HLA-B44-restricted cytotoxic T lymphocytes recognizing an epitope on hepatitis C virus nucleocapsid protein. *Hepatology* **18**,1039-1044.

16. Erickson, A. L., Houghton, M., Choo, Q. L., Weiner, A. J., Ralston, R., Muchmore, E., and Walker, C. M. (1993) Hepatitis C virus-specific CTL responses in the liver of chimpanzees with acute and chronic hepatitis C. *J. Immunol.* **151**,4189-4199.

17. Shirai, M., Akatsuka, T., Pendleton, C. D., Houghten, R., Wychowski, C., Mihalik, K., Feinstone, S., and Berzofsky, J. A. (1992) Induction of cytotoxic T cells to a cross-reactive epitope in the hepatitis C virus nonstructural RNA polymerase-like protein. *J. Virol.* **66**,4098-4106.

18. Paul, W. E. and Seder, R. A. (1994) Lymphocyte responses and cytokines. *Cell* **76**,241-251.

19. Sher, A. and Coffman, R. L. (1992) Regulation of immunity to parasites by T cells and T-cell derived cytokines. *Annu. Rev. Immunol.* **10**,385-409.

20. Doherty, P. C., Allan, W., Eichelberger, M., and Carding, S. R. (1992) Roles of ab and gd T cell subsets in viral immunity. *Annu. Rev. Immunol.* **10**,123-151.

21. Unutmaz, D., Pileri, P., and Abrignani, S. (1994) Antigen indipendent activation of naive and memory resting T cells by a cytokine combination. *J. Exp. Med.* **180**,1159-1164.

22. Bertoletti, A., D'Elios, M. M., De Carli, M., Zignego, A. L., Durazzo, M., Boni, C., Missale, G., Penna, A., Fiaccadori, F., Del Prete, G. F., and Ferrari, C. (1996) Different cytokine profiles of intrahepatic T cells in chronic hepatitis B and hepatitis C virus infections. *Submitted.*

23. Moretta, A., Pantaleo, G., Moretta, L., Mingari, M. C., and Cerottini, J. C. (1983) Quantitative assessment of the distribution of cytolytic T lymphocytes within human resting or alloactivated peripheral blood T cell populations. *J. Exp. Med.* **158**,571-577.

24. Napoli, J., Bishop, G. A., McGuiness, P. H., Painter, D. M., and McCaughan, G. W. (1996) Progressive liver injury in chronic hepatitis C infection correlates with increased intrahepatic expression of Th1-associated cytokines. *Hepatology* In press.

25. Ferrari, C., Mondelli, M. U., Penna, A., Fiaccadori, F., and Chisari, F. V. (1987) Functional characterization of cloned intrahepatic, hepatitis B virus nucleoprotein-specific helper T cell lines. *J. Immunol.* **139**,539-544.

26. Barnaba, V., Franco, A., Alberti, A., Balsano, C., Benvenuto, R., and Balsano, F. (1989) Recognition of hepatitis B envelope proteins by liver-infiltrating T lymphocytes in chronic HBV infection. *J. Immunol.* **143**,2650-2655.

27. Ferrari, C., Penna, A., Bertoletti, A., Valli, A., Antoni, A. D., Giuberti, T., Cavalli, A., Petit, M. -A., and Fiaccadori, F. (1990) Cellular immune response to hepatitis B virus-encoded antigens in acute and chronic hepatitis B virus infection. *J. Immunol.* **145**,3442-3449.

28. Jung, M. C., Spengler, U., Schraut, W., Hoffman, R., Zachoval, R., Eisenburg, J., Eichenlaub, D., Riethmuller, G., Paumgartner, G., Ziegler-Heitbrock, H. W. L., Will, H., and Pape, G. R. (1991) Hepatitis B virus antigen-specific T-cell activation in patients with acute and chronic hepatitis B. *J. Hepatol.* **13**,310-317.

29. Penna, A., Chisari, F. V., Bertoletti, A., Missale, G., Fowler, P., Giuberti, T., Fiaccadori, F., and Ferrari, C. (1991) Cytotoxic T lymphocytes recognize an HLA-A2-restricted epitope within the hepatitis B virus nucleocapsid antigen. *J. Exp. Med.* **174**,1565-1570.

30. Simmonds, P. (1995) Variability of hepatitis C virus. *Hepatology* **21**,570-581.

31. Moskophidis, D., Lechner, F., Pircher, H., and Zinkernagel, R. M. (1993) Virus persistence in acutely infected immunocompetent mice by exhaustion of antiviral cytotoxic effector T cells. *Nature* **362**,758-761.

32. Rocha, B., Grandien, A., and Freitas, A. A. (1995) Anergy and exhaustion are independent mechanisms of peripheral T cell tolerance. *J. Exp. Med.* **181**,993-1003.

33. Burstein, H. J. and Abbas, A. K. (1993) In vivo role of interleukin 4 in T cell tolerance induced by aqueous protein antigen. *J. Exp. Med.* **177**,457-463.

CHAPTER 25

THE EPIDEMIOLOGICAL AND CLINICAL ASPECTS OF HEPATITIS C IN ITALY

F. Morisco, I. Falzarano, G. Del Vecchio Blanco and N. Caporaso
Dipartimento di Internistica Clinica e Sperimentale
"F. Magrassi" II Università di Napoli
Via Pansini 5, II Policlinico 80131, Napoli

Summary
Overt parenteral transmission of HCV infection justifies only a portion of new cases. After the introduction of anti-HCV screening performed on blood donors the incidence of post-transfusional C hepatitis in Italy has decreased. Indeed, it is probable that other routes of diffusion (intrafamilial spreading) are relevant. In our experience the anti-HCV+ prevalence (determined on 1670 family members of 578 anti-HCV+ subjects) is 15.6% in spouses and 2.1% in offspring ($p < 0.01$). It is even higher in subjects older than 50 years compared to younger ones. These results indicate a prevalent horizontal trasmission which happened in the past when poor sanitary conditions facilitated the intrafamilial diffusion. This determined a cohort effect interrupted by the enhanced knowledge of transmission mechanisms of HCV infection.

The epidemiology of viral hepatitis is changing in Italy.
Through the course of the years, there has been a documented reduction of cases of acute hepatitis A amongst infants and adolescents. This age-group was more widely affected, but recently there is an increase of cases in adult subjects (1).
The incidence of acute hepatitis B and Delta, and the HBsAg prevalence in the general population have had a marked decline, even before the active immunoprophylaxis introduction, and is probably due to improved socio-economic conditions and expanded knowledge of transmission mechanisms (1). Presently, viral infection from hepatitis C (HCV) is widely spread throughout Italy. Studies performed on blood donors indicate a prevalence of 1-2% (2,3) even though this category of subjects cannot be considered representative of the general population. As a matter of fact, in the selection, subjects from some age-groups and/or those belonging to risk groups

P. Gentilini and M. U. Dianzani. New Trends in Hepatology, 227-223

(injection drug users, thalassemics, etc.) were excluded. The prevalence of antibodies to hepatitis C virus (anti-HCV) in the general population is decisively higher when appropriate epidemiological criteria are used.
In the study performed on the inhabitants of Valentano (province of Viterbo), the overall anti-HCV prevalence proved to be 8.4% with an even greater percentage (18.2%) in those subjects aged 60-70 years (4). The observation that HCV infection does not involve subjects during the first two decades of life was confirmed by a series of studies performed on a large number of young subjects who showed a prevalence of 0.4% and 0.5% (5,6). This is contrary to what happens in HBV infection, where greater incidence is found in subjects 12-14 years old.
It is widely documented that HCV is mainly transmitted by means of parenteral exposure such as receipt of blood and blood products, dental and medical surgery, intravenous drug use, use of glass syringes and infected instruments (7). In fact, when subjects belonging to these categories were separately studied, an elevated prevalence was found to be:
a) 60-80% in intravenous drug users (with or without HIV positivity).
b) 60-90% in hemophiliacs.
c) approx. 60% in thalassemics requiring blood transfusions.
Parenteral transmission justifies only a portion (approx. 50%) of newly infected cases (8). Furthermore, due to the introduction of anti-HCV screening (ELISA I in '91 and ELISA II in '92) performed on blood donors, the incidence of post-transfusional hepatitis in Italy has decreased from 7.5 cases per 10(blood transfusions in 1986 to 0.4 cases in 1993 (9). Thus, it is probable that other routes of transmission are epidemiologically relevant.

Intrafamilial Transmission

Familial environment must be considered epidemiologically as a place that contains numerous ways of transmitting viral hepatitis infections:
1) vertical transmission - mother-to-infant and perinatal
2) horizontal transmission - sexual behavior, unapparent parenteral exposure, and cohabitation in general
The role of household contact in the spreading of hepatitis C viral infection has not yet been well defined. Anyway, it is documented that:

a) in relatives of chronic HCV carriers, the prevalence of anti-HCV positivity is decisively higher compared to the general population (10,11).
b) HCV infection can be transmitted by means other than parenteral, but with less efficiency than B and Delta infections.
c) positive family members often have liver damage (11).
In 1994, we conducted a study on 1670 family members for 578 anti-HCV+ subjects, selected homogeneously throughout Italy (12). The anti-HCV prevalence resulted decisively higher in spouses than in offspring (Table 1), and in subjects older than 50 years compared to younger ones. The low prevalence of anti-HCV positivity in the first decades of life indirectly proves the scarce relevance of the vertical transmission of this infection. Although it is known that the passive transmission of anti-HCV from mother to child is habitual (13), the risk in transmitting the infection is generally associated with the presence of elevated viral levels (>10() in the mother's blood (14). This event is more common in mothers who are contemporarily HIV positive (15).
The age-specific prevalence observed between the older population and the younger one (whether or not they are spouses or offspring) suggests a particular modality of transmission.
Presently, we are observing subjects that became HCV infected when poor sanitary conditions and scarse knowledge of transmission mechanisms facilitated the horizontal intrafamilial diffusion. Subsequently, improvements in environmental conditions have interrupted the epidemiologic chain; thus, reducing the risk of infection in the younger generations (cohort effect). This epidemiologic mechanism is confirmed by logistic regression analysis used to evaluate all the possible risk factors correlated with C virus infection (7). Such a study has demonstrated that the independent risk factors of HCV infection are blood transfusions, drug abuse, previous use of glass syringes, previous tuberculosis infection and a prolonged hospital stay before 1970). Meanwhile, it is reasonable to think that the diffusion of HCV infection in Italy happened several decades ago (prior to 1970) when mono-use materials began being used) and when parenteral-type transmission, especially the unapparent type, was not yet known. Recently, HCV epidemiology has changed and the infection almost exclusively affects the high risk categories, i.e. drug abusers, which fortunately represent only a small portion of the general population. Therefore, it is very likely that new cases of infection and carriers of chronic HCV will progressively decrease in Italy in the future.

Quite often, family members of anti-HCV+ subjects have chronic liver damage. In our experience, we have found that the prevalence of chronic liver disease in this category is 53.1% (11). Generally, subjects who are affected by chronic liver disease either have light clinical picture or are completely asymptomatic. The way chronic hepatitis presents itself emerged from a recent study we held. From observations of 357 consecutive patients, from January 1993 to December 1994, we found that 90% of cases diagnosed were discovered unexpectedly (through blood donations, general population and/or family member screening, etc) (Table 2).

The following must be considered:

1) Even though there are no symptoms, liver disease could exist. As a matter of fact, most of the anti-HCV+ subjects we observed had slight increases in transaminase levels (which is the laboratory "spy" for detecting liver disease at various stages of evolution).

2) A slight increase in, or persistent normality of serum transaminase levels does not signify absence of liver damage. Damage, often severe, is frequently found, even when subjects have a normal clinic and laboratory picture. It is possible that our present laboratory test (transaminases) is not the most indicated parameter to evidentiate the damage induced by HCV. It seems that elevations in γ–Gt values can represent a more sensitive index to evidentiate the liver damage caused by chronic HCV infection. The pathogenic mechanism of chronic damage caused by C virus is not well defined and it probably differs from that caused by HBV.

3) Normality of the histological and biochemical parameters does not indicate the absence of viral replication. In these cases, the determination of HCV-RNA is necessary to individuate eventual "healthy carriers". We prospectively observed for 2 years, 10 HCV-RNA+ subjects with persistently normal transaminase values and we regularly determined viremia levels and indexes of necrosis (16). The purpose of our study was to evaluate the natural history and to determine how the infection evolves in these subjects. It is not known if the presence of the virus is compatible with a prolonged "healthy" status. The average of viremia levels resulted discretely elevated and stable throughout the 2-year follow-up period (Table 3). This result is difficult to explain since there was a continued biochemical absence of liver damage. Therefore, we hypothesize that there might be a particular host-virus interaction which renders the infection less damaging.

TABLE 1: Prevalence of anti-HCV positivity in our patients' population in regards to type of relationship.

	n.	%
Spouses	72/494	15.6
Offspring	19/906	2.1

$p < 0.01$

TABLE 2: Modality of presentation of chronic hepatitis HCV+ in 311 cases.

	n.
Subicterus	3
Itching	1
Asthenia	18
Occasional results	
anti-HCV+	17
HBsAg+	-
ALT	268
gammaglobulin	4

TABLE 3: Mean $\pm$ SE (x 10^5 Eq/ml) of HCV-RNA levels in 10 patients with persistently normal ALT values during the 2-year follow-up period.

Basal	1 year	2 years
21.7 ± 7.4	23.09 ± 4.7	23.9 ± 4.7

References

1. Mele, A., Ferrigno, L., Stasi, MA., et al. (1990) Sistema epidemiologico integrato dell' epatite virale acuta. Rapporto annuale 1989 e risultati 1985-1989. Rapporti ISTAT: 24

2. Sirchia, G.,Bellobuono, A., Giovannetti, A., Marconi, M. (1989) Antibodies to Hepatitis C virus in Italian blood donors, Lancet i, 797.

3. Chiaramonte, M., Stroffolini, T., Caporaso, N., et al. (1991) Hepatitis C virus infection in Italy: a multicentric seroepidemiological study. Ital J Gastroenterol 23, 555-558.

4. Stroffolini, T., Menchinelli, M., Taliani, G., et al. (1995) High prevalence of hepatitis C virus infection in a small central Italian town: lack of evidence of parenteral exposure, Ital J Gastroenterol 27, 235-238.

5. D' Amelio, R., Stroffolini, T., Matricardi, PM., et al. (1994) Low prevalence of anti-HCv antibody among Italian air force recruits, Scand J Infect Dis in press.

6. Romanò, L., Azara, A., Chiaramonte, m., et al. (1994) Low prevalence of anti-HCV antibody among Italian children, Infection 22, 350-351

7. Chiaramonte, M., Stroffolini, T., Lorenzoni, U., et al. (1996) Risk factors in community-acquired chronic hepatitis C virus infection: a case-control study in Italy, J Hepatol 24, 129-134.

8. Alter, MJ., Hadler, SC., Judsan, FN., et al. (1990) Risk factors for acute non A, non B hepatitis in the United States and association with hepatitis C virus infection, J.A.M.A. 264, 2231-2235.

9. Mele, A., Stroffolini, T., Catapano, R., et al. (1995) Incidence of transfusion associated B and non A, non B hepatitis in Italy, B M J 311, 846-847.

10. Buscarini., E., Tanzi, E., Zanetti, AR., et al. (1993) High prevalence of antibodies to hepatitis C virus among family members of patients with anti-HCV positive chronic liver disease, Scand J of Gastroenterol 28, 343-346.

11. Coltorti, M., Caporaso, N., Morisco, F., et al. (1994) Prevalence of hepatitis C virus infection in the household contacts of patients with HCV-related chronic liver disease, Infection 22, 183-186.

12. Caporaso, N., Ascione, A., D' Antonio, M., et al. (1995) Prevalence of anti-HCV among spouses and offspring of anti-HCV positive subjects: an Italian multicentre study, Ital J Gastroenterol 27, 5-7.

13. Wejstal, R., Hermodsson, S., Iwarson, S., et al. (1990) Mother-to-infant transmission of hepatitis C virus infection, J Med Virol 30, 178-180.

14. Ohto, H., Terazawa, S., Sasaki, N., et al. (1994) Transmission of hepatitis C virus from mother to infant, N Engl J Med 330, 744-750.

15. Zanetti, AR., Tanzi, E., Paccagnini, S., et al. (1995) Mother-to-infant transmission of hepatitis C virus, Lancet 345, 289-291.
16. Morisco, F., Tuccillo, C., Del Vecchio Blanco, G., et al. (1996) Levels of viremia in subjects without clinical and biochemical signs of liver damage: two years of follow-up, Ital J Gastroenterol in press).

CHAPTER 26

DIAGNOSTIC EVALUATION OF PATIENTS WITH CHRONIC HCV INFECTION

S. NARDIELLO, G. PASQUALE, G.B. GAETA, G. GIUSTI
Clinica Malattie Infettive, Seconda Università di Napoli

Summary

Since the HCV genome and polyprotein were identified in recent years, a large number of laboratory tests for the diagnosis and assessment of HCV infection have been created. Moreover, the usefulness of needle liver biopsy in the assessment of chronic HCV infection has been revisited. In this survey we have reviewed the new techniques and procedures mainly on the basis of the research of the Italian Project on Liver Cirrhosis and Viral Hepatitis and of our own experiences, so as to suggest their optimal use in diagnosing and monitoring chronic HCV infection.

1. Introduction

Following the cloning of the first antigen of the hepatitis C virus (HCV) in 1989 (1), several tests for the detecting of anti-HCV antibodies were created, and tests for the detection of serum HCV-RNA have also become available in recent years. Moreovoer, liver biopsy has been re-evaluated in the study of chronic HCV infections.

In this paper we review the diagnostic possibilities offered by the tests for the detection of anti-HCV and HCV-RNA, and the new systems for grading and staging the histological liver lesions. We also report our suggestions for a rational use of all these diagnostic procedures in the clinical evalutation of patients with chronic HCV infection.

P. Gentilini and M. U. Dianzani. New Trends in Hepatology, 234-243

2. Tests for detection of anti-HCV antibodies

Antibodies to structural and non-structural proteins, expressed by different regions of the HCV genome, are detected by ELISA or RIA tests. The earliest ELISA test created in 1989, which detected antibodies to the first immunogenic cloned HCV antigen, c100-3 (2), although lacking optimal sensitivity, demonstrated the very high prevalence of anti-HCV antibodies in patients suffering from the previously named cryptogenic chronic liver disease. In addition, this early test showed that HCV infection is also frequent in patients with no history of blood transfusion or parenteral exposure (3). The 2nd and 3rd generation ELISA tests, which detect antibodies to new or modified HCV antigens, offer satisfactory sensitivity and specificity for chronic HCV infections. However, they are not suitable for an early diagnosis of acute type C hepatitis, and may give false-positive results in subjects with high serum levels of gammaglobulins due to autoimmune diseases. Supplemental immunoblotting assays were introduced to detect the pattern of positivity of the antibodies against individual structural and non-structural antigens and are used to check doubtful results of the ELISA or RIA tests. In a recent review of ours, we reported the antigens utilized for all ELISA, RIA and supplemental tests licensed in Italy (4).

3. Tests for detection of HCV-RNA

As yet HCV viremia can be assessed only by seeking serum HCV-RNA. The most sensitive technique is nested PCR, which can identify about ten copies of HCV-RNA per ml of serum (5). It requires complex laboratory facilities and highly skilled personnel. However, despite complete adherence to the strict protocols, false positive results are at times observed, due to sample contamination by amplicons generated during previous tests. A commercial kit designed to prevent sample contamination by amplicons is now available for the detection of HCV-RNA by single-step PCR (Amplicor HCV, Trade Name). The Amplicor HCV test has a sensitivity of about 1,000 genome equivalents of HCV-RNA per ml of serum (6, 7). A new PCR technique (Amplicor HCV Monitor, Trade Name) has been designed to give a quantitative evaluation of HCV-RNA in serum in the range from 10^3 to 10^6 genome equivalents per ml. This test doses PCR products at different dilutions of the amplified sample by comparison with the optical density of a co-amplified internal standard. Serum HCV-RNA can also be detected without PCR amplification by direct hybridization of viral RNA with specific probes and by the use of branched DNA molecules as a signal amplifier in a chemiluminescence assay (Quantiplex, Trade Name) (8). The lesser sensitivity of the branched DNA assay prevents its use as an appropriate test for the qualitative detection of serum HCV-RNA. However this method is simpler than PCR and gives a satisfactory and reproducible quantification of HCV-RNA concentrations in the range of $2x10^5$ to $12x10^7$ copies per ml of serum.

4. Tests for identificafion of HCV genotypes

Epidemiological surveys have identified at least 6 major genotypes and several subtypes of HCV, and a recent consensus conference (9) has suggested adopting the Simmonds classification. For clinical purposes the analysis of the HCV genome is based on selective PCR, which utilizes home-made primers complementary to the type-specific regions of HCV (10). A commercial genotyping method is based on the hybridization of the PCR products with different deoxynucleotide oligomers, which recognize the HCV types and subtypes (11). Typing of HCV may be achieved also by serotyping; however, complete concordance between genotyping and serotyping has not yet been reached, although a recent report claims to have achieved satisfactory concordance (12). The studies on HCV genotypes have substantially contributed to the knowledge on HCV epidemiology worldwide. However, the recent consensus report (13) from the Italian Association for the Study of the Liver has pointed out that the clinical usefulness of HCV typing is still under evaluation.

5. Needle liver biopsy

The percutaneous liver biopsy remains an important procedure in the diagnosis as well as in the management of patients with chronic liver diseases. Moreover, the occurrence of major complications is very exceptional provided this procedure is performed in hospitalized patients after or during ultrasound examination and after the exclusion of any contraindications (14, 15).

In chronic HCV infection the liver biopsy is necessary to establish the diagnosis of chronic hepatitis on the basis of the intralobular necroinflammatory lesions, portal and periportal inflammation, fibrosis and architectural changes. In two preliminary papers we described the histological pictures of chronic hepatitis due to different viral infections (16, 17). In Table 1 we report our experience on the main histological lesions observed in more than one thousand needle liver biopsies carried out during the 1990-95 period on patients suffering from HBV, HDV or HCV chronic hepatitis without cirrhosis. In agreement with the enlighteningobservations made by Scheuer (18), these data clearly indicate that portal follicular lymphoid aggregates, fatty change, naked eosinophilic bodies and

TABLE 1. Occurrence of different histological lesions in 1078 consecutive needle liver biopsies from patients with chronic viral hepatitis. Cases with a histological activity index of <4 or the presence of cirrhosis were excluded. All the specimens were examined by the same pathologist (G.P.), who was unaware of the etiology.

Type of lesion	HBV 128 cases n°	%	HDV 97 cases n°	%	HCV 853 cases n°	%
Portal lymphoid follicles	13	(10)	43	(44)	768	(90)
Fatty change[a]	13	(10)	17	(18)	665	(78)
Rhomboid-shaped hepatocytes	86	(67)	48	(49)	708	(83)
Naked acidophilic bodies	17	(13)	17	(18)	478	(56)
Focal necrosis ≥1[b]	102	(80)	76	(78)	665	(78)
Bridging necrosis	51	(40)	53	(55)	307	(36)
Lymphocytic infiltration of sinusoids	74	(58)	80	(82)	512	(60)
Giant hepatocytes	42	(33)	38	(39)	102	(12)
Bile duct damage	5	(4)	11	(11)	384	(45)
Fibrosis from 1 to 3[c]	90	(70)	90	(93)	682	(80)

[a] in more than 10% of hepatocytes
[b] according to the Knodell scoring system (ref. 19)
[c] according to the Scheuer scoring system (ref. 20)

biliary duct damage are the prominent lesions of chronic hepatitis due to HCV.

The histological examination may also show the coexistence of a concomitant liver disease due to another etiological factor, by detecting either tissue viral markers or lesions indicative of a primary biliary tract disease or of an inherited metabolic disorder.

Besides its nosological usefulness, the liver biopsy is essential for the grading and staging of chronic hepatitis. Grading is a measurement of the intensity of the necroinflammatory activity, staging is a measurement of the extent of fibrosis and architectural alterations. Several authors have proposed methods which attribute numerical scores to both grading and staging, thus providing a semiquantitative assessment of the histological lesions. For the grading we prefer to utilize the system proposed by Knodell, whose wide range allows a more precise assessment of lesions (19), and for the staging the system proposed by Scheuer (20).

A new classification of chronic hepatitis has recently been proposed on the basis of Knodell's Histological Activity Index (HAI), resulting from the sum of the scores for necrosis and inflammation (21). Therefore, the old classification of chronic hepatitis (lobular, persistent or active) has been replaced by the following: minimal chronic hepatitis (an HAI score from 1 to 3); mild chronic hepatitis (HAI from 4 to 8); moderate chronic hepatitis (HAI from 9 to 12); severe chronic hepatitis (HAI from 13 to 18). To obtain a more complete evaluation of the histological picture, we suggest reporting independently both the Knodell score for the grading and the Scheuer score for the staging. In fact the measurement of necroinflammatory activity should be assessed separately from the measurement of fibrosis and architectural distortions, which are the consequence of the necroinflammatory process and indicate the progression of chronic hepatitis to cirrhosis.The scoring systems have proved to be useful in assessing the histological lesions during the spontaneous evolution of chronic HCV infection or in evaluating the effects of therapy in clinical trials.

Immunohistochemical staining of HCV antigens in the liver of patients or of experimentally infected chimpanzees has been obtained using antibodies from convalescent sera (22) or monoclonal antibodies against structural and non-structural HCV antigens (23). The HCV presence is revealed by a granular immunostaining in the hepatocyte cytoplasm. Despite the interesting data obtained, the usefulness of these techniques in clinical practice has not yet been fully assessed.

Recent research has detected HCV-RNA in liver tissue using intracellular amplification of HCV-RNA by PCR, or in situ hybridization of the HCV-RNA sequences with probes of c-DNA. The majority of studies report a cytoplasmic localization of HCV-RNA, but nuclear staining has also been observed (24, 25).

These techniques have also made the identification possible of extrahepatic sites of HCV replication, such as peripheral blood mononuclear cells (26, 27), salivary glands, etc. They are not yet in routine use, but their use in the future might contribute to verifying any residual HCV replication after the disappearance of plasma HCV-RNA, spontaneously or after antiviral treatment.

6. Diagnostic approach to patients with chronic HCV infection

Measuring ALT levels and performing the ELISA test for anti-HCV are the first steps to be taken in the diagnostic assessment of patients with a possible chronic HCV infection (4). Further diagnostic tests to be utilized vary according to the association of the results of these tests, i.e. positive ELISA test and raised ALT, positive ELISA test and normal ALT, negative ELISA test and raised ALT.

6.1 PATIENTS WITH A POSITIVE ELISA TEST AND RAISED ALT

For patients who have a positive ELISA test for anti-HCV and long lasting hypertransaminasemia, even slight or fluctuating, a diagnosis of chronic hepatitis due to HCV infection is reasonable, and in our experience an anti-HCV supplemental assay is not mandatory. In fact we have observed that in anti-HCV positive patients suffering from chronic liver diseases, the RIBA test is virtually always positive. As soon as 2nd generation tests for anti-HCV were available, we performed a RIBA test on 98 randomly selected ELISA-positive patients with chronic liver disease. The RIBA test gave positive results in all patients (28). Later a 100% concordance between the ELISA and RIBA tests was found in about 200 anti-HCV positive liver cirrhosis patients we studied to be included in a multicentre Italian study (29).

As regards whether serum HCV-RNA should be sought in anti-HCV positive hypertransaminasemic patients, a recent consensus report (13) has stated that the PCR test is not mandatory for these patients, as viremia is almost invariably present.

In anti-HCV positive patients with a chronic liver disease, HCV may not be the only etiological factor, and this infection may be associated to some other pathogenic factor, such as alcohol abuse, inborn errors of metabolism or a concomitant viral infection. As a consequence, additional etiological factors should be sought on the basis of the geographical prevalence of the single factors or when the clinical and histological picture is not fully consistent with an HCV infection. The frequent association of chronic HCV infection to other pathogenic factors has clearly been found in an Italian multicentre study on liver cirrhosis, the promoting group of which included two of the authors (G.B.G. and G.G.). In this study the pathogenic factors of 1829 cases of liver cirrhosis were studied, and anti-HCV antibodies were found in 1328 cases with both the ELISA and supplemental RIBA test. HCV infection was the only etiological factor in 65.7% of them, in a further 29.2% it was associated to alcohol abuse, and in the remaining 5.1% it was associated to a chronic HBV infection, with or without HDV (29).

There is general agreement by the experts that in patients with an anti-HCV positive chronic liver disease, the liver biopsy is indicated as a rule for the grading and staging of the disease. In fact in chronic HCV infection there is no strict correlation between the results of the biochemical tests and the degree of liver damage (17). In our opinion a biopsy is not necessary when a diagnosis of cirrhosis has been established from an unequivocal clinical picture and imaging technique results.

6.2 PATIENTS WITH A POSITIVE ELISA TEST AND NORMAL ALT

For patients who show a positive ELISA test for anti-HCV and persistently normal levels of serum ALT the diagnostic approach is somewhat more complex. For these patients we suggest performing a supplemental immunoblotting assay for anti-HCV and a qualitative detection of HCV-RNA using PCR. A PCR positive/RIBA positive result suggests the presence of a chronic HCV infection, and a PCR negative/RIBA positive result suggests a past infection, either fully resolved or associated to a residual non-active liver disease. In PCR positive/RIBA positive cases, the liver biopsy is indicated and often a histological picture of mild or minimal hepatitis is found (30). However, when the histological picture is normal, a diagnosis of healthy carrier can be put forward, but a long lasting follow-up is advisable.

6.3 PATIENTS WITH A NEGATIVE ELISA TEST AND RAISED ALT

The diagnosis of chronic HCV infection should be suspected in some categories of long lasting hypertransaminasemic patients, even in the presence of a negative result of the anti-HCV ELISA test. In fact, the anti-HCV test may be negative due to the low antibody synthesis in immunocompromised hosts or in the offspring of HCV-infected mothers. Moreover, serum anti-HCV antibodies may be undetectable due to their sequestration in immunocomplexes in patients with cryoglobulinemia. In all these categories of patients, a search for HCV-RNA using PCR should always be included in the diagnostic protocol; the liver biopsy may be advisable in HCV-RNA positive cases.

For anti-HCV negative patients not belonging to the above-mentioned categories, we suggest seeking serum HCV-RNA after the exclusion of all other known causes of long lasting hypertransaminasemia.

References

1. Choo, Q.L., Kuo, G., Weiner, A.J., Oberby, L.R., Bradley, D.W., Houghton, M. (1989). Isolation of a cDNA clone derived from a blood borne non-A, non-B hepatitis genome. Science **244**, 359-362.

2. Kuo, G., Choo, Q.L., Alter, J., et al. (1989). An assay for circulating antibodies to a major etiologic virus of human nonA-nonB hepatitis. Science **244**, 362-364.

3. Gaeta, G.B., Rapicetta, M., Sardaro, C., et al. (1990). Prevalence of anti-HCV antibodies in patients with chronic liver disease and its relationship to HBV and HDV infections. Infection **18**, 277-279.

4. Nardiello, S., Pasquale, G., Gaeta, G.B., Rapicetta, M., Giusti, G. (1996). Diagnostic flow chart in chronic HCV infection. A proposal. Giorn. It. Mal. Inf. **2**, 8-17.

5. Garson, J.A., Tedder, R.S., Briggs, M., et al. (1990). Detection of hepatitis C viral sequences in blood donations by "nested" polymerase chain reaction and prediction of infectivity. Lancet **335**, 1419-1422.

6. Longo, M.C., Berninger, M.S., Hartley, J.L. (1990). Use of uracil DNA glycosilase to control carry-over contamination in polymerase chain reaction. Gene **93**, 125-128.

7. Young, K.K.Y., Resnick, R.M., Myers, T.W. (1993). Detection of hepatitis C virus RNA by a combined reverse transcription-polymerase chain reaction assay. J. Clin. Microbiol. **81**, 882-886.

8. Urdea, M., Horn, T., Fultz T., et al. (1991). Branched DNA amplification multimers for the sensitive, direct detection of human hepatitis viruses. Nucleic Acids Research Symposium **24**, 197-200.

9. Simmonds, P., Alberti, A., Alter, H.J., et al. (1994). A proposed system for the nomenclature of hepatitis C viral genotypes. Hepatology **19** (suppl.), 1323-1324.

10. Okamoto, H., Sugiyama, Y., Okada, S., et al. (1992). Typing hepatitis C virus by polymerase chain reaction with type-specific primers: application to clinical surveys and tracing infectious sources. J. Gen. Virol. **73**, 673-679.

11. Stuyver, L., Rossau, R., Wyseur, A., et al. (1993). Typing of hepatitis C virus isolates and characterization of new subtypes using a line probe assay. J. Gen. Virol. **74**, 1093-1102.

12. Dixit, V., Quan, S., Martin, P., et al. (1995). Evaluation of a novel serotyping system for hepatitis C virus: strong correlation with standard genotyping methodologies. J. Clin. Microbiol. **33**, 2978-2983.
13. AISF Report (1995). Diagnostica molecolare nell'infezione da virus dell'epatite C: applicazioni nella pratica clinica. A cura della Commissione: "Tecnologie molecolari nella diagnostica delle epatopatie".
14. Piccinino, F., Sagnelli, E., Pasquale, G., Giusti, G. (1986). Complication following percutaneous liver biopsy. A multicentre retrospective study on 68,276 biopsies. J. Hepatol. **2**, 165-173.
15. Caremani, M., Benci, A, Tacconi, D., et al. (1994). La biopsia epatica negli anni '90: indicazioni e metodi. Giorn. Mal. Inf. Parass. **46**, 423-434.
16. Pasquale, G., Sagnelli, E., Filippini, P., et al. (1992). Alterazioni istologiche nella epatite cronica da virus dell'epatite C (HCV). In: Le epatiti croniche virali, storia naturale e terapia (Eds. G. Giusti, F. Piccinino, B. Galanti , G.B. Gaeta), Masson, pag. 53-63.
17. Piccinino, F., Sagnelli, E., Pasquale, G., Piccinino, R. (1993). La morfologia nella clinica delle epatiti croniche virali. Giorn. Mal. Inf. Parass. **45**, 516-522.
18. Scheuer, P., J., Ashrafzadeh, P., Sherlock, S., Brown, D., Dusheiko, G.M. (1992). The pathology of hepatitis C. Hepatology **15**, 567-571.
19. Knodell, R.G., Ishak, K.G., Black, W.C., et al. (1981). Formulation and application of a numerical scoring system for assessing histological activity in asymptomatic chronic active hepatitis. Hepatology **1**, 431-435.
20. Scheuer, P.J. (1991). Classification of chronic viral hepatitis: a need for reassessment. J. Hepatol. **13**, 372-374.
21. Desmet, V.J., Gerber, M., Hoofnagle, J.H., Mamms, M., Scheuer, P.J. (1994). Classification of chronic hepatitis: diagnosis, grading and staging. Hepatology **19**, 1513-1520.
22. Krawczynski, K., Beach, M., Bradley, D., et al. (1992). Hepatitis C virus antigen in hepatocytes: immunomorphologic detection and identification. Gastroenterology **103**, 622-629.
23. Yap, S.-H., Willems, M., Van den Oord, J., et al. (1994). Detection of hepatitis C virus antigen by immuno-histochemical staining: a histological marker of hepatitis C virus infection. J. Hepatol. **20**, 275-281.
24. Negro, F., Pacchioni, D., Shimizu, Y. et al. (1992). Detection of intrahepatic replication of hepatitis C virus RNA by in situ hybridization and comparison with histopathology. Proc. Natl. Acad. Sci. USA 89, 2247-2251.
25. Blight, K., Trowbridge, R., Rowland, R., Gowans, E. (1992). Detection of hepatitis C virus RNA by in situ hybridization. Liver **12** (Spec. issue), 286-289.
26. Bresters, D., Cuypers, H.T.M., Reesink, H.W., et al. (1992). Detection of hepatitis C viral RNA sequences in fresh and paraffin-embedded liver biopsy specimens of non-A, non-B hepatitis patients. J. Hepatol. **15**, 390-395.
27. Ferri, C., Monti, M., La Civita, L., et al. (1993). Infection of peripheral blood mononuclear cells by hepatitis C virus in mixed cryoglobulinemia. Blood **82**, 3301-3304.
28. Giusti, G., Pasquale, G., Galante, D., et al. (1993). Clinical and histological aspects of chronic HCV infection and cirrhosis. Hepato-Gastroenterol. **40**, 365-369.
29. De Bac, C., Stroffolini, T., Gaeta, G.B., Taliani, G., Giusti, G. (1994). Pathogenic factors in cirrhosis with and without hepatocellular carcinoma: a multicenter italian study. Hepatology **20**, 1225-1230.

30. Naito, M., Hayashi, N., Hagiwara, H., et al. (1994). Serum hepatitis C virus RNA quantity and histological features of hepatitis C virus carrieirs with persistently normal ALT levels. Hepatology **19**, 871-875.

CHAPTER 27

CORRELATION BETWEEN HEPATITIS C VIRUS RNA LEVELS IN SERUM, LIVER AND PERIPHERAL BLOOD MONONUCLEAR CELLS AND SEVERITY OF LIVER DISEASE IN CHRONIC HEPATITIS C PATIENTS

L.E. ADINOLFI, R. UTILI, A. ANDREANA, R. ZAMPINO, G. MORMONE, G. RUGGIERO.

Institute of Medical Therapy, Second University of Naples, Via Cotugno 1, 80135 Napoli - Italy.

Summary
Hepatitis C virus (HCV) can infect and replicate in extrahepatic sites, like peripheral blood mononuclear cells (PBMC); this could lead to a reduced response to interferon (IFN) therapy, or to a relapse after interferon is discontinued. The detection of HCV RNA using polymerase chain reaction (PCR) or branched-DNA (bDNA) assay is of clinical usefulness since serum HCV RNA levels seem to predict response to interferon, while further studies are necessary to better define the importance of HCV RNA measurement in liver and PBMC.

HCV RNA is a marker of hepatitis C virus infection and can be detected in serum and liver of more than 95% of chronic hepatitis patients whose serum tests positive for serum HCV-Ab (1). It is well known that HCV can infect extrahepatic sites and replicate in them. In particular, HCV infection of peripheral blood mononuclear cells has been documented (2, 3). Extrahepatic HCV infection may be less responsive to interferon treatment than liver infection thus representing the source of HCV reactivation in patients who relapse after interferon is discontinued (4).

Serum HCV RNA levels may be estimated with the polymerase chain reaction (PCR) or with the branched-DNA (bDNA) assay (Chiron, Emeryville, CA). The former procedure is not highly reproducible (1) whereas the bDNA assay is reproducible and can be performed on serum samples directly, since target amplification is not needed. Quantitation of serum HCV RNA is of clinical usefulness since serum HCV RNA levels seem to predict response to

P. Gentilini and M. U. Dianzani. New Trends in Hepatology, 244-250

interferon (5), although further studies are needed to assess the issue. Less is known about the clinical significance of HCV RNA levels in liver and PBMC. Recently, Dailey and coworkers at the Chiron Corporation have developed a method for quantitation of HCV RNA in liver biopsy specimens as well as in PBMC using a bDNA assay (6-8). The method is based on the extraction of the RNA from liver tissue and PBMC according to a modification of the method of Cox (9). The liver and PBMC specimens are homogenized in guanidine HCl and sarcosyl. RNA in the homogenized samples is selectively precipitated overnight at -20°C with ethanol. The precipitate is resolubilized in sample buffer containing protease K and SDS and added directly to the 96-well microplate for the bDNA assay. From this point on, the sample is processed in the same manner as serum samples. The results of liver HCV quantitation are calculated based on the weight of processed tissue and are expressed as HCV Eq/gram of liver tissue. The results of PBMC HCV quantitation are expressed as HCV Eq/10^7 cells. Using the above mentioned methods the authors studied 23 patients with chronic hepatitis C (CHC) and different histological activity. They found a significant correlation between serum and liver HCV RNA levels (6). The mean levels of HCV RNA in serum and liver were higher in patients with chronic active hepatitis than in those with mild chronic hepatitis or with cirrhosis. In another study, Campbell et al. (8) studied the relationship between the HCV RNA levels in PBMC and the response to interferon. They observed no relationship between PBMC HCV RNA levels and basal ALT values in untreated patients. The authors found that patients with high levels of HCV RNA in PBMC appeared to respond less frequently to IFN treatment, whereas responder patients tended to have low or undetectable HCV RNA levels in their PBMC at baseline. With the use of the above mentioned procedure, we were able to quantitate the HCV RNA levels in paired samples of serum and liver tissue and in PBMC the latter being representative of an extrahepatic site of viral infection (10). In agreement with previous observations (6-8) the method which we used was found to be reliable and reproducible for quantitation of HCV RNA in liver specimens and PBMC. We investigated 18 consecutive patients (M/F 12/6; median age, 53 years, range 38-63) seen at the Institute of Medical Therapy, 2nd University of Naples, for CHC. All patients were Italian-born heterosexuals. None of the patients had a history of blood transfusion or was an intravenous drug abuser. The diagnosis of CHC was based on elevation of serum ALT levels for at least 6 months and presence of HCV-Ab and HCV RNA in serum. Liver biopsy was performed in all patients and the histological features were those of minimal changes in 6 patients, chronic active hepatitis (CAH) in 9 patients and cirrhosis in 3 patients. Patients with neoplastic disorders, auto-immune diseases, excessive alcohol intake, HBV or HIV infections and Child B or C liver cirrhosis were excluded from the study. Analysis of HCV genotypes, using the reverse hybridization with line probe assay (INNO LiPA HCV; Immunogenetics, Belgium), showed that 12 patients (64%) were infected by genotype 1b and 6 patients (36%) by genotype 2a.

The results of HCV RNA quantitation in serum, liver and PBMC of patients with chronic hepatitis C are summarized in table 1. HCV RNA levels were assayed by bDNA on serum and liver specimens of all 18 patients studied and on PBMC of 12 subjects whose PBMC were available. Data were analyzed according to the severity of histological activity (11): group 1, minimal changes, 6 patients (HAI, mean score, 2.1); group 2, CAH, 9 patients (HAI, mean score, 7.1); and group 3, cirrhosis, 3 patients (HAI, mean score, 10). Mean levels of HCV RNA in serum and liver were higher in group 2 (CAH) than in group 1 ($P < 0.01$).

TABLE 1. HCV RNA levels in serum, liver and PBMC of CHC patients according to the severity of histological damage.

HISTOLOGY	HCV RNA CONCENTRATION (Mean $\pm$ s.e. x 10^5)		
	SERUM (Eq/ml)	LIVER (Eq/g)	PBMC ($Eq/10^7$cells)^
Minimal changes (6)* HAI score = 2.1	10 ± 6	473 ± 92	0.23 ± 0.1
CAH (9) HAI score = 7.1	$144 \pm 36^{\lozenge}$	$5378 \pm 1680^{\lozenge}$	$0.71 \pm 0.2^{\lozenge}$
Cirrhosis (3) HAI score = 10	$54 \pm 16^{+}$	$1591 \pm 391^{+}$	$1.05 \pm 0.2^{+}$

^ 12 patients tested (4, minimal changes; 5, CAH; 3, cirrhosis); * Number of patients; $^{\lozenge}$ $P< 0.01$ and $^{+}$ $P< 0.02$ vs minimal changes.

HCV RNA levels detected in serum and liver of cirrhotics were higher than those found in minimal changes ($P < 0.01$) and lower than those found in CAH, though the difference did not reach statistical significance. HCV RNA levels in PBMC increased with the severity of histological activity. Patients with cirrhosis showed the highest amount of HCV RNA as compared to the other two groups (Table 1).
There was a strong correlation ($r = 0.88$, $p < 0.001$) between serum (Eq/ml) and liver (Eq/g liver) HCV RNA levels (Fig.1). The mean liver to serum HCV RNA ratio was 34 (range: 8 - 68). This result is similar to that found by Coelho-Little et al. (6) who reported a mean ratio of liver to serum HCV RNA levels of 36 (range 1 - 138). On the contrary, there was no correlation between serum or liver and PBMC HCV RNA levels.

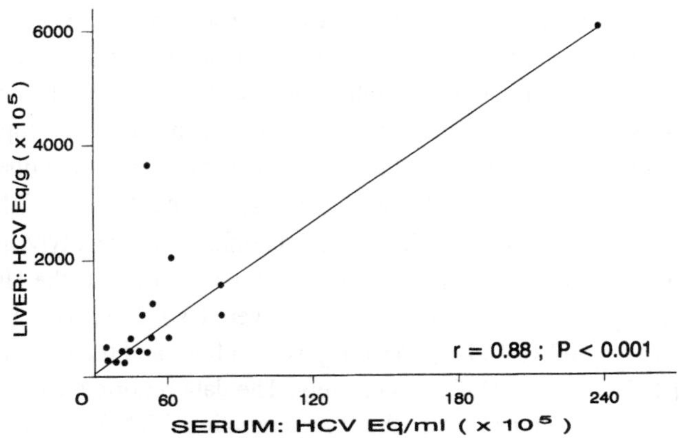

FIGURE 1. Correlation between serum and liver HCV RNA levels.

Although these results need to be confirmed on a larger series of patients, they seem to indicate that the serum HCV RNA level reflects the hepatic viral burden. Thus, the hepatic HCV RNA quantitation could be considered unnecessary in the evaluation of a chronic hepatitis C patient considering the high cost and the complexity of the procedure. The observation of lower HCV RNA levels in livers of cirrhotic patients as compared to those found in livers of CAH patients may be accounted for, at least in part, by the presence of fibrosis since data are expressed on a liver weight basis. If this is true, one could hypothesize a correlation between amount of HCV in liver and progression of hepatic damage as due to a direct effect of the virus. On the other hand, the inverse correlation between serum HCV RNA levels and hepatic disease duration, also reported by Magrin et al. (12), suggests that, besides the virus other factors, i.e host immune response, may modulate the HCV replication in liver and influence the progression of the liver disease. It is interesting to note that HCV-host relationship may be different in the Asiatic population, which in general is more tolerant to hepatitis viruses due to the acquisition of infection early in the life. Indeed, two different studies (13,14) performed in such patients found that serum HCV RNA levels tended to increase with the progression of histopathological changes of the liver. The authors (13, 14) reported that patients with cirrhosis and hepatocellular carcinoma had the highest HCV RNA serum levels and hypothesized a direct role of the virus in the progression of the liver disease. Detection of HCV RNA in PBMC has been demonstrated by several investigators (2, 3, 8) and active viral replication seems to occur in these cells (2). The presence of HCV in PBMC has been related with the extrahepatic manifestations of HCV infection, such as mixed cryoglobulinemia (15, 16); with the development of lymphoproliferative disorders (17); and with the recurrence of the disease after response to IFN treatment (4). We have demonstated that the HCV RNA levels detected in serum, liver and PBMC of patients infected by genotype 1b did not differ from those of patients infected by genotype 2a. In fact, the HCV RNA levels according to HCV genotype 1b and 2a were 83 $\pm$ 29 vs 47.6 $\pm$ 26 Eq/ml in serum; 2767 $\pm$ 507 vs 1642 $\pm$ 343 Eq/g liver in liver and 0.85 $\pm$ 0.17 vs 0.72 $\pm$ 0.24 Eq/107 cells in PBMC, respectively. The data reported above for HCV genotype 2 were obtained with the 1st generation bDNA assay, therefore results were corrected by multiplying the obtained value for a factor of 3 as suggested by Lau et al. (18). These results seem to indicate that the different response to interferon between the two HCV genotypes in patients with CHC in the various stages of liver disease cannot be explained on the basis of different viral load either in liver or in extrahepatic sites of infection. Further studies on the relationship between HCV RNA levels in serum, liver and PBMC at different stages of chronic hepatitis C as well as under interferon treatment are warranted. These studies may shed light on the pathogenesis of chronic HCV hepatitis and elucidate the virological basis of response to interferon therapy.

ACKNOWLEDGMENT This work was supported by a grant by MURST, Rome, Italy; targeted project "Liver cirrhosis and viral hepatitis".

References

1) Shindo, M., Di Bisceglie, A.M., Cheung, L., Shih, W.-K., Cristiano, K., Feinstone, S.M., and Hoofnagle, J.H. (1991) Decrease in serum hepatitis C viral RNA during alpha-interferon therapy for chronic hepatitis C, Ann. Intern. Med. 115, 700-704.

2) Zignego, A.L., Macchia, D., Monti, M., Thiers, V., Mazzetti, M., Foschi, M., Maggi, E., Romagnani, S., Gentilini, P., and Bréchot, C. (1992) Infection of peripheral mononuclear blood cells by hepatitis C virus, J. Hepatol. 15, 382-386.

3) Bouffard, P., Hayashi, P.H., Acevedo, R., Levy, N., and Zeldis, J.B. (1992) Hepatitis C virus is detected in a monocyte/macrophage subpopulation of peripheral blood mononuclear cells of infected patients, J. Infect. Dis. 166, 1276-1280.

4) Gurakar, A., Fagiuoli, S., Faruky, H., De Maria, N., Balkan, M., Van Thiel, D.H., and Friedlander, L. (1995) Utility of hepatitis C virus RNA determinations in hepatic tissue as an end point for interferon treatment of chronic hepatitis C, Hepatology 22, 1109-1112.

5) Hagiwara, H., Hayashi, N., Mita, E., Takehara, T., Kasahara, A., Fusamoto, H., and Kamada T. (1993) Quantitative analysis of Hepatitis C virus RNA in serum during interferon alfa therapy, Gastroenterology 104, 877-883.

6) Coelho-Little, E., Jeffers, L.J., Bartholomew M, Rajender Reddy, K., Schiff, E.R., and Dailey P J. (1995) Correlation of HCV-RNA levdels in serum and liver of patients with chronic hepatitis C, J. Hepatol. 22, 248-249.

7) Dailey, P., Collins, M., Wright, T., Wilber, J., Neuwald, P., and Urdea, M. (1993) Development of a method to prepare liver tissue samples for quantification of HCV RNA using a branched DNA (bDNA) signal amplification assay, Gastroenterology 104, A20, Abs. 78.

8) Campbell, C., Dailey, P.J., Urdea, M.S., Wilber, J., Collins, M.A., Mason, A.L., Bodicky, C., and Perrillo, R.P. (1994) HCV RNA in peripheral blood mononuclear cells of chronic hepatitis C patients treated with interferon alfa-2b: another possible indicator of response?, Gastroenterology 106, A148, Abs. 592.

9) Cox, R.A. (1968) The use of guanidinium hydrochloride in the isolation of nucleic acids, Methods Enzymol. 12B, 120-122.

10) Andreana, A., Adinolfi, L.E., Mormone, G., Zampino, R., Utili, R., Ragone, E., Ruggiero, G. (1995) Correlazione tra livelli di HCV RNA nel siero, nel fegato e nei linfomonociti del sangue periferico: possibile ruolo predittivo di risposta all'interferone. Atti del XCVI Congresso Società Italiana di Medicina Interna, Roma 12-15 ottobre. Abs. Pag. 401.

11) Knodell, R.G., Ishak, K.G., Black, W.C., Chen, T.S., Craig, R., Kaplowitz, N., Kiernan, T.W., and Wollman J. (1981) Formulation and application of a numerical scoring system for assessing histologic activity in asymptomatic chronic active hepatitis, Hepatology 1, 431-435.

12) Magrin, S., Craxì, A., Fabiano, C., Simonetti, R.G., Fiorentino, G., Marino, L., Diquattro, O., Di Marco, Vito., Loiacono, O., Volpes, R., Almasio, P., Urdea, M.S., Neuwald, P., Sanchez-Pescador, R., Detmer, J., Wilber, J.C., and Pagliaro, L. (1994) Hepatitis C viremia in Chronic liver disease: relationship to interferon-a or corticosteroid treatment, Hepatology 12, 273-279.

13) Kato, N., Yokosuka, O., Hosoda, K., Ito, Y., Ohto, M., and Omata, M. (1993) Quantification of hepatitis C virus by competitive reverse transcription-polymerase chain reaction: increase of the virus in advanced liver disease, Hepatology 18, 16-20.

14) Hagiwara H., Hayashi, N., Mita M., Naito M., Kasahara A., Fusamoto H., and Kamada T. (1993) Quantitation of hepatitis C virus RNA in serum of asymptomatic blood donors and patients with type C chronic liver disease, Hepatology 17, 545-550.

15) Adinolfi, L.E., Utili, R., Attanasio, V., Zampino, R., Ragone, E., Tripodi, M.F., and Ruggiero, G. (1996) Epidemiology, clinical spectrum and prognostic value of mixed cryoglobulinemia associated to hepatitis C virus infection: a prospective study, Ital.J. Gastroenter. 28, 1-9.

16) Ferri, C., Monti, M., La Civita, L., Longobardo, G., greco, F., Pasero, G., gentilini, P., Bombardieri, S., Zignego, A.L. (1993) Infection of periferal blood mononuclear cells by hepatitis C virus in mixed cryoglobulinemia. Blood 82,3701-3704.

17) Ferri, C., Caracciolo, F., Zignego, AL., La Civita, L, Monti, M., Longobardo, G., Lombardini F., Greco, F., Capochiani, E., Mazzoni, A. Et al. (1994) Hepatitis C virus infection in patients with non-Hodgkin's lymphoma, Br. J Haematol. 88,392-394.

18) Lau J.Y. N:, Simmonds P., and Urdea M. S. (1995) Implications of variations of "conserved" regions of hepatitis C virus genome, Lancet 346, 425-426.

CHAPTER 28

HEPATITIS C VIRUS LYMPHOTROPISM AND POSSIBLE PATHOGENETIC IMPLICATIONS.

ANNA LINDA ZIGNEGO[1], CARLO GIANNINI[1], MONICA MONTI[1], GRAZIA CARECCIA[1], FRANCESCA GIANNELLI[1], M. EUGENIA MARROCCHI[1], CLODOVEO FERRI[2], PAOLO GENTILINI[1].

1) Istituto di Medicina Interna; University of Florence, Florence,Italy.

2) Rheumatology and Clinical Immunology Units, Istituto di Patologia Medica I, Pisa, Italy.

Summary

Hepatitis C virus (HCV) is a virus that contains a single-stranded positive-sense RNA genome and is distantly related to the flaviviruses and pestiviruses. Following its discovery, the identification at a structural level of existing analogies between HCV and Pesti- and Flavivirus, has become a basis for research in evaluating whether common aspects in the natural history of such infections exist. One of these analogies is the possibility to infect elements of the lymphatic system (lymphotropism). This viral characteristic is of interest in regards to possible clinical and pathological consequences. In particular, one of the most intringuing hypotheses concerns the possibility that HCV lymphotropism may represent at least one of the "missing links" between HCV infection and some lymphoproliferative disorders frequently observed in association with this infection. Studies performed in this field are in agreement with this hypothesis. However the direct demonstration is still lacking and clarification of the mechanisms eventually in play deserves further study.

Natural infection of lymphatic cells.

The existence of HCV lymphotropism was suspected due to research carried out prior to the discovery of HCV demonstrating that it is possible to transmit NANB hepatitis to a monkey through infusion of lymphatic cells (1). HCV lymphotropism was then initially shown following studies of peripheral blood mononuclear cells (PBMC) withdrawn from subjects affected by chronic HCV infection (2-4). It was also demonstrated that PBMC originating from subjects

P. Gentilini and M. U. Dianzani. New Trends in Hepatology, 251-259

who were co-infected by HIV had particularly high levels of infection. HCV infection of cells of the mononuclear-phagocytic type was also shown in studies performed on liver and bone marrow sections, as well as in different lymphoid organs (5, 6).

Infection of PBMC does not seem to be an invariable phenomenon in HCV chronically infected patients. In a recent study of chronic anti-HCV antibody carriers with varying degrees of liver damage, HCV infection of PBMC was found in 60% of cases (7). In our experience, PBMC infection appeared to be very frequent in the course of chronic evolutive hepatitis or cirrhosis, whereas it was very rare in autoresolving forms and in healthy carriers of antibodies or the virus (chronic carriers of anti-HCV antibodies or HCVRNA and antibodies without apparent hepatic damage at histological examination). Consequently, HCV lymphotropism does not seem to completely justify the existence of "healthy" HCV carriers (8). The results obtained following in vitro studies of lymphatic cells withdrawn from subjects with chronic HCV infection provides further interesting data. Indeed, it was possible to demonstrate that stimulation of lymphatic cells by polyclonal activators in vitro (therefore, very likely by antigenic stimuli in vivo) causes the increase of intracellular replication of HCV. This is indirectly confirmed by experiments in which the detection of HCV sequences significantly increased after culture in presence of PHA\PMA (2, 7). Such data is in favour of the hypothesis that a "latent" HCV infection of lymphatic cells in vivo may be activated following activation of lymphatic cells through significant antigenic stimulus. Consequently, important reflections concerning the interpretation of mechanisms for transmission of the infection could be made. Possible explanations could also be made regarding the repetition of hepatitis C infection in liver transplant subjects, the exacerbation of an enduring asymptomatic hepatitis or the repetition of exacerbation of the virus following an apparently successful treatment with interferon. Indeed, recent studies showed that among "responder" patients (subjects experiencing ALT level normalization and/or disappearance of HCV viremia following treatment with interferon), those with persistent PBMC infection tended to relapse after varying periods of time following the interruption of treatment (9).

A final important aspect revealed by studies of "natural" infection of lymphatic cells is the infection of mononuclear cells directly involved in intrahepatic inflammatory infiltrate and therefore in immunomediated liver damage. In our experience, the analysis of T cell-clones, withdrawn from the hepatic biopsies of subjects with chronic hepatitis, demonstrated that about one intrahepatic T lymphocyte in three was infected by the C virus (7). These data, especially in comparison to the results of studies demontrating a scarce percentage of infected PBMC (less than 1/10) in patients with analogous hepatic pathology, support the hypothesis that infected lymphocytes are higly concentrated at the site where valid immune-mediated viral clearance would be necessary. In light of this ascertainment, a marked HCV infection of lymphatic cells could diminish the lymphatic system's ability to put efficient viral clearance into effect, consequently facilitating the persistence of the virus in the host and chronic evolutive illness. Furthermore, the same chronic infection of the liver may facilitate the infection of lymphatic cells which are present in the area of liver damage with mechanisms of cell-cell transmission of infection in preferential hepatic-lymphatic and lymphatic-lymphatic cell directions. Instead of being "antithetical", these events may co-operate and mutually reinforce each other.

As previously addressed, like T lymphocytes, B lymphocytes and monocytes-macrophages have been implicated in hosting infection as well. This is substantiated by the analysis of infection in freshly withdrawn cells in single separated populations, the study of T cell clones obtained from peripheral blood samples (see above) (2, 7), and experimental infection in vitro in single B or T cell populations obtained from healthy subjects as will be shown in the following paragraph.

Artificial infection of lymphatic cells.

A number of laboratories have ascertained that it is possible to infect both B and T human lymphocytes in vitro with highly viremic sera (7, 10). In particular, Shimizu and coworkers first showed that certain human lymphocytic cell lines were susceptible to HCV infection and that the viral replication in a human T-cell line was productive for infectious HCV. The infection of T cells by HCV appears to be the most effective in case of cells also infected by retrovirus, which is in agreement with what has been observed in vivo (see above). Interestingly, infection of human cells in vitro was easier and more rapidly carried out by using lymphatic cells rather than cells originating from the liver (10). Successively, human B-cell lines were also shown to be capable of supporting a productive infection of HCV and long-term, persistently infected cultures of these lymphoid cell cultures have been established (11, 12) Infection of cultured cells can be verified by the polymerase chain reaction (PCR) technique, immunofluorescence and cytofluorimetry as well as by in situ hybridization. More recently, the use of standard thin-section electron microscopy (EM) and immunoperoxidase EM allowed the observation of 50 nm virus-like particles in the cytoplasm of both in vitro infected human T and B cell lines. Interestingly,in comparison to liver samples taken from an infected chimpanzee, these lymphoid cultured cells contained a higher amount of virus-like HCV particles (13).

Lymphotropism of HCV and HCV-associated lymphoproliferative disorders

One of the most intriguing hypotheses suggested by the observation of HCV lymphotropism is that it may be the "missing link" between HCV infection and some autoimmune-lymphoproliferative disorders frequently observed in association with this infection .

Amongst these disorders, mixed cryoglobulinaemia (MC), which was previously defined as "essential", has proven to be accompanied by HCV infection in a large majority of cases (14-19).

The observation that HCV infection of lymphoid cells is present in a high number of MC patients (20) could suggest that HCV lymphotropism plays a role in the pathogenesis of such disease. In globally considering patient populations with MC who were studied for the presence of infection in lymphatic cells, it is possible to state that HCV genomic sequences were detected in about 80% of uncultured PBMC taken from MC patients and antigenomic sequences in about 50% of MC patients and in 80% after mitogenic stimulation. Finally, HCV genotyping showed that, on one hand, there was no MC-specific genotype in that all commonly observed types were also detectable in MC patients. On the other hand, genotype 2 was more significantly represented in patients with MC (classical or evoluted into a NHL) than in patients with chronic hepatitis and no evidence of MC.

These data, which were obtained in patients characterized by a "benign" lymphoproliferative disorder, although in some cases the disorder had evolved into a malignant lymphoma, have been confirmed and expanded in studies performed in patients affected by a clinically overt B-cell type NHL. Only in a minority of these patients, NHL complicated MC. In synthesis, ongoing HCV replication was established in about 30% and in 90% of the unselected subjects with idiopathic NHL consecutively admitted to the hospital (haematological units) or also having MC, respectively. Infection of PBMC (fresh or cultured with mitogens) was determined in all the patients having at least one HCV serum marker (anti-HCV antibodies and /or HCV RNA). In addition, the most frequent HCV genotype observed in serum samples from HCV positive patients were again 1b (about 50%) and 2 (a or c) (35%). The percentage of this latter genotype was higher when 1b+2 coinfections in serum or lymphoid cells/tissues (neoplastic tissues: bone marrow or lymph-node) were included. Interestingly, in those HCV-positive NHL patients in which it was possible to know the date of infection, this latter preceded the appearance of the haematological malignancy by many years (medially 9) (21-27)

In synthesis, data obtained from the different studies performed until now suggest that HCV plays a role both in the immediate pathogenesis of MC, related to the vascular and tissue deposition of HCV containing immune complexes, and in B-cell lymphoproliferation which may be regarded as the remote disorder of this disease. In particular, the significantly higher HCV RNA titers observed in cryoprecipitates (28) or in whole sera, rather than in supernatants (personal observation),suggests that HCV antigens may directly participate in the composition of circulating immune complexes of MC with important pathogenetic implications. On the other hand, data collected indicate that HCV infection in MC patients, particularly in those evolved into a NHL, significantly affects the immune system. An active (minus-strand HCV RNA positive) or latent replication (detection of minus strand HCV RNA only in mitogen-stimulated cells) demonstrated in the majority of MC patients, especially in those with NHL, reinforce the hypothesis that HCV lymphotropism may be involved in the pathogenesis of a chronic immunological disorder which may vary from benign lymphoproliferation to malignant lymphoma (18, 20, 29) even if, of course, the fact that HCV infection of lymphatic cells may also be observed in patients without evidence of lymphoproliferative disorders suggests that additional factors may co-operate (16, 30). Therefore, it has been suggested that MC itself may be the expression of a low-grade malignant lymphoma (18, 31, 32) in light of the detection of lymphoid aggregates in the liver, bone marrow and spleen of these patients, as well as by the presence of a monoclonal rheumatoid factor in the cryoprecipitates and clonal expansion of IgMK-bearing B cells in peripheral blood. Finally, the higher prevalence of type 2 in MC patients than in chronic HCV carriers without MC suggests that this genotype, considered as a "benign" variant of HCV with respect to severity of liver damage, may tend more than other genotypes to trigger lymphoproliferative disorders. Subsequently, the observation of a latent type 2 coinfection in lymphatic cells-tissues from MC with different genotypes detected in serum may be of interest.

In conclusion, data obtained from virological analysis of patients with MC/NHL suggest that HCV, possibly through its lymphotropism and with the cooperation of several different factors (viral, environmental and/or constitutional), may be responsible for chronic lymphoprolipheration which may switch over to a B-cell malignancy. Preliminary data concerning the high frequency of HCV infection also in different B-cell lymphoproliferative disorders such as MGUS (monoclonal gammopaties of undetermined significance) and CLL (chronic lymphatic leukemia), seem to be consistent with this hypothesis. Further studies at the cellular and molecular level will be important in order to clarify the pathogenetic role played by HCV in determining these disorders and the mechanisms eventually involved.

Acknowledgements:

This work was supported by the National Research Council (CNR) Targeted Project "Prevention and Control Disease Factors" Subproject "SP3", Contract No. 91.00168 and by the Italian Liver Foundation. We gratefully acknowledge Dr Jean-Paul Bonn and Dr Franco Boretti (Chiron Diagnostics, Lyon, France and Milan, Italy), who kindly provided bDNA, and Prof. Giampiero Buzzelli for helpful discussion.

REFERENCES

(1) Hellings JA, Veen-du Prie V, Boender P. Trasmission of non-A, non-B hepatitis by leucocytes preparations. in: Zuckerman AJ, ed. Viral Hepatitis and Liver Disease. New York: Alan R. Liss, 1988:543-9.

(2) Zignego AL, Macchia D, Monti M, Thiers V, Mazzetti M, Foschi M, Maggi E, Romagnani M, Gentilini P, Brechot C. Infection of peripheral mononuclear blood cells by hepatitis C virus. J Hepatol 1992: 15 (3) :382-6

(3) Muller HM, Pfaff E, Goeser T, Kallinowsky B, Solbach C, Theilman L. Peripheral blood leucocyte serve as a possible extrahepatic site for hepatitis C virus replication. J Gen. Virol. 1993; 74: 669-676

(4) Artini M, Natoli G, Avantaggiati ML, Balsano G, Chirillo P, Costanzo A, Bonavita MS, Levrero M. Detection of replicative intermediates of viral RNA in peripheral blood mononuclear cells from chronic hepatitis C virus carriers. Arch Virol 1993; S8: 23-9.

(5) Blight K, Trowbridge R, Rowland R, Gowans E. Detection of hepatitis C virus RNA by in-situ hybridization. Liver 1992; 12: 286-9

(6) Manzin A, Candela M, Paolucci S, Caniglia ML, Gabrielli A, Clementi M. presence of hepatitis c virus (HCV) genomic RNA and viral replicative intermediates in bone marrow and peripheral blood mononuclear cells from HCV-infected patients. Clin Diag Lab Immunol, 1994;1:160-163

(7) Zignego AL, De Carli M, Monti M, Careccia G, La Villa G, Giannini C, Mario Milco D'Elios, Del Prete G, Gentilini P. Hepatitis C virus infection of mononuclear cells from peripheral blood and liver infiltrates in chronically infected subjects. J. Med. Virol. 1995; 47 (1):58-64

(8) Brillanti S, Foli M, Gaiani S, Masci C, Miglioli M, Barbara L : Persistent hepatitis C viraemia without liver disease [letter]. Lancet, 1993 i: 464

(9) Quian C, Camps J, Maluenda MD, Civeira MP, Prieto J. Replication of hepatitis C virus in peripheral blood mononuclear cells. Effect of alpha interferon therapy. J. Hepatol. 1992; 19: 380-83.

(10) Shimizu YK, Iwamoto A, Hijikata M, Purcell RH, Yoshikura H. Evidence for in vitro replication of hepatitis C virus genome in a human T-cell line. Proc Natl Acad Sci USA 1992; 89:5477-5481

(11) Shimizu YK, Purcell RH, Yoshikura H. Correlation between the infectivity of hepatitis C virus in-vivo and its infectivity in-vitro. PNAS 1993; 90: 6037-41
(12) Shimizu YK, Yoshikura H. Evidence for multicycle infection of hepatitis C virus and inhibition by interferons alpha and beta. J Virol 1994; 68: 8406-8
(13) Shimizu YK, Feinstone SM, Kohara M, Purcell RH, Yoshikura H. Hepatitis C virus: detection of inrtacellular virus particles by electron microscopy. Hepatology 1996; 23 (2): 205-9
(14) Ferri C, Marzo E, Longombardo G, Lombardini F, La Civita R , Liberati AM, Gerli R , Greco F, Monti M, Gentilini P, Bombardieri S , Zignego AL. Interferon-alpha in mixed cryoglobulinemia patients: a randomized crossover controlled trial. Blood 81: 1132-1136,1993.
(15) Ferri C, La Civita L, Longombardo G, Zignego AL. Hepatitis C virus and mixed cryoglobulinaemia. Br J Rheumatol 33:301, 1994.
(16) AL Zignego, C Ferri, M Monti, L La Civita, G Careccia, G Longombardo, F Lombardini, S Bombardieri, P Gentilini. Hepatis C virus genotype analysis in patients with type II mixed cryoglobulinemia. Ann. Intern Med 1996;124: 31-34.
(17) C Ferri, L La Civita, AL Zignego. Lymphoproliferation and hepatitis C virus infection. Ann. Intern Med in press.
(18) Pozzato G, Mazzaro C, Crovatto m, Modolo ML, Ceselli S, Mazzi G et al. Low-grade malignant lymphoma, hepatitis C virus infection and mixed cryoglobulinemia. Blood 1994; 84(9):3047-53.
(19) Monti G, Galli F, Invernizzi F, Pioltelli P, Saccardo F, Monteverde A et al. Cryoglobulinemias: a multi-centre study of the early clinical and laboratory manifestations of primary and secondary disease. QJM 1995; 88(2): 115-26
(20) Ferri C, Monti M, La Civita L, Longombardo GF, Gentilini P, Bombardieri S, Zignego AL. Infection of peripheral blood mononuclear blood cells by hepatitis C virus in mixed cryoglobulinemia. Blood, 1993; 82: 3701-04.
(21) Ferri C, La Civita L, Mazzoni A, Zignego AL. Hepatitis C virus infection in patients with B-cell Non Hodgkin's lymphoma. JAMA , 272:355-356, 1994.
(22) Ferri C, La Civita L, Longombardo G, Lombardini F, Gentilini P, Pasero G, Zignego AL, Monti M, Mazzaro C, Greco F, Mazzoni A. Hepatitis C virus in mixed cryoglobulinemia and B cell lynphoma. Clin Exp Rheum, 12:89-90, 1994;
(23) Ferri. C, Caracciolo F, Zignego AL, La Civita L, Monti M, Longombardo G, Lombardini F, Greco F, Capochiani E, Mazzoni A, Mazzaro C, Pasero G. Hepatitis C virus infection in patients with non-Hodgkin's lymphoma. Brit J Haematol., 88: 392-4, 1994..
(24) Ferri C, Caracciolo F, Zignego AL , La Civita L, Monti M, G Longombardo, F Lombardini, F Greco, E Capochiani, A Mazzoni, C Mazzaro, G Pasero. Hepatitis C virus infection in patients with B-cell non-Hodgkin's lymphoma. Eur J Cancer, 30:1591-1592, 1994.
(25) C Ferri, M Monti, L La Civita, G Careccia, C Mazzaro, G Longombardo, F Lombardini, F Greco, G Pasero, S Bombardieri, AL Zignego. Hepatitis C virus infection in non-Hodgkin's B-cell lymphoma complicating mixed cryoglobulinaemia. Eur J Clin Invest,24:781-784,1994.
(26) C Ferri, L La Civita, C Giannini, R Cecchetti, G Longombardo, AL Zignego. Type C chronic hepatitis complicated by B-cell lymphoma. Am J Gastroenterol 1995; 90: 2071-72.

(27) C Ferri, L La Civita, M Monti, G Longombardo, F Greco, G Pasero, AL Zignego. Can type C hepatitis be complicated by B-cell malignant lymphoma? Lancet 346: 1426-1427, 1995.

(28) Agnello V, Chung RT, Kaplan LM. A role for hepatitis C virus infection in type II cryoglobulinemia. N Engl J Med 1992; 327: 1490-1495.

(29) (B) Franzin F, Efremov DG, Pozzato G, Tulissi P, Batista F, Burrone OR. Clonal B-cell expansions in peripheral blood of HCV-infected patients. Br J Haematol 1995; 90: 548-52.

(30) (A) De Vita S, Sansonno D, Dolcetti r, Ferraccioli G, Carbone A, Cornacchiulo V et al. Hepatitis c virus within a malignant lymphoma lesion in the course of type II mixed cryoglobulinemia. Blood 1995; 86(5): 1887-92

(31) Perl A, Gorevic PD, Ryan DH, Condemi JJ, Ruszkowski RJ, Abraham GN. Clonal B cell expansion in patients with essential mixed cryoglobulinemia. Clin Exp Immunol 1989; 76: 54-60.

(32) Monteverde A, Rivano MT, Allegra GC, Monteverde AJ, Zigrossi P, Baglioni P, Gobbi M, et al. Essential mixed cryoglobulinemia type II: a manifestation of low-grade malignant lymphoma? Clinical morphological study of 12 cases with special reference to immunohistochemical findings. Acta Haematol 1988; 79: 20-25.

CHAPTER 29

HCV-INDUCED CRYOGLOBULINEMIC VASCULITIS: PATHOGENESIS AND THERAPEUTIC IMPLICATIONS

DOMENICO SANSONNO, VITO CORNACCHIULO, FRANCO DAMMACCO

Department of Biomedical Sciences and Human Oncology, Section of Internal Medicine and Clinical Oncology, University of Bari Medical School, Bari, Italy

Summary

Leucocytoclastic vasculitis is the dominant lesion of mixed cryoglobulinemia (MC). The high prevalence of antibodies to hepatitis C virus (HCV) in association with the higher concentration of HCV RNA genomic sequences in the cryoglobulins and analysis of the composition of immune complexes (ICs) suggest a close relation between MC and HCV infection and strongly supports the view that this virus plays a key role in causing vascular damage. Our data indicate that endothelial cells are fully susceptible to infection of HCV, and support the contention that they serve as sufficient targets for the binding of HCV proteins expressed on the cell surface to serum immunoglobulins. The *in situ* demonstration of IgM RF WA cross-idiotype (XId) adds further evidence that RF of the WA group participates in the development of vasculitis, and probably stabilizes the binding of ICs. Lymphomonocytes may be crucial in the infection of endothelial cells by acting as a circulating viral reservoir. The efficacy of interferon in the treatment of MC, has been shown in more than 50% of patients and includes improvement of cutaneous vasculitis and renal function. However, almost 80% of responders have a clinical and biochemical relapse after treatment withdrawal.

P. Gentilini and M. U. Dianzani. New Trends in Hepatology, 260-272

Introduction

Cryoglobulins are immunoglobulins (Igs) that become insoluble at temperatures below 37°C and give rise to high molecular weight aggregates. They are found in small quantities in normal serum, but in large concentrations in many pathological conditions (1).

Leukocytoclastic, often necrotizing vasculitis is the dominant lesion of cryoglobulinemia. Cryoglobulins are thought to form immune complexes (ICs) that activate inflammatory effectors and complement factors to induce vascular lesions characterized by neutrophil infiltration, deposition of ICs and necrosis of the vessel wall. It is well established that cryoglobulinemia mainly produces vasculitis in small and medium-sized arteries (2). Conventionally, cryoglobulins are classified on the basis of their Ig composition as type I consisting of a monoclonal Ig alone, type II as a mixture of monoclonal and polyclonal Igs, and type III of polyclonal Igs. In mixed cryoglobulinemias (MC), IgM typically has rheumatoid factor (RF) activity.

MC is found in association with several infections, collagen-vascular and lymphoproliferative diseases. Patients without identifiable underlying diseases are considered to have "essential" MC (EMC).

Cutaneous vasculitis is most frequently the first evidence of cryoglobulinemia and provides an early opportunity to recognize it and foresee systemic complications. The most common histopathologic pictures are vasculitis, inflammatory and noninflammatory purpura without vasculitis, and hyaline thrombosis.

Vasculitis is characterized by inflammatory infiltrates involving the blood vessel wall and associated with fibrinoid necrosis and hemorrhage. Usually, there is a negative correlation between the presence of vasculitis and the cryocrit values. Furthermore, purpura, petechiae, livedo reticularis and ulcers seem more frequent in types II and III than type I cryoglobulinemia.

The clinical features of cutaneous vasculitis may vary in function of advanced age, corticosteroid therapy, thrombocytopenia and blood vessel fragility.

Hepatotropic Viruses and EMC

EMC is definitely associated with chronic liver disease (CLD). Impaired liver function has been reported (3) in approximately 2 patients out of 3. CLD has been occasionally regarded as a direct consequence of IC-mediated damage. Whether cryoglobulins are promoted by the liver damage itself, owing to reticuloendothelial system impairment in the blood clearance of circulating ICs, is still a matter for speculation.

Indirect evidence suggests that MCs are antigen-antibody ICs, in which it is frequently possible to identify the specificity of IgG antibody, whereas the detection of the primary antigen(s) in the cryoprecipitate nearly always has proved to be remarkably difficult (4). Hepatitis C virus (HCV) has recently been incriminated in the pathogenesis of EMC. Many investigators have reported a 30% to 100% prevalence of HCV antibodies in the sera of MC patients (5-8).

HCV is an enveloped virus with a diameter of 30-60 nm and a ~10-Kb positive-stranded RNA genome (9). It appears to be a distant relative of the human Flaviviruses and animal Pestiviruses, and shares their genetic organization. Like them, it encodes a long polyprotein precursor that is co-translationally and post-translationally cleaved into structural and nonstructural proteins by viral and host-encoded proteases. Significant nucleotide and amino acid heterogeneity is present throughout the HCV genome, with a well-characterized hypervariable region in the E2 envelope glycoprotein domain. This has led to the recognition of six HCV subtypes based on differences in the nucleotide for NS5 (10).

The most definitive test for diagnosing active HCV infection is the reverse polymerase chain reaction (RT-PCR), which measures the presence of viral RNA. HCV RNA occurs in more than 80% of MC patients, and a higher concentration is always found in the cryoprecipitates than in the supernatants (6, 11-13). In our own experience (14), HCV RNA has been found to be entirely confined to the cryoprecipitates in 18/26 (69.2%) patients, and 10^3 to 10^7 times more concentrated in the remaining 8 cases.

ICs and WA Cross-Reactive Idiotype (XId) in EMC

The WA cross-idiotype (XId) is the major XId among mRF in EMC (15). It is almost always associated with the light chain XId 17-109 and the heavy chain XId G6 postulated as the products of the restricted expression of germline genes with few or no somatic mutations (16). Our recent data (17) on the composition of soluble ICs in acute and chronic HCV infection without cryoglobulinemia show that HC virions are bound to IgG molecules with specific anti-HCV activities, which in turn are linked to IgM bearing the 17-109 XId. The 17-109 XId was detected on IgM in sera without cryoglobulins, even at low concentrations consistent with the range indicated for "natural" antibodies and with the amount reported for polyclonal RFs occurring in patients with RA (18).

The observation that these ICs are uniquely associated with HCV infection supports the view that in this situation WA XId RF derives from a specific antigen-driven response. The demonstration of WA XId-positive, RF-negative cells in normal individuals seems compatible with the suggestion that their physiological role is the secretion of "natural" antibodies to common pathogens, and that RF activity is a cross-reaction that develops with somatic mutations accompanying their proliferation (19).

HCV RNA and HCV-related proteins in damaged tissues

Suggestive evidence for the direct role of HCV in the pathogenesis of vasculitis is the demonstration of HCV RNA and proteins in the vessel walls of HCV-infected MC patients (20). Studies on skin biopsies with monoclonal antibodies to structural and nonstructural HCV antigens (i.e., c22-3, c33c, c100-3) have demonstrated that specific immune deposits are preferentially located in the intima of small dermal blood vessels. Two main immunohistochemical patterns were established: 1) coarse deposits that were sometimes very prominent and almost completely filled the microvascular spaces; 2) HCV antigens deposition within vessel walls and in perivascular spaces with no other lumen alteration. Viral proteins were deposited either in homogeneous or in fibrillar array. Positivity confined to the vessel walls was detected in apparently normal skin, without inflammatory infiltrates, intravascular deposition of hyaline material, and with intact vessel walls. HCV antigen-positive signals were shown within and between endothelial cells up to the layers of the basal lamina, in the absence of perivascular deposition. Similar pictures were found for HCV RNA sequences in skin tissue by *in situ* hybridization (ISH). However, although in most instances HCV RNA was confined to the dermal vessel walls, in other cases a strong signal not associated with cell structures, but diffused to connective tissue was detected.

Active cutaneous vasculitis was strikingly associated with the presence of HCV in the blood vessels. We have demonstrated (21) HCV RNA sequences *in situ* in 94.7% of MC patients with cutaneous vasculitis, and in 18.2% of patients with noninflammatory changes ($p < 0.001$). In the adjacent sections, viral proteins were found in 78.9% of patients with vasculitis and in 27.3% of those without ($p < 0.005$). The ability of sense strand probes to display a skin tissue signal strongly suggests that replicative intermediates of antigenomic HCV RNA are present within endothelial cells, which may represent another extrahepatic HCV replication site. It is suggested that, by analogy with Flaviviruses, HCV lacking reverse transcriptase proliferates by cytoplasmic RNA replication. Although the demonstration of HCV antigens in the vessel walls of MC patients suggests a pathogenetic role for this virus in the induction of vasculitis, the lack of direct correlation between vascular HCV antigen reactivity and inflammation indicates that further mechanisms are likely to be involved in the pathogenesis of vasculitis, and that HCV antigen deposition precedes and possibly triggers tissue damage (20).

Evidence for the role of cryoproteins in the pathogenesis of vasculitis is the demonstration of IgM and IgG and complement fractions at the sites of vascular damage. However, failure to demonstrate a direct relation with the amount of circulating cryoproteins argues against their direct role in the production of vasculitis, and suggests that peculiar characteristics of ICs and/or local environment are crucial factors in the endothelial damage. The extent of cryoglobulin deposition may be the result of a critical antigen/antibody ratio in circulating ICs, in that high molecular weight ICs are rapidly cleared from the circulation, whereas low molecular weight material containing dissociated IgG and IgM is trapped within tissues (22). This strongly suggests that tissue specific ICs are formed *in situ* through the binding of HCV proteins expressed on endothelial cells to serum immunoglobulins.

It has been reported (23) that HCV replicates in peripheral and bone marrow mononuclear cells. We have shown (24) that either B and T lymphocytes or monocytes sustain HCV replication irrespective of the type and severity of liver disease. Furthermore, it was shown that a close relation exists between endothelial cells and HCV-infected circulating mononuclear cells, which were found both within the lumen in close contact with apparently noninfected cells and in some instances fixed to the vessel wall areas positive for HCV antigens (fig. 1, A-D). These different patterns suggest that circulating mononuclear cells may operate as an extrahepatic HCV reservoir capable of infecting endothelial cells.

There is also indirect evidence that HCV is an important cause of cryoglobulinemic nephropathy (25, 26), usually consisting of a membranoproliferative glomerulonephritis (MPGN) with subendothelial deposits. Johnson *et al.* (27) have reported a strict association between MPGN and HCV infection. They hypothesized that renal damage could be the result of an immune-mediated reaction, in that a tissue antigen released by the virus or a neoantigen induced by viral infection may act as the main target in the cytopathogenetic mechanism(s). This hypothesis is also in keeping with many examples of animal and human models of IC disease, in which glomerular

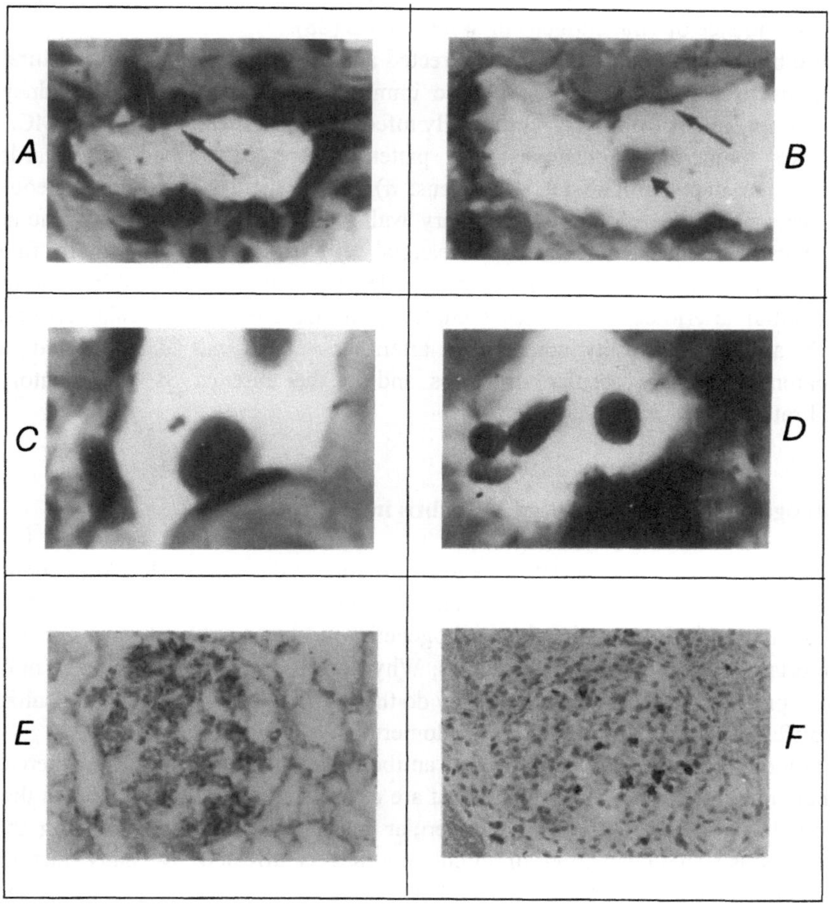

Figure 1. Simultaneous demonstration of HCV deposits in dermal vessel wall and within circulating cells. In panels (A-B) HCV immunoreactants are revealed in a limited area or along the vessel walls (long arrows) and in a circulating mononuclear cell (short arrow). In (C), an infected blood mononuclear cell can be found in strict contact with an apparently uninfected endothelial cell. In (D) a negative reaction is demonstrated in HCV-unrelated skin biopsy.

HCV-related proteins are detected in unfixed cryostat kidney sections from patients with cryoglobulinemic MPGN. In (E) immune reactants were solely detected in glomerular capillaries, whereas in (F) they were found as granular bead-like deposits within glomerular area.

damage has been strictly associated with viral infection despite the lack of a direct evidence of viral antigens in tissue lesions (28).

We have used a panel of moAbs directed against structural and nonstructural proteins to demonstrate HCV-specific immunoreactive deposits in 9 kidney biopsy specimens from HCV-chronically infected patients with MPGN and MC.

Two main immunohistochemical patterns were established as regards glomerular deposition of HCV antigens: *a*) heavy, diffuse and homogeneous deposits along the glomerular capillary walls (fig. 1, E); *b*) diffuse granular deposits in the mesangial and paramesangial cells (fig. 1, F). Furthermore, fine as well as coarse HCV immunoreactive deposits were found within tubulo-interstitial arterioles, sometimes completely filling the microvascular spaces. HCV antigens reactivity confined to arteriolar vessels was also detected in apparently normal vascular structures and in the absence of inflammatory infiltrates.

Pathogenesis of HCV-Induced Vasculitis in MC

The demonstration of HCV-related proteins and/or HCV RNA genomic sequences at the site of vascular damage both in skin and renal vasculitis in MC does not entirely explain the pathogenetic mechanisms, and raises many important questions for further studies. Why does IC vasculitis develop in only some patients with HCV viremia? Why do these virally induced deposits localize to different regions of the skin or the glomerulus?

Some individuals may produce little antibody capable of forming ICs, whereas others may produce circulating ICs that are cleared extrarenally. It is known that some ICs are handled by the glomerular mesangium without damaging the glomerulus. The deposition of circulating ICs is affected by many factors, including their size, antigen and antibody charge and ability to dissociate and reassociate. Our findings indicate that IC deposits are formed *in situ* by the HCV antigens expressed by endothelial cells or mesangial cells, followed by the binding of circulating anti-HCV antibodies linked in turn by IgM RF. The *in situ* demonstration of IgM RF 17-109 XId as massive intraluminal deposition adds evidence that RF of WA group participates in the formation of vascular immune deposits and the development of vasculitis.

Once ICs are fixed to endothelial cell expressing HCV proteins, a series of events ensue in which recruitment of leukocytes from the blood is one of the most dramatic cellular responses to tissue damage and inflammation, and is central to the physiologic trafficking of lymphocytes. These events occur through activation of endothelium, including the transient expression of endothelial surface molecules that promote leukocyte adherence. The adhesion molecules include intracellular adhesion molecule 1, vascular cell adhesion molecule 1, endothelial-leukocyte adhesion molecule 1 (ELAM-1). In chronic inflammation of the skin, binding of lymphocytes to cytokine-stimulated endothelial cells involves the expression of ELAM-1 (29, 30). In this context, HCV-infected circulating mononuclear cells may infect and/or reinfect endothelial cells, which constitute a strategically important barrier against virus spread.

The persistence of HCV in damaged glomeruli together with IgM, IgG and C3 deposition is in keeping with an immune-mediated pathogenetic mechanism, in that the virus expressed on endothelial cells may be the target for circulating ICs, with subsequent complement activation and production of cytokines and other inflammatory factors as schematically reported in fig. 2.

Therapeutic Approaches

Recognition of cryoglobulinemic vasculitis and MPGN as HCV-related disorders lends support to the rational use of antiviral agents, such as IFN, in their treatment. Following several studies (31-33) on the efficacy of recombinant IFNα (rIFNα) in patients with EMC, our long-term, randomized, controlled study (34) with the use of natural IFNα (nIFNα, 3 MU thrice weekly for 1 year) confirmed that it helps to reduce disease activity in more than half of HCV-positive patients with MC. Interestingly, our results demonstrated that, although the combination of nIFNα plus prednisone (PDN, 16 mg/day on non-IFN days) did not increase the rate of clinical response, it induced a more prompt response, stabilized its beneficial effect and delayed the relapse. A possible synergistic mechanism could be envisaged for combined nIFNα plus PDN, in that PDN could act directly by regulating IFN-induced proinflammatory cytokines. Conversely, the remission rate induced by PDN alone significantly differ from that occurring spontaneously in untreated patients.

It was demonstrated that the therapeutic effect of nIFNα was closely related to inhibition of HCV replication. Clinical remission was associated with undetectable levels of HCV RNA that preceded normalization of ALT and a significant decrement of cryocrit levels. Decrement of cryoglobulin precipitation in patients receiving nIFNα therapy may conceivably be ascribed to several mechanisms, namely: *a*) inhibition of virogenesis, resulting in a lower amount of

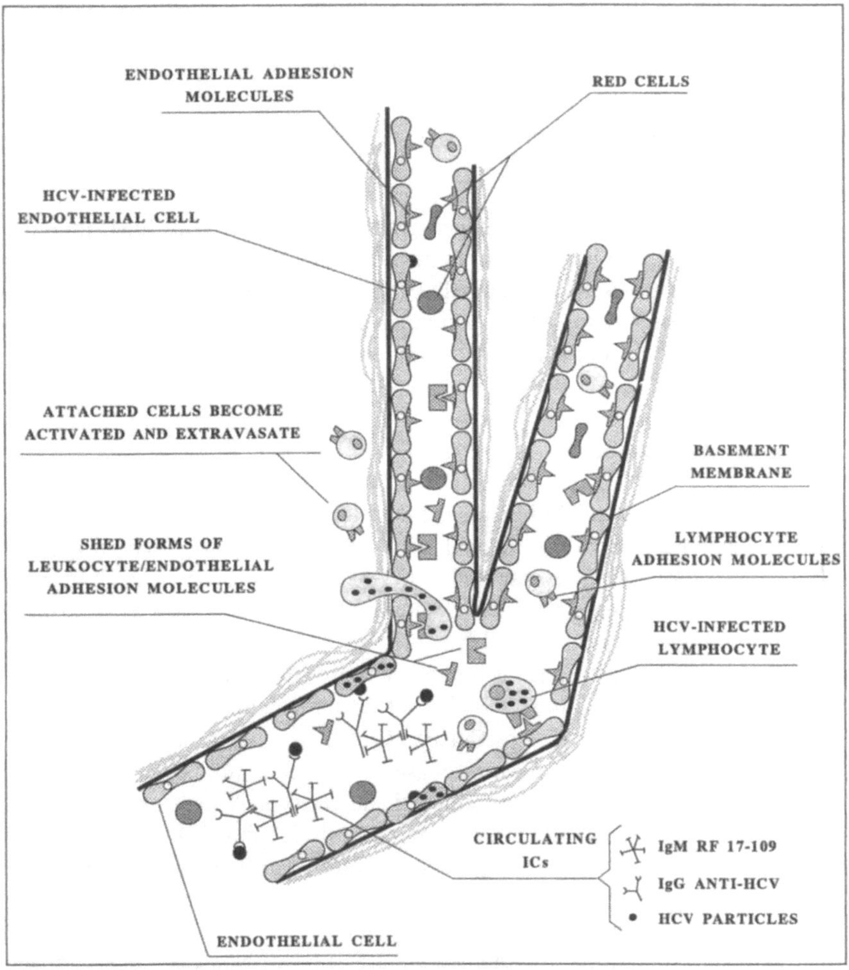

Figure 2. Scheme of hypothetical pathogenetic mechanism of vascular damage in mixed cryoglobulinemia. ICs formed of HCV, IgG anti-HCV and IgM RF bearing 17-109 XId are targeted to infected endothelial cells. Activated endothelial cells induce leukocyte/endothelial adhesion molecules, which play a key role in sustaining acute and chronic inflammation. HCV infected circulating mononuclear cells may in turn form a viral reservoir capable of infecting or reinfecting endothelial cells.

viral antigens available for specific IC formation; *b*) a more efficient clearance of circulating ICs by the reticuloendothelial system secondary to improvement of liver function; *c*) inhibition of IgM RF synthesis; *d*) immunoregulation of T-cell function; and *e*) increased expression of HLA antigens.In terms of rate of clinical response, efficacy of nIFNα treatment of MC associated with HCV infection matches that reported in studies performed in HCV-induced CLD (35, 36), suggesting that the occurrence of cryoproteins does not modify the probability of response of MC patients to this treatment. It was also noted that mean serum HCV RNA levels increased in almost 40% of patients treated with PDN alone. This is reminiscent of the putative immune-mediated enhancement of hepatitis B viremia during immunosuppressive therapy. It was not demonstrated in the group of patients receiving nIFNα plus PDN, possibly because of the prevailing inhibition of virogenesis by nIFNα.

IFN is a significant improvement in the therapy of MC. Even so, the probability of relapse within 6 months after treatment is almost 80%. This implies that optimal doses and/or duration of IFN schedule treatment should be considered in future studies.

Acknowledgment

This work was supported in part by Italian Ministry of University and Scientific and Technological Research, Group "Liver Cirrhosis and Viral Hepatitis" and by Italian Foundation for the Study of the Liver.

References

1. Maire, M.A., Mittey, M. and Lambert, P.H. (1989) The presence of cryoprecipitable immunoglobulins in normal human sera may reflect specific molecular interactions, *Autoimmunity* **2**, 155-164.
2. Jennette, J.C., Falk, R.J., Andrassy, K., Bacon, P.A., Churg, J., Gross, W.L., Hagen, E.C., Hoffman, G.S., Hunder, G.G., Kallenberg, C.G.M., McCluskey, R.T., Sinoco, R.A., Rees, A.J., van Es, L.A., Waldherr, R. and Wiik, A. (1994) Nomenclature of systemic vasculitides, *Arthritis Rheum.* **37**, 187-192.
3. Levo, Y., Gorevic, P.D., Kassab, H.J., Tobias, H. and Franklin, E.C. (1977) Liver involvement in the syndrome of mixed cryoglobulinemia, *Ann. Intern. Med.* **87**, 287-92.

4. Appel, G.B. (1993) Immune-complex glomerulonephritis. Deposits plus interest, *N. Engl. J. Med.* **328**, 505-506.
5. Ferri, C., Greco, F., and Longombardo, G. (1991) Hepatitis C virus antibodies in mixed cryoglobulinemia patients, *Arthritis Rheum.* **34**, 1606-1610.
6. Agnello, V., Chung, R.T. and Kaplan, L.M. (1992) A role for hepatitis C virus infection in type II cryoglobulinemia, *N. Engl. J. Med.* **327**, 1490-1495.
7. Dammacco, F. and Sansonno, D. (1992) Antibodies to hepatitis C virus in essential mixed cryoglobulinemia, *Clin. Exp. Immunol.* **87**, 352-356.
8. Pechère-Bertschi, A., Perrin, L., De Saussure, P., Widmann, J.J. and Shifferly, J.A. (1992) Hepatitis C: a possible ethiology for cryoglobulinemia type II, *Clin. Exp. Immunol.* **89**, 419-422.
9. Choo, Q.L., Kuo, G., Weinre, A.J., Overby, L.R., Bradley, D.W. and Houghton, M. (1989) Isolation of a cDNA clone derived from a blood-borne non-A, non-B viral hepatitis genome, *Science* **244**, 359-362.
10. Simmonds, P. (1995) Variability of hepatitis C virus, *Hepatology* **21**, 570-583.
11. Dammacco, F., Sansonno, D., Cornacchiulo, V., Mennuni, C., Carbone, R., Lauletta, G., Iacobelli, A.R. and Rizzi, R. (1993) Hepatitis C virus infection and mixed cryoglobulinmeia: a striking association, *Int. J. Clin. Lab. Res.* **23**, 45-49.
12. Ábel, G., Zhang, Q-X. and Agnello, V. (1993) Hepatitis C virus infection in type II mixed cryoglobulinemia, *Arthritis Rheum.* **36**, 1341-1349.
13. Ferri, C., La Civita, L., Longombardo, G., Greco, F. and Bombardieri, S. (1993) Hepatitis C virus and mixed cryoglobulinemia, *Eur. J. Clin. Invest.* **23**, 399-405.
14. Sansonno D., Cornacchiulo, V., Iacobelli, A.R. and Dammacco F. (1993) New clinical and molecular features of essential mixed cryoglobulinemia, in A.G. Dalgleish, A. Albertini and R. Paoletti (eds.), *The Impact of Biotechnology on Autoimmunity,* Kluwer Academic Publishers, Dordrecht, pp. 27-36.
15. Gorevic, P.D. and Frangione B. (1991) Mixed cryoglobulinemia cross-idiotype: implications for the relationship of MC to rheumatic and lymphoproliferative diseases. *Semin. Hematol.* **28**, 79-84.

16. Andrews, D.W., and Capra, J.D. (1981) Complete aminoacid sequence of variable domains from two human monoclonal anti-gamma globulins of the WA cross-idiotypic group: suggestion that the J segments are involved in the structural correlate of the idiotype, *Proc. Natl. Acad. Sci. USA* **78,** 3799-3803.
17. Sansonno, D., Iacobelli, A.R., Cornacchiulo, V., Lauletta, G., Di Stasi, M.A., Gatti, P. and Dammacco, F. (In press) Immunochemical and biomolecular studies of circulating immunecomplexes isolated from patients with acute and chronic hepatitis C virus infection, *Eur. J. Clin. Invest.*
18. Fong, S., Chen P.P., Gilbertson T.A., Weber J.R., Fox R.I., and Carson D.A. (1986) Expression of three cross-reactive idiotypes on rheumatoid factor autoantibodies from patients with autoimmune diseases and seropositive adults, *J. Immunol.* **137,** 122-128.
19. Martin T., Duffy S.F., Carson D.A. and Kipps T.J. (1992) Evidence for somatic selection of natural autoantibodies, *J. Exp. Med.* **175**, 983-991.
20. Sansonno D., Cornacchiulo V., Iacobelli A.R., Di Stefano R., Lospalluti M. and Dammacco F. (1995) Localization of hepatitis C virus antigens in liver and skin tissues of chronic hepatitis C virus-infected patients with mixed cryoglobulinemia, *Hepatology* **21**, 305-312.
21. Sansonno, D., Cornacchiulo, V., Iacobelli, A.R. and Dammacco, F. (Submitted) In situ demonstration of HCV RNA and HCV-related proteins in skin and liver of patients with mixed cryoglobulinemia..
22. Theophilopoulos A.N. and Dixon, F.J. (1990) Immune Complexes in Human Diseases, *Am. J. Pathol.* **100**, 531-594.
23. Moldvay, J., Deny, P., Pol, S., Brechot, C. And Lamas E. (1994) Detection of hepatitis C virus RNA in peripheral blood mononuclear cells of infected patients by *in situ* hybridization. *Blood* **83**, 269-73.
24. Sansonno, D., Iacobelli, A.R., Cornacchiulo, V., Iodice, G., and Dammacco, F. (1996) Detection of hepatitis C virus (HCV) proteins by immunofluorescence and HCV RNA genomic sequences by nonisotopic in situ hybridization in bone marrow and peripheral blood mononuclear cells of chronically HCV-infected patients, *Clin Exp Immunol.* **103**, 414-421
25. Roth, D. (1995) Hepatitis C virus: the nephrologist's view, *Am. J. Kidney Dis*. **25**, 3-16.
26. D'Amico, G. and Fornasieri, A. (1995) Cryoglobulinemic glomerulonephritis: a membranoproliferative glomerulonephritis induced by hepatitis C virus, *Am. J. Kidney Dis*. **25**, 361-369.

27. Johnson, R.J., Gretch, D.R., Yamabe, H., Hart, J., Bacchi, C.E., Hartwell, P., Couser, W.G., Corey, L., Wener, M.H., Alpers, C.E. and Willson, R. (1993) Membranoproliferative glomerulonephritis associated with hepatitis C virus infection, *N. Engl. J. Med.* **328**, 465-470.
28. Fornasieri, A., Li, M., Armelloni, S., Pinerolo De Septis, C., Schiaffino, E., Sinico, R.A., Schmid, C. and D'Amico, G. (1993) Glomerulonephritis induced by human IgMK-IgG cryoglobulins in mice, *Lab. Invest.* **5**, 531-540.
29. Oppenheimer-Marks, N. and Lipsky, P.E. (1994) Transendothelial migration of T-cells in chronic inflammation, *The Immunologist* **2,** 58-64.
30. Gesualdo, L., Di Paolo, S., Milani, S., Pinzani, M., Grappone, C., Ranieri, E., Pannarale, G. and Schena, F.P. (1994) Expression of platelet-derived Growth Factor Receptors in normal and diseased human kidney, *J. Clin. Invest.* **94**, 50-58.
31. Bonomo, L., Casato, M., Afeltra, A. and Caccavo, D. (1987) Treatment of idiopathic mixed cryoglobulinemia with alpha interferon, *Am. J. Med.* **83**, 726-730.
32. Ferri, C., Marzo, E., Longombardo, G., Lombardini, F., La Civita, L., Vanacore, R., Liberati, A.M., Gerli, R., Greco, F., Moretti, A.., Monti, M., Gentilini, P., Bombardieri, S. and Zignego, A.L. (1993) Interferon-α in mixed cryoglobulinemia patients: a randomized crossover-controlled trial, *Blood* **81**, 1132-1136.
33. Misiani, R., Bellavita, P., Fenili, D., Vicari, O., Marchesi, D., Sironi, P.L., Zilio, P., Vernocchi, A., Massazza, M., Vendramin, G., Tanzi, E. and Zanetti, A. (1994) Interferon alpha-2a therapy in cryoglobulinemia associated with hepatitis C virus, *N. Engl. J. Med.* **330**, 751-756.
34. Dammacco, F., Sansonno, D., Han, J.H., Shyamala, V., Cornacchiulo, V., Iacobelli, A.R., Lauletta, G. and Rizzi, R. (1994) Natural interferon alpha vs its combination with 6-methyl-prednisolone in the therapy of type II Mixed cryoglobulinemia. A long-term, randomized, controlled study, *Blood* **84**, 3336-3343.
35. Terrault, N. and Wright, T. (1995) Interferon and hepatitis C, *N. Engl. J. Med.* **332**, 1509-1511.
36. Perrillo, R.P. (1994) The management of chronic hepatitis B, *Am. J. Med.* **96**, 1A 34-40.

Section V

CLINICAL ASPECTS OF CHRONIC LIVER DISEASE

CHAPTER 30

CIRRHOSIS ASSOCIATED CONGESTIVE GASTROPATHY

Physiopathological aspects

R. PETRINO, A. DI NAPOLI, S. AVIGNONE, M. MESTRINER, C. MARINONE, L. CHIANDUSSI

Division of Internal Medicine, University of Turin. S. Vito Hospital, via. S. Vito 34, 10133 Turin, Italy.

Summary

Cirrhosis associated congestive gastropathy (CG) is an endoscopic and histological condition located in gastric mucosa, characterized mainly by vascular alterations. While the endoscopic picture, although well classified by Mc Kormack description, is not specific, the histological findings are typical, and comprehend initially inflammatory lesions, and in more advanced stages microvascular lesions. The supposed pathogenesis of such alterations is a deregulated release of vasoactive substances, with prevalence of vasodilators. The main factor implicated seems to be nytric oxyde (NO), overproducted by inducible NO-syntase, related to endotoxemia. In this study we have tried to better define the prevalence of vascular and inflammatory lesions in CG and to relate them to the pathogenetic process. We have considered the endoscopic and histologic observations in a cirrhotic population, grading each parameter in an attempt to find significant association. The results obtained show that both inflammatory and vascular lesions are present in about 80% of cases, and that also in 78% of patients there was a bacterial pollution that is significantly related to esophageal varices, vascular and inflammatory histological damage but not to endoscopic evidence of GC. We conclude that the possible pathogenic mechanism may start from blood stasis with vasodilatation, followed by bacterial pollution which causes mucosal damage and an inflammatory reaction.

1. Gastric Modifications in Hepatic Cirrhosis

Gastric alterations associated to hepatic cirrhosis are located both in submucosa, like gastric varices and, more frequently, in mucosa layer, configuring the real

P. Gentilini and M. U. Dianzani. New Trends in Hepatology, 275-285

endoscopy. It is possible to make a staging of the disease, according to the classification of the lesions found (4, 5). Gastric varices are classified in Stage 1 (suspected) in case of "big folds" or dilated veins; Stage 2 (sure) when the aspect is convoluted (6, 7). CG is described according the McCormack classification (8):

TABLE 1. McCormack Classification of congestive gastropathy

Mild or Moderate	Red spots, scarlatiniform Superficial reddening of mucosal folds Mosaic pattern of mucosal surface
Severe	Cherry red spots Erosions and hemorrage

With the exception of the "mosaic pattern" that is a specific picture of congestive gastropathy, the other endoscopic lesions are common to many other pathogen noxae, like biliary reflux, NSAID, alcohol and Helicobacter pylori infection. It is evident that histological evaluation is necessary to well define CG. The available literature data show that the endoscopic aspect is similar in gastritis and CG, whereas in the latter case the pathological lesions are mainly of vascular origin. In fact, while in chronic gastritis the most peculiar aspect is a lymphocitic and polymorphonuclear infiltrate (9), and vascular alterations are seldom observed, in course of CG there is almost always the evidence of mucosal vessel dilatation and ultrastructural alteration of endothelial cells (8, 10). In submucosa we can find artero-venous shunts, vessel dilatations and haemorragic soffusions (10, 11). An inflammatory component is seldom described in the histologic picture of CG, but it seems more frequent and evident in early stages of the pathology (12-14).

1.1 Etiopathogenetic hypothesis

The mucosal vascular damage observable in CG is the expression of haemodynamic alterations, proper of hepatic cirrhosis. An increment of whole blood flow in stomach is described (15). With regard to the perfusion of mucosa layer the literature data are discordant, since in different studies an increment of flow (15-17) or a reduction (18, 19) has been observed. Panes et al. (20) studied the mucosal flow by Laser Doppler Fluximetry and Spectrophotometry, observing an increment of gastric blood flow. The authors explained such observation with an initial vascular congestion followed by a hyperdynamic state, generalized, proper of severe hepatic cirrhosis. The cause of the systemic hyperdynamic state seems to be due to a deregulated release or production of vasoactive substances, with a prevalence of vasodilators (21). The substances implicated are prostacycline (PGI_2), glucagon, bradykinin, substance P, atrial natriuretic peptide (ANP) and, more recently, NO. NO is a potent vasodilator synthetized in endothelial cells from L-arginine, by NO-synthase, an enzyme existing in two forms: constitutive and inducible. The inducible NO-synthase is responsive to many stimuli, like some cytokines and bacteric endotoxins (22-24). Piqué et al. (25) suggest that NO plays an important role in regulating gastric mucosa integrity. Studies on rats show that such substance acts on mucosal microcirculation both in basal conditions and as a mediator of vasodilatation after acid stimulus (26). Lopez et all. have suggested a possible interaction between NO and tumor necrosis factor alpha (TNFα) in causing the haemodynamic alterations observed in hepatic cirrhosis, and its relation to endotoxemia (27). It seems in fact, that the release of TNFα by monocytes, spontaneous or endotoxin induced, causes the induction of NO-synthase (28-30). The described vascular alterations lead to a weakness of gastric mucosa, documented by a decrease of membrane potentials. This causes an increased sensitivity to lesive agents, strictly related to severity of cirrhosis. Nevertheless it is not known whether cirrhotic patients are more susceptible than normal population to H. pylori infection and the pathogenetic role of the bacteria in CG (31, 32).

2. Aim of the study

We have tried to better define the role and the prevalence of vascular, inflammatory or trophic lesions in determining CG on the basis of the controversial data available on its real histologic picture. In particular we propose to correlate endoscopic and histologic observations in a cirrhotic population with the aim to describe the pathogenetic process to the end stage lesions. We recently studied 87 consecutive patients affected by hepatic cirrhosis. Diagnosis was made by biochemical and clinical evaluation, classifying the patients by Child-Pugh score within 3 days from enrollment.

TABLE 2. Clinical data of the 87 patients included in the study

Mean age	55 (range 34-67)
Males/females	58/29
HBV/HCV	10/27
Alcohol	40
Cryptogenic	8
Biliary	2
Child-Pugh score	A 51, B 27, C 9

All patients were submitted to upper endoscopy, recording the parameters reported in Table 3. For histological evaluation, 4 gastric biopsies were obtained, 2 antral and 2 fundic. Bioptic specimens were paraffin embedded, stained by Haematoxylin-Eosin and Giemsa and were blindly observed by two pathologists. Each parameter was expressed using a numeric score, to obtain semiquantitative variables. The parameters were pair-matched and analyzed by Chi-square test. Statistical significance was for $p < 0.05$, but sure results were considered for $p < 0.01$.

TABLE 3. Endoscopic and histologic parameters recorded

<u>Endoscopic</u>		
Esofageal and Gastric Varices	F1, F2, F3	
Congestive Gastropathy	Mild	Grade 1
	Severe	Grade 2
Peptic Ulcer	Present	Grade 1
	Absent	Grade 0
<u>Histologic</u>		
Chronic Gastritis	Grade 0 - 3 according to severity of infiltrate and atrophy	
Microvasculopathy	Grade 0 - 3 according to the presence of congestion, dilatation or neoangiogenesis	
Helicobacter pylori	Grade 0 - 3 according to density	
Bacteric pollution	Grade 0 - 3 according to density	

2.2 Results

About 2/3 of the patients studied showed an endoscopic picture of CG, 54% mild and 13% severe. Esophageal varices F1 were observed in 35% of cases, F2 in 16% and F3 in 6%. Peptic ulcer was observed in 9 patients (1%).With regard to histologic picture, we observed inflammatory lesions, generally mild, in 80% of cirrhotic patients, while vascular lesions were present in 76% of cases (figure 1). H. pylori were found in 69% of patients, while unexpectedly, in 78% of patients we observed a bacterial pollution different from H. pylori. (figures 2 and 3). No significant differences were observed among cirrhotic patients of different etiology. The mean score of endoscopic and histologic parameters is shown in the graph of figure 4. These results, analyzed by chi-square test, showed some statistical correlation as schematically represented in figure 5, and synthesized in Table 4. In particular, we did not observe a relation between the presence of the endoscopic picture of congestive gastropathy and histological lesions, both inflammatory and vascular. On the other hand microvascular lesions correlated significantly both with oesophageal varices and with bacterial pollution (H. pylori and different bacteria). Bacterial colonisation seemed to be related also with inflammatory lesions.

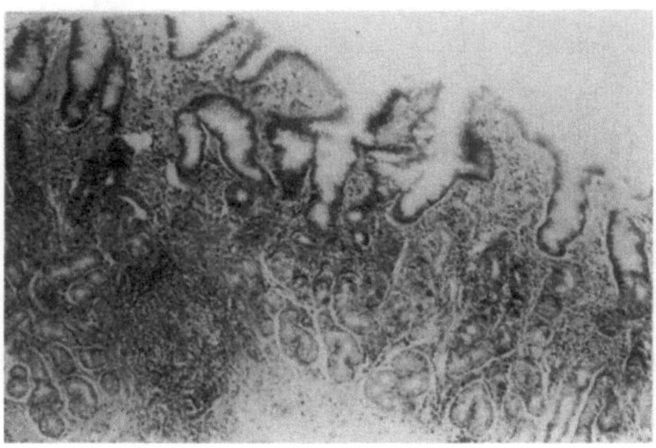

Figure 1. Gastric antral biopsy. Inflammatory infiltration in the mucosa, vessel congestion and dilatation are evident. Giemsa 10x.

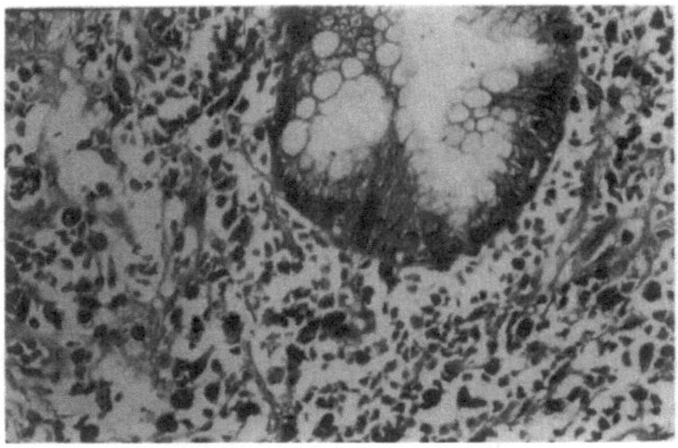

Figure 2. Gastric antral biopsy. Microvessels dilatation and congestion and H. pylori colonisation in the gland lumen. Giemsa 40x.

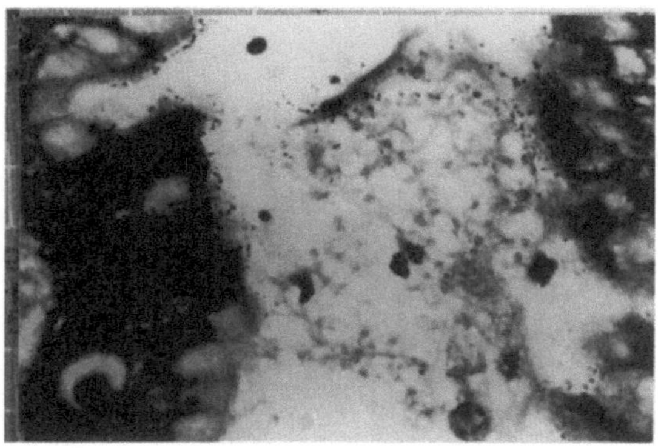

Figure 3. Gastric antral biopsy. Bacterial colonies on mucosal surface. Giemsa 20x.

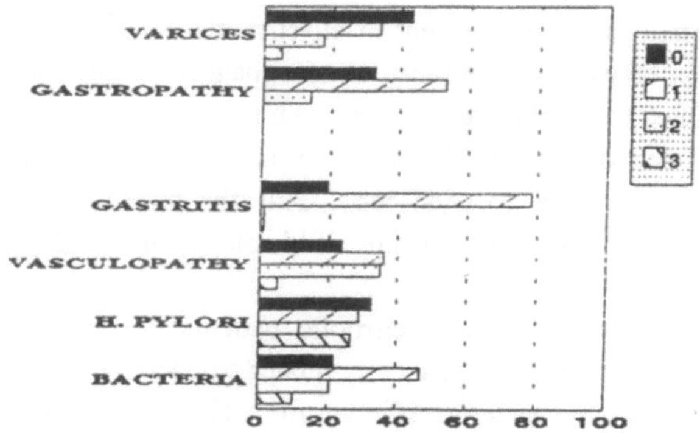

Figure 4. Grading of the severity of endoscopical and histological findings. Varices F1, F2 and F3 are quantified as 1, 2, 3. Values are expressed as % of the total number (87 patients).

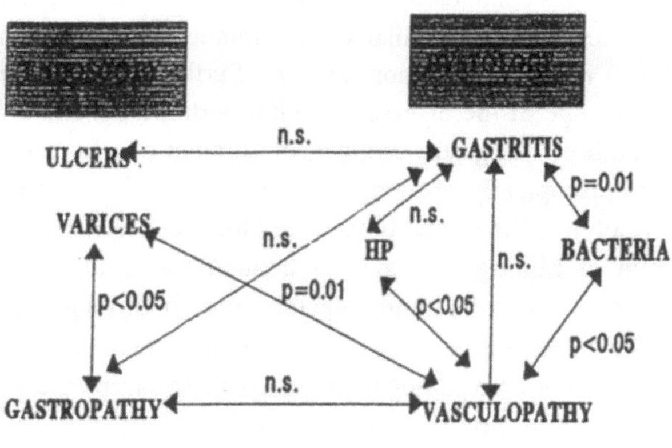

Figure 5. Schematic presentation of Chi-square test between endoscopic and histological parameters pair matched.

DISCUSSION

The results previously shown allow to formulate the following considerations.

1. Endoscopic alterations are not present in all cirrhotic patients; nevertheless, there is a correlation between the presence of oesophageal varices and CG. This data, besides, is related to the clinical stage of disease.

2. All the patients, showing either altered or normal endoscopic pattern, show histological lesions not related to endoscopy. Only the presence of varices is linked to the evidence of microvasculopathy at histology, in a highly statistical way.

3. The gastric histological lesions in cirrhotic patients are of vascular and inflammatory origin, and both are statistically related to bacterial pollution. This is caused predominantly by bacteria different from H. pylori, probably cocci originating from saliva.

On the basis of these data and of that available in literature we can affirm that our results surely confirm the vascular pathogenesis of endoscopic gastric lesions; in fact CG and varices are more frequent in advanced stages of cirrhosis, when portal hypertension and the related hyperdynamic state is more severe. With this clinical picture the more evident histological alterations are of vascular type, such as vessel dilatation, congestion and microvessels neoformation in gastric mucosa. At this point it is important to underline that our observation is confined to mucosa, while the studies conducted on the animal showed that the alterations interest the entire gastric wall, particularly the submucosa, where congestion, hemorrages and shunts formation are more evident. Furthermore, our data show that there is a clinical stage of the disease in which portal hypertension has not yet caused any alteration on gastro-esophageal circulation. In this stage a mucosal damage, microscopically observable, is no longer always present. We believe it is important to define the physiopathological mechanism of such lesions, with the aim of finding strategies of treatment able to prevent more severe lesions. In the first stages the implied factors cause both inflammatory and vascular damage. The factor statistically related to such damage seems to be bacterial proliferation. A possible pathogenetic mechanism can be the following: hyperdynamic state linked to cirrhosis causes an initial blood flow increase of gastric mucosa with dilatation and microvessel neoformation. As many studies demonstrate, this condition leads to vasoactive peptides production by endothelial cells, such as glucagone, atrial natriuretic peptide and NO. It was also observed that bacteria toxins can stimulate NO production directly or mediated by TNFα and other cytokines. A final sequence could be the following:

vasodilatation, neoangiogenesis, blood stasis, weakness of mucosal barrier caused by H. pylori and other bacteria, mucosal damage, inflammatory answer. Such lesions are certainly more evident in this stage, when there is only modest vascular damage. In conclusion, we believe it is useful to submit all cirrhotic patients, with or without evident endoscopic lesions, to mucosal hemodynamic and histological study, to define the precise pathogenetic sequence of vascular lesions. We propose to study a wide population of patients with Laser-Doppler flussimetry, mucosal NO determination and histological evaluation to confirm our hypothesis and to give statistical weight to our observations.

References

1) Payen, J.L., Cales, P.: Modifications gastriques au cours de la cirrhose, Gastroenterol. Clin. Biol. 15 (1991), 285-295.

2) Vigneri, S., Termini, R., Piraino, A., Scialabba, A., Pisciotta, G., Fontana, N.: The stomach in liver cirrhosis. Endoscopic morphological and clinical correlations, Gastroenterology 101 (1991), 472-478.

3) Lingenfelser, T., Krige, J.E.: The stomach in cirrhosis. The legend of Proteus retold, J. Clin Gastroenterol 17 (1993), 92-96.

4) Cales, P., Buscail, L., Bretagne, J.F., Champigneulle, B., Bourbon, P., Duclos, B., Dapoigny, M., Dumas, R., Pierrugues, R., Davion, T., Cenni, J.C., Pariente, E.A.: Concordance inter-observateurs inter-centres des signes endoscopiques gastro-esophagiens au cours de la cirrhose. Resultats d'une étude prospective multicentrique, Gastroenterol. Clin. Biol. 13 (1989), 967-973.

5) Cales, P., Zabotto, B., Meskens, C., Caucanas, J.P., Vinel, J.P., Desmorat, H., Fermanian, J., Pascal, J.P.: Gastroesophageal endoscopic features in cirrhosis. Observer variability, interassociation and relationship to hepatic dysfunction, Gastroenterology 98 (1990), 156-162.

6) Hashizume, M., Kitano, S., Hamaga, H., Koyanagi, N., Sugimachi, K.: Endoscopic classification of gastric varices, Gastrointest. Endosc. 36 (1990), 276-280.

7) Misra, S.P., Dwivedi, M., Misra, V., Agarwal, S.K., Gupta, R., Gupta, S.C., Mital, V.P.: Endoscopic and histologic appearance of the gastric mucosa in patients with portal hypertension, Gastrointest. Endoscopy 36 (1990), 575-579.

8) McCormack, T.T., Sims, J., Eyre-Brook, I., Kennedy, H., Goepel, J., Johnson, A.G., Triger, D.R.: Gastric lesions in portal hypertension: inflammatory gastritis or congestive gastropathy, Gut 26 (1985), 1226-1232.

9) Di Napoli, A., Petrino, R., Boero, M., Bellis, D., Chiandussi, L.: Quantitative assessment of histological changes in chronic gastritis after eradication of Helicobacter pylori, J. Clin Pathology 45 (1992), 796-798.

10) Papazian, A., Braillon, A., Dupas, J.L., Sevenet, F., Capron, J.P.: Portal hypertensive gastric mucosa: an endoscopic study. Gut 27 (1986), 1199-1203.

11) Phelps, T.O., Mullone, J.: Portal hypertension and gastric erosions in the rat. Arch. Surg. 111 (1976), 190-194.

12) Iwao, T., Toyonaga, A., Sumino, M., Takagi, K., Oho, K., Nishizono, M., Ohkubo, K., Inoue, R., Sasaki, E., Tanikawa, K.: Portal hypertensive gastropathy in patients with cirrhosis, Gastroenterology 102 (1992), 2060-2065.

13) Gianelli, C., Gioineni, A., Graziani, M.G., Luminari, M.: Gastric damage in cirrhotic patients: endoscopic and histological findings, Gastroenterology 96 (1989), 600.

14) McCormick, P.A., Sakey, E.A., Dhillon, A.P., Kaye, G., McIntyre, N., Burroughs, A.K.: Portal hypertensive gastropathy or Campylobacter pylori associated gastritis, J. Hepatology 9 (1989), 563.

15) Benoit, J.N., Womack, W.A., Korthuis, R.J., Wilborn, W.H., Granger, D.N.: Chronic portal hypertension effects on gastrointestinal blood flow distribution, Am. J. Physiology 250 (1986), 535-539.

16) Gerahty, J.G., Angersin, W.S., Carter, D.C.: Autoradiographic study of the regional distribution of gastric blood flow in portal hypertensive rats, Gastroenterology 97 (1989), 1108-1114.

17) Leung, F.U., Slodownik, E., Jensen, D.M., Vendeventer, G., Guth, P.H.: Gastroduodenal mucosal hemodynamics by endoscopic reflectance spectrometry, Gastrointest. Endoscopy 37 (1987), 284-288.

18) Moreau, R., Lee, S., Soupison, T., Roche Sicot, J., Sicot, C.: Abnormal tissue oxygenation in patients with cirrhosis and liver failure, J. Hepatology 7 (1988), 98-105.

19) Sarfeh, J., Tarnawaski, A.: Gastric mucosal vasculopathy in portal hypertension, Gastroenterology 93 (1987), 1129-1131.

20) Panes, J., Bordas, J.M., Pique, J.M., Bosch, J., Garcia-Pagan, J.C., Feu, F., Casadevall, M., Terés, J., Rodés, J.: Increased gastric mucosal perfusion in cirrhotic patients with PGH, Gastroenterology 103 (1992), 1875-1882.

21) Wu, Y., Cartland Burns, R., Sitzman, J.V.: Effects of Nitric Oxide and glocoxigenase inhibition of splanchnic hemodinamics in portal hypertension, Hepatology 18 (1993), 1416-1421.

22) Guarner, C., Soriano, G., Tomas, A., Bulbena, O., Novella, M.T., Balanzo, J., Vilardell, F., Mourelle, M., Moncada, S.: Increased serum nitrate levels in patients with cirrhosis: relationship to endotoxemia, Hepatology 18 (1993), 1139-1143.

23) Blei, A.T.: Portal hypertension, Current Opinion in Gastroenterology 10 (1994), 295-302.

24) Vallance, P., Moncada, S.: Hyperdynamic circulation in cirrhosis: a role of nitric oxyde?, Lancet 337 (1991), 776-778.

25) Pique, J.M., Esplugnes, J.V., Witthle, B.J.R.: Endogenous NO as a mediator of gastric mucosal vasodilatation during acid secretion, Gastroenterology 102 (1992), 168-174.

26) Whittle, B.J.R., Lopez-Belmonte, J., Moncada, S.: Regulation of gastric mucosal integrity by endogenous NO: interactions with prostanoids and sensory neuropeptides in the rat. Br. J. Pharmacology 99 (1990), 607-611.

27) Lopez-Talavera, J.C., Merrill, W.W., Groszmann, J.: Tumor necrosis factor alpha: a major contributor to the hyperdynamic circulation in prehepatic portal hypertensive rats. Gastroenterology 108 (1995), 761-767.

28) Garcia-Tsao, G., Albillos, A., Barden, G.E., West, A.B.: Bacterial translocation in acute and chronic portal hypertension, Hepatology 17 (1993), 1081-1085.

29) Sorell, W.T., Quigley, E.M.M., Jin, G., Johnson, T.J., Rikkers, L.F.: Bacterial translocation in the portal hypertensive rat: studies in basal conditions and on exposure to hemorragic shock, Gastroenterology 104 (1993), 1722-1726.

30) Genecin, P., Groszman, P.J.: Portal hypertension. Disease of the Liver 7th ed. Shiff, E., Shiff, L. Eds. Lippincott, Philadelphia 1993, 935-973.

31) D'Amico, G., Montalbano, L., Traina, M., Pisa, R., Menozzi, M., Spanò, C., Pagliaro, L., and The Liver Study Group of V. Cervello Hospital: Natural history of congestive gastropathy in cirrhosis, Gastroenterology 99 (1990), 1558-1564.

32) Guslandi, M., Sorghi, M., Foppa, L., Tittobello, A.: Congestive gastropathy versus chronic gastritis: a comparison of same pathophysiological aspects, Digestion 54 (1993), 160-162.

CHAPTER 31

TREATMENT OF ASCITES IN CIRRHOSIS

PAOLO GENTILINI, GIORGIO LA VILLA, VINCENZO CASINI RAGGI, ANTONIO DELLO SBARBA, ROBERTO GIULIO ROMANELLI, PIERO TICALI, FRANCESCO GAMBILONGHI, DONATO RICCARDI, MASSIMO PINZANI, GIACOMO LAFFI

Istituto di Medicina Interna, Facolta' di Medicina e Chirurgia - Universita' degli Studi di Firenze, viale Morgagni 85, I-50134 Firenze.

SUMMARY

The authors discussed the principal criteria for a correct medical treatment of ascites in liver cirrhosis. A therapeutical approach to ascites, based on a standardized sequential or stepped-care treatment was then considered, together with the available strategies for the management of diuretic resistant ascites. Finally, preliminary data on the efficacy of albumin infusion in ascitic patients undergoing a diuretic treatment were reported.

Introduction

Ascites, which eventually occurs in more than ¾ of cirrhotic patients, is a major complication of liver cirrhosis, since it adversely affects survival (1-2). In fact, the development of ascites is associated with profound disturbances of systemic and splanchnic hemodynamics and of renal function that play a key role in the pathogenesis of this complication and contribute to the poor prognosis of these patients. Until the 1980's, the probability of survival at one year in patients affected by liver cirrhosis after the first occurrence of ascites was 56% (3). Today, accurate therapy of ascites itself and the other major complications of cirrhosis results in a longer survival. Indeed, in a series of 405 patients with compensated cirrhosis observed at out Institution, 65% of them were still alive at 3 years and 40% at 5 years after the first episode of ascites (2).

The accumulation of a great amount of fluid in the peritoneal cavity induces a further increase in portal pressure, favouring bleeding from esophageal varices. Other complications strictly linked to the presence of ascites include hernias, respiratory impairment and, more importantly, spontaneous bacterial peritonitis and hepatorenal syndrome (HRS) (4). The pathogenesis of ascites is

P. Gentilini and M. U. Dianzani. New Trends in Hepatology, 286-295

complex and still not completely understood: nevertheless, present evidence indicates that in patients with cirrhosis, sinusoidal portal hypertension triggers renal sodium and water retention and the retained fluid accumulates in the peritoneal cavity as ascites.

Medical treatment of ascites is therefore aimed at determining a negative sodium balance to induce the translocation of fluid from the peritoneal cavity to the intravascular space and thus its excretion into urine. This is usually accomplished with bed rest, low-sodium diet and the administration of diuretics. Among these drugs, aldosterone antagonists such as spironolactone and potassium canrenoate proved to be the first choice agents to relieve ascites in non-azotemic cirrhotic patients. In fact, several reports indicate that activation of the renin-angiotensin-aldosterone (RAA) system is of major importance in the pathogenesis of sodium retention in cirrhosis. When anti-aldosteronic drugs are no longer effective in inducing a negative sodium balance, a loop diuretic must be added. Patients not responding to these drugs are said to have refractory (diuretic resistant) ascites. As discussed later, administration of plasma-expanders may also be useful, especially in patients requiring high-dose diuretics or not responding at all, similarly to those undergoing paracentesis (3, 4)

When treating cirrhotic patients with ascites, it is necessary to consider that net translocation of ascitic fluid from the abdominal cavity into systemic circulation is a rather limited phenomenon; it has been found to be highly variable from one patient to another, being lower than 500 ml per day in some of them (5). Diuretic treatment produces a loss of fluids, followed by the passage of ascitic fluid to the intravascular compartment. However, the repeated administration of diuretics eventually leads to a contraction of circulating blood volume, accompanied by arterial hypotension, further activation of the RAA system and the sympathetic nervous system (SNS) and a possible decrement of renal function. Thus, if the loss of body weight during the administration of diuretics is greater than 500 g per day, patients are at risk of developing complications due to the depletion of intravascular volume, such as prerenal azotemia and hyponatremia. On the other hand, patients also having peripheral edema are somehow protected from plasma volume depletion due to the preferential and rapid mobilization of fluid accumulated as edema (6).

Other complications of an inappropriate diuretic therapy include hyperkalemia and acidosis in patients receiving aldosterone antagonists, hyponatremia, alkalosis and hepatic encephalopathy in those receiving loop diuretics (4).

Sequential medical treatment

From a practical point of view, a standardized stepped-care medical treatment of ascites based on the following scheme proved to be useful:
1) *First step*: bed rest and sodium-restricted diet. Assumption of the standing posture exerts favourable hemodynamic effects in patients with cirrhosis and ascites: in fact, this manoeuvre leads to an increase in central volume and cardiac output, so reducing the degree of activation of the SNS and the RAA system. Therefore, bed rest together with a low sodium diet favours the disappearance of ascites (7,8). Restriction of sodium intake should be limited to 40 mmol per day. A lower sodium intake makes meals unappetizing and may lead to pre-renal azotemia or dilutional hyponatremia (4). On the other hand, an unrestricted sodium intake (or the lack of compliance to the prescribed diet) may lead to diuretic resistance (9). Bed rest and low-sodium diet induce the disappearance of ascites in about 10% of patients: a favourable response to this treatment is more likely to occur in patients who have not previously had ascites, who have an urinary sodium excretion higher than 10 mmol per day, and who have a normal renal function (10). In the remaining patients, bed rest and low sodium diet improve the response to diuretics.
2) *Second step*: addition of aldosterone antagonists. Patients who do not respond to bed rest and sodium-restricted diet must be treated with anti-aldosteronic drugs, such as spironolactone or potassium canreonate (8, 9). These compounds have high intestinal absorption (about 70%) and a good bioavailability due to an extensive binding to plasma proteins. The diuretic response to spironolactone or potassium canreonate, another aldosterone antagonist with a lesser anti-androgenic activity (11), is delayed so that these drugs are effective only after 3-4 days of treatment. The natriuretic potency of aldosterone antagonists is very low especially when compared to loop diuretics. Nevertheless, these drugs are more effective than loop diuretics in relieving ascites in cirrhosis. This assumption was established by the only controlled study comparing the diuretic effectiveness of spironolactone and furosemide (12). The natriuretic response to aldosterone antagonists depends on plasma aldosterone concentrations, patients with higher plasma aldosterone levels requiring higher doses of the drug up to 500-600 mg/day. On the other hand, a recent multicentric trial indicates that administration of aldosterone antagonists up to a maximum of 400 mg/day is effective in about 70% of patients, and that higher doses provide only a relatively small increase in the success rate, but hospitalization is prolonged and

side effects are more frequent. Therefore, in patients not responding to 200 mg/day of an aldosterone antagonist, addition of a loop diuretic is probably more useful than increased doses of those drugs (4,13).

3) *Third step*: addition of loop diuretics. Furosemide is the most widely experimented loop diuretic, and it is also active in patients with renal impairment (14). Furosemide is rapidly absorbed by the intestinal tract with a bioavailability of about 60% and binding to plasma proteins. It is secreted by the epithelial cells of the proximal renal tubule and inhibits sodium reabsorption in the ascending limb of Henle's loop, interfering with the Na^+,K^+/$2Cl^-$ cotransport system. In comparison to spironolactone and analogues, furosemide has a shorter half-life and its biological effects last between 3 and 6 hours (14). The addition of 25-50 mg of furosemide daily to an aldosterone antagonist drug leads to a good diuretic response in about 30% of patients (8). Ethacrynic acid, bumetanide and piretanide have similar effectiveness as furosemide but side effects are more frequent, especially with ethacrynic acid (15). Torasemide is a recently introduced sulfonyl-urea derivative with greater bioavailability and longer half-life than furosemide (16). When administered to cirrhotic patients with ascites in equipotent doses as furosemide, this drug induced a two-fold greater diuretic and natriuretic response, with similar effects on kaliuresis (17).

4) *Fourth step*. About 10% of patients do not respond to aldosterone antagonist plus loop diuretics. A small number of these latter patients showed a satisfactory natriuresis with higher diuretic doses up to 400 mg spironolactone and 160 mg furosemide per day (9). In our experience, the addition of 100 ml of 25% of human albumin is also useful, leading to a diuretic and natriuretic response in about another 7% of all patients (8). Most of them, however, either do not respond to high dose diuretics or develop severe side effects (hepatic encefalopathy, hyponatremia and renal impairment) which preclude the use of effective doses of diuretics. These patients have the so-called refractory ascites, either of the diuretic-resistant or the diuretic-intractable type (18).

The mechanism(s) responsible for the development of refractory ascites is still poorly understood. One explanation may be related to an impairment in renal hemodynamics, so that the filtered sodium load is decreased and sodium reabsorption in the proximal tubule, where diuretics are not effective, is increased (9). An impaired pharmacokinetics of loop diuretics also contributes to diuretic resistance, at least in some patients (19). Both torasemide and furosemide, show a reduced elimination rate through renal and non-renal routes, and a larger distribution to body fluids. Consequently, the half-life of these drugs is longer than in healthy subjects, but urinary excretion of pharmacologically active metabolites is quantitatively unchanged after torasemide administration, whereas it is reduced after furosemide. Therefore, torasemide induces greater diuretic and natriuretic effects than furosemide, probably related to a maintained urinary excretion of its active metabolites (20). Finally, the renal response of cirrhotic patients with ascites to diuretic treatment also depends on the patients' age, since in our experience patients with refractory ascites, on average, are older then those who responded to diuretics (4).

Diuretic-resistant ascites

The treatment of diuretic resistant ascites is, for some aspects, similar to that of patients with HRS. Patients with refractory ascites always have a marked decrease in effective arterial blood volume (EABV), which is further impaired by all the manoeuvres forcing diuresis. Moreover, in cirrhotic patients, normal BUN and serum creatinine levels are often associated with some degree of renal impairment as indicated by simultaneous measurement of glomerular filtration rate (21).

Today, the most exploited therapeutic approaches for patients with refractory ascites are:

1) repeated paracentesis with administration of human albumin
2) peritoneovenous (Le Veen) shunt
3) transjugular intrahepatic portosystemic shunt (TIPS)
4) portosystemic surgical shunts
5) orthotopic liver transplantation.

Repeated paracentesis, with the infusion of albumin (6-8 g per liter of ascitic fluid removed) and standard medical treatment (as outlined above), can be easily performed also in outpatients, thereby shortening or eliminating hospital stay, improving the quality of life (22). The insertion of a peritoneovenous Le Veen shunt, on the other hand, may lead to more frequent and serious side effects such as acute pulmonary edema, disseminated intravascular coagulation, hemorrhage from rupture of gastroesophageal varices, local and systemic infection, without improving survival rate (9). A multicentric randomized study comparing repeated large-volume paracentesis associated with intravenous albumin infusion and Le Veen shunt demonstrated that these procedures are equally effective in relieving refractory ascites, but shunt occlusion is common and survival is not improved (23). Transjugular intrahepatic portosystemic shunt (TIPS) is an accepted treatment for recurrent variceal hemorrhage. TIPS placement also results in an improvement in renal sodium excretion, in a reduction of portal hypertension, plasma renin activity, plasma aldosterone and plasma norepinephrine concentrations, together with a reduction or disappearance of ascites. However, deterioration of liver function, hepatic encephalopathy, infections and stent occlusion were often observed, and mortality from underlying diseases is substantial (24).

Some drugs have been tried in patients with ascites, more with the aim of better understanding the pathophysiology of this disorder than with the purpose of eliminating ascites. Administration of atrial natriuretic peptide (ANP) to cirrhotic patients with ascites induced an heterogeneous natriuretic response (25), patients with refractory ascites usually showing no improvement in sodium excretion (26). Administration of vasodilating prostaglandins also failed to reverse refractory ascites and HRS (27), whereas administration of thromboxane synthase inhibitors or TxA_2 antagonists led to an improvement in free water excretion and the renal sensitivity to furosemide, but with the possible occurrence of more pronounced bleeding tendency (28-30).

Preliminary controlled study using albumin infusion

Patients with liver cirrhosis, usually show an increase in plasma volume and cardiac output. In these patients, however, effective central blood volume and EABV are reduced, according to the peripheral arterial vasodilation hypothesis (31) and clearly indicated by the finding of a striking activation of SNS and the RAA system. All these hemodynamics and endocrine abnormalities are even more marked in patients with advanced liver disease and are favoured and/or worsened by the use of diuretics. All the above considerations provided a rationale for the use of plasma expanders, in the treatment of ascites in cirrhosis. Among plasma expanders, human albumin has the advantage of being safe, since it is a physiological component, having a long half-life (about 20 days) and functioning as a carrier for diuretics. Dextran and haemaccel, instead, show shorter half-lives and may be responsible for idiosyncratic reactions. Human albumin, moreover, may increase circulating plasma volume and improve systemic and renal dynamics and response to the diuretic regimen. Indeed, the safety and utility of albumin infusion has been suggested by previous uncontrolled studies (32).

To better define the role of albumin in the medical treatment of ascites and in improving the response to diuretic regimen, we studied 113 patients with cirrhosis (60 men, 53 women, mean age 61.1 ± 0.9, range 36 - 80 years) admitted to our Institution for the treatment of decompensated liver cirrhosis. All subjects were submitted to the above described stepped-care medical treatment. 11 patients (9.7 %) eliminated ascites with bed rest and a sodium restricted diet. The remaining 102 patients were randomly allocated to receive human albumin (100 ml of a 25% solution, 51 patients) or no plasma expanders. All patients were given up to 200-300 mg of oral potassium canrenoate and up to 50 mg of furosemide or 20 mg of torasemide per day. 44 patients included in the albumin group and 36 patients receiving only diuretics showed a satisfactory response, the rate of natriuretic response being significantly different between the two groups ($p < 0.05$) (figure 1).

<u>113 PATIENTS</u>

bed rest and sodium-restricted diet

↙ ↘

11 RESPONDERS | 102 NON-RESPONDERS

↙ ↘

51 receive diuretics | 51 receive diuretics + albumin

↙ ↘ ↙ ↘

36 responders (70.6%) | 15 non-responders (29.4%) | 44 responders (86.3%) | 7 non-responders (13.7%)

($p < 0.05$)

Figure 1. Stepped-care medical treatment of ascites: albumin infusion improves the natriuretic response to diuretic administration

Moreover, the subsequent administration of albumin to 10 out of 15 non-responders in the diuretic group led to a good response in 7 patients. These results indicate that addition of human albumin is a useful tool in the medical treatment of ascites and support theoretical considerations about the importance of the reduction in EABV as a determinant of a poor response in several patients.

References

1) Ginès P, Quintero E, Arroyo V, Teres J, Bruguera M, Rimola A, Caballeria J, et al. Compensated cirrhosis: natural history and prognostic factors. Hepatology 1987;7:122-128.

2) Gentilini P, Laffi G, La Villa G, Romanelli RG, Buzzelli GP, Casini Raggi V, Melani L, et al. Long course and prognostic factors of virus-induced liver cirrhosis. 1996, submitted for publication.

3) Arroyo V, Ginès P, Planas R, Panes J, Rodès J. Management of patients with cirrhosis and ascites. Semin Liver Dis 1986;6:353-369.

4) Gentilini P, Laffi G. Pathophysiology and treatment of ascites and the hepatorenal syndrome. Baillière's Clin Gastroenterol 1992;6(3):581-607.

5) Shear L, Ching S, Gabuzda GJ. Compartimentalization of ascites and edema in patients with hepatic cirrhosis. Gastroenterology 1970;282:1391-1396.

6) Pockros PJ, Reynolds TB. Rapid diuresis in patients with ascites from chronic liver disease: the importance of peripheral edema. Gastroenterology 1986;90:1827-1833.

7) Ring-Larsen H, Henriksen JH, Wilken C, Clausen J, Pals H, Christensen NJ. Diuretic treatment in decompensated cirrhosis and congestive heart failure: effects of posture. Br Med J 1986;292:1351-1353.

8) Gentilini P, La Villa G, Laffi G, Buzzelli G, Pinzani M, Cominelli F, Moscarella S, Birardi A. Sodium retention in cirrhosis: aspects of pathophysiology and treatment. Front Gastrointest Res 1986;9:203-218.

9) Arroyo V, Epstein M, Gallus G, Gentilini P, Ring-Larsen H, Salerno F. Refractory ascites in cirrhosis: mechanism and treatment. Gastroenterol Int 1989;2:195-207.

10) Rocco VK, Ware AJ. Cirrhotic ascites. Pathophysiology, diagnosis, and management. Ann Int Med 1986;105:573-585.

11) Gentilini P. *Hepatology Elsewere*: spironolactone and canrenoate: different antialdosteronic diuretic agents. Hepatology 1991;13:999-1000.

12) Perez Ayuso RM, Arroyo V, Planas R, Gaya J, Bory F, Rimola A, Rivera F, Rodès J. Randomized comparative study of efficacy of furosemide versus spironolactone in non-azotemic cirrhosis with ascites. Relationship between the diuretic response and the activity of the renin-angiotensin-aldosterone-system. Gastroenterology 1983;84:961-968.

13) Bernardi M, Laffi G, Salvagnini M, Azzena G, Bonato S, Marra F, Trevisani F, et al. Efficacy and safety of the stepped care medical treatment of ascites in liver cirrhosis: a randomized controlled clinical trial comparing two diets with different sodium content. Liver 1993;13:156-162.

14) Weiner IM. Diuretics and other agents employed in the mobilization of edema fluid. In Gilman AG, Rall TW, Nies AS & Taylor P (eds): Goodman & Gilman's The pharmachological basis of therapeutics, 8th edn, pp 713-731. New York: Pergamon Press, 1990.

15) Laffi G, La Villa G, Carloni V, Foschi M, Bartoletti L, Quartini M, Gentilini P. Loop diuretic therapy in liver cirrhosis with ascites. J Cardiovasc Pharmacol 1993;22(3): S51-S58.

16) Lesne M. Comparison of the pharmacokinetics of torasemide and furosemide in healthy volunteers. Arzneimittelforschung 1988;38:160-163.

17) Laffi G, Marra F, Buzzelli GP, Azzena G, Meacci E, De Feo ML, La Villa G, Gentilini P. Comparison of the effects of torasemide and furosemide in nonazotemic cirrhotic patients with ascites: a randomized, double-blind study. Hepatology 1991;13:1101-1105.

18) Arroyo V, Ginès P, Gerbes AL, Dudley FJ, Gentilini P, Laffi G, Reynolds TB, et al. Definition and diagnostic criteria of refractory ascites and hepatorenal syndrome in cirrhosis. Hepatology 1996;23:164-176.

19) Pinzani M, Daskalopoulos G, Laffi G, Gentilini P, Zipser RD. Altered furosemide pharmacokinetics in chronic alcoholic liver disease with ascites contributes to diuretic resistance. Gastroenterology 1987;92:294-298.

(20) Gentilini P, La Villa G, Marra F, Carloni V, Melani L, Foschi M, Quartini M, et al. Pharmacokinetics and pharmacodynamics of torasemide and furosemide in patients with diuretic resistant ascites. J Hepatol 1996; in press.

21) Papadakis MA, Arieff AI. Unpredictability of clinical evaluation of renal function in cirrhosis. Am J Med 1987;82:945-952.

22) Ginès P, Arroyo V, Quintero E, Planas R, Bory F, Cabrera J, Rimola A, et al. Comparison of paracentesis and diuretics in the treatment of cirrhotics with tense ascites. Results of a randomized study. Gastroenterology 1987;93: 234-241.

23) Ginès P, Arroyo V, Vargas V, Planas R, Casafont F, Panes J, Hoyos M, et al. Paracentesis with infusion of albumin as compared with peritoneovenous shunting in cirrhosis with refractory ascites. N Engl J Med 1991;325:829-835.

24) Wong F, Blendis L. Transjugular intrahepatic portosystemic shunt for refractory ascites: tipping the sodium balance. Hepatology 1995;22:358-364.

25) Laffi G, Pinzani M, Meacci E, La Villa G, Renzi D, Baldi E, Cominelli F, et al. Renal hemodynamic and natriuretic effects of human atrial natriuretic factor infusion in cirrhosis with ascites. Gastroenterology 1989;96:167-177.

26) Laffi G, Marra F, Pinzani M, Meacci E, Tosti-Guerra C, De Feo ML, Gentilini P. Effects of repeated atrial natriuretic peptide bolus injections in cirrhotic patients with refractory ascites. Liver 1989;9:315-321.

27) Laffi G, La Villa G, Gentilini P. Hepatorenal syndrome pathogenesis and treatment. Seminars in Liver Diseases 1994;14:71-81.

28) Pinzani M, Laffi G, Meacci E, La Villa G, Cominelli F, Gentilini P: Intrarenal thromboxane A_2 generation reduces the furosemide-induced sodium and water diuresis in cirrhosis with ascites. Gastroenterology 1988;95:1081-1087.

29) Gentilini P, Laffi G, Meacci E, La Villa G, Cominelli F, Pinzani M, Buzzelli G. Effects of OKY 046, a thromboxane synthase inhibitor, on renal function in non-azotemic cirrhotic patients with ascites. Gastroenterology 1988;94:1470-1477.

30) Laffi G, Marra F, Carloni V, Azzena G, De Feo ML, Pinzani M, Tosti-Guerra C, Gentilini P. Thromboxane receptor blockade increases water diuresis in cirrhotic patients with ascites. Gastroenterology 1992;103:1017-1021.

31) Schrier RW, Arroyo V, Bernardi M, Epstein M, Henriksen JH, Rodès J. Peripheral vasodilation hypothesis: a proposal for the initiation of renal sodium and water retention in cirrhosis. Hepatology 1988;8:1151-1157.

32) Moller S, Bendtsen F, Henriksen JH. Effects of volume expansion on systemic hemodynamics and central and arterial blood volume in cirrhosis. Gastroenterology 1995;109:1927-1925.

CHAPTER 32

SPECTRAL EEG MONITORING OF HEPATIC ENCEPHALOPATHY.

P. AMODIO, F. DEL PICCOLO, A. GATTA.
SplenoEpatologia, University of Padova, Italy

SUMMARY
Automatic quantitative analysis of digital EEG tracing has given the opportunity to obtain more repeatable data. However, great care in technical details concerning EEG signal amplification, filtration, sampling and quantisation is mandatory. Also the technical features of spectral analysis of EEG tracing, a kind of quantitative analysis, need accurate standardisation to have comparable results. Correctly standardised spectral EEG monitoring of hepatic encephalopathy may give useful data in therapeutic trials.

Abnormalities of EEG tracing in hepatic encephalopathy are known since 1950, when Foley (1) described the slow high-voltage delta discharges in the EEG of patients with hepatic coma. In 1955, Bickford and Butt (2) showed a link between the clinical stages and the EEG findings in hepatic encephalopathy: they reported that theta activity is present in confused cirrhotic patients, whereas in more severe stages the so-called "triphasic waves" appear and, finally, delta rhythm follows in patients with deep coma. The authors emphasised the importance of "triphasic waves" which are similar to eyeblink artefact, but with a front-occipital delay. Triphasic waves are constituted by a deep downward (positive) deflection preceded and followed by low-amplitude upward (negative) deflections, giving the whole complex a triphasic contour. The "triphasic wave pattern" was later recognised to be an unspecific feature of metabolic encephalopathies (3, 4).

In 1957 Parsons-Smith et al. (5) clearly described and staged the EEG features of cirrhotic patients in comparison with mental and neurological conditions (tab. 1). The Parsons-Smith's classification, however, is merely qualitative, so that inter and possibly intra observers errors may limit its applicability.

Such a limit of Parsons-Smith's classification was clearly perceived, in fact the subsequent studies regarding the EEG signs of hepatic encephalopathy tried to provide some kinds of objective quantitation of EEG alterations.

At the beginning of the sixties, Laidlaw and Read (6) tried to quantify the dominant EEG frequency of cirrhotic patients and controls by a kind of

P. Gentilini and M. U. Dianzani. New Trends in Hepatology, 296-305

electronic wave analyser. Data were used to assess the sensitivity of these patients to morphine. Even if it was a pioneer work performed with an obsolete and not-well described technology, it clearly indicated the future developments of research: 1) the need to quantify the EEG signs of encephalopathy, 2) the need of quantitative EEG to explore pharmacodynamic properties of drugs used in hepatic encephalopathy.

Table 1: Parsons-Smith's grading of the EEG features in liver disease (5).

A:	Generalised suppression of the alpha rhythm and its frequent replacement by faster potentials in all leads.
B:	The alpha rhythm is very unstable and disturbed by random waves at 5-7 per sec. over both hemispheres. The rhythms are most often seen over the temporal lobes. In many cases there is an underlying fast activity.
C:	An alpha rhythm is still seen, but is disturbed over both hemispheres by medium-voltage 5-6 per sec. waves. The rhythms occur in runs, are not paroxysmal, and do not usually block to eye opening, though in some of the records blocking does occur. The rhythms are seen particularly well over the temporal and the frontal lobes.
D:	The 5-6 per sec rhythms seen in grade C are now constant in all areas and replace all other cortical activity recorded on the electroencephalogram.
E:	The 5-6 per sec. rhythms are replaced by frontally preponderant bilateral synchronous 2 per sec. rhythms which spread backwards over the hemispheres. At times the 6 per sec. rhythms may reappear.

Later, automatic quantitative analysis of EEG tracings performed with various kinds of technology were utilised in cirrhotic patients to assess the presence of latent encephalopathy by provocative or resolutive tests (7, 8).

The still used Conn's grading of EEG alterations in hepatic encephalopathy, which was proposed in the seventies (9), is a kind of quantitative classification based on the dominant frequency criterion (table 2).

Table 2: Conn's grading of EEG alterations in hepatic encephalopathy (10).

grade 0:	normal alpha rhythm: 8.5-12 Hz
grade 1:	7-8 Hz rhythm
grade 2:	5-7 Hz rhythm
grade 3:	3-5 Hz rhythm
grade 4:	≤ 3 Hz rhythm

It was the realisation that brain waves can be modelled as a (quasi-stationary) stochastic process which provided theoretical support for the mathematical analysis of EEG tracings. In this respect, a relevant contribution was given by the work of Cooley and Tekey (10) who developed the fast Fourier transform algorithm (FFT): a mathematical trick which allows rapid computer solutions to

the problem of Fourier analysis. This is a frequency-domain analysis translating wave form, which are voltage magnitudes as a function of time, into spectra, which are magnitudes as a function of frequency (fig 1).
This kind of conversion has its mathematical roots in the work of Baron Jean-Baptiste Joseph Fourier (1768-1830), who, studying ocean tides, discovered that any arbitrary wave form could be decomposed into a series of pure sine waves of different frequency, amplitude and phase.

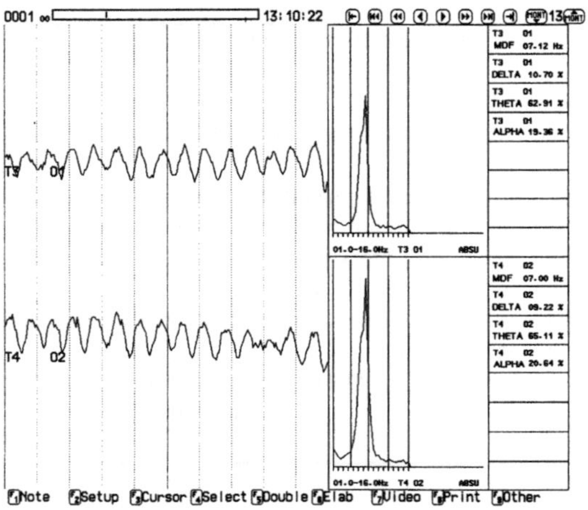

Figure 1: On the left the EEG signal is shown in function of time (conventional way). On the right the same signal is shown in function of frequency (spectral analysis). Frequency range 1-25.5 Hz, sampling rate 128 Hz, conversion resolution 400 μV/8 bits. Patient with mild hepatic encephalopathy. Recording in the SplenoEpatologia of the University of Padova. Equipment: Brain Quick, Micromed, Italy.

An example of this resolution is given by the rainbow, where light diffraction occurs, so that the single component colours (wavelength) of white light are visualised.
However, not only the theoretical achievements by Cooley and Tekey (10) were important, but also the technological developments permitting the transformation of the analogical continuous shape of EEG tracing into a series of discrete digits. This technological feature deserves to be considered for its importance in the evaluation of the quality of any quantitative EEG analysis which, obviously, first needs the digital conversion of EEG recording, assuming that an adequate EEG is performed with low impedence and without muscle contraction artefacts or sleeping effect.
There are three main steps to obtain digital data from EEG recording on the scalp:
1) signal amplification and filtration, 2) signal sampling, 3) signal quantitation.

Amplification. Amplification is common to all kinds of EEG equipment. It is needed to enhance 5,000-10,000 times the scalp EEG signals, ranging about tens μVolt, to the range of Volt, needed to the functioning of any electronic converting system. The amplification should be the most linear possible for the frequency range of 0.5-70 Hz which is important from a neurophysiologic point of view.
Eventually, another important feature of the acquisition system is filtration (i.e. the exclusion of the contribution of specific frequencies while preserving others), because the analogical signal to convert should not contain frequencies higher than half of the sampling frequency, for the reasons explained below.
Sampling. Sampling refers to the number of times the potential differences are measured in a second. It is a critical point of the process, because the reconstruction of a wave contour depends on the number of points describing such a wave. In detail, the reconstruction is not based on linear interpolation, but on the Shannon theorem which allows the exact reconstruction of the wave contour provided that sampling frequency is at least twice the wave frequency.
Quantisation. Signal quantisation refers to the number of discrete intervals (quanta) into which the sampled signal can be converted by the computer. The higher the number of intervals, the higher the measurement accuracy. The magnitude expressing the accuracy (conversion resolution) is given by the ratio of the maximal convertible signal (expressed in Volt) over the number of intervals (expressed in bits, i.e. 2^{bits}).
Once a reliable digital EEG is obtained, fractions of EEG tracing (called epochs) can be transformed by FFT as follows:

$$s(t)=\Sigma A_n \sin (ft + \phi_n) \quad (1)$$

where: s=signal; A= amplitude; f=wave frequency; ϕ= phase

The above equation means that at any time the signal is given by the sum of n pure sine waves of different frequency, amplitude and phase.
Spectral EEG analysis based on FFT has been extensively employed in the study of hepatic encephalopathy by van der Rijt et al. (11), in Rotterdam. They obtained the EEG tracing from temporo-occipital dipoles (T3-O1 and T4-O2), filtering signals at 25.6 Hz. The sampling frequency was 51.2 Hz, the conversion resolution 5 mV/11 bits. Spectral analysis in the frequency range 1-25.6 Hz was performed in a period of 100 sec. subdivided in ten epochs of 10 sec. each. Mean values of single estimates were automatically calculated. The neurophysiological parameters considered were: 1) the mean dominant frequency (MDF), 2) the relative powers of delta, theta and alpha rhythms, i.e. the percentage power of each rhythm over the power of the total frequency range analysed. Power, a

magnitude expressed as V^2, reflects the amplitude of EEG waves. Mean dominant frequency is a single value synthesising the overall EEG frequency. It is defined by the following equation:

$$MDF = \Sigma_i (f_i S_i) / \Sigma_i S_i \qquad (2)$$

where f_i= frequency i; S_i= power of frequency i

Analysing the EEG of 55 controls and 66 cirrhotic patients with hepatic encephalopathy ascertained and graded by two independent physicians, Van der Rijt et al. (11) found that MDF, at a cut-off of 6.4 Hz, clearly discriminate controls from cirrhotics with at least grade 2 hepatic encephalopathy (sensitivity 100% -$CI_{95\%}$=86-100%-, specificity 100% -$CI_{95\%}$=93-100%-). However, when MDF was higher than 6.4 Hz, it could not discriminate cirrhotics with grade 1 hepatic encephalopathy from those without encephalopathy, or controls. Moreover, no other cut-off lower than 6.4 Hz could be found to differentiate grade 2 from grades 3 and 4. On the other hand, a relative power of theta rhythm ≥ 35% was constantly found in grade 1 hepatic encephalopathy, and in 38% ($CI_{95\%}$=22-56%) of cirrhotics without overt hepatic encephalopathy. A relative power of delta rhythm ≥ 70% was found only in grades 3 and 4 hepatic encephalopathy with spectrum power which is ≥ 250 μV^2 in grade 3 hepatic encephalopathy (12).

Therefore, taking into account also the criterion of the percentages of the single rhythms, van der Rijt proposed a quantitative classification of EEG alterations in hepatic encephalopathy (tab 3) which maintained some features characterising Parsons-Smith's EEG classification which had been lost in those classifications based only on the criterion of the main EEG frequency, as, for instance, Conn's EEG grading of hepatic encephalopathy .

Table 3: Van der Rijt's grading of EEG alterations in hepatic encephalopathy based on spectral EEG analysis (12).

Grade	MDF (Hz)	theta %	delta %	Power (μV^2)
0	≥ 6.4	< 35		
1	≥ 6.4	≥35		
2	< 6.4		< 70	
3	< 6.4		≥ 70	≥250
4	< 6.4		≥ 70	<250

The various grades of hepatic encephalopathy identified by Van der Rijt's classification were later found to have predictive value on the survival of cirrhotic patients: studying 60 cirrhotic patients, the mortality within one year of grade 3-4 was 82%, that of grade 1-2 was 30% and that of grade 0 was about 27% (13).

There are 2 other points worth considering: 1) is spectral EEG analysis useful to detect and quantify mild and subclinical hepatic encephalopathy and, in particular, what is its value in comparison with evoked potentials and event related responses? 2) does quantified EEG analysis give more repeatable information than visual EEG reading? Few studies considered these points.

In 1987 Levy et al. (14) studied 49 cirrhotic patients without overt hepatic encephalopathy to compare the prevalence of central nervous system dysfunction detected by flash evoked VEP, spectral EEG analysis according to Van der Rijt and NCT. They found significant prolongation of N3 latency in 29% ($CI_{95\%}$=17-43%) of cirrhotics, whereas the relative power of theta wave was increased (>35%) in 10% ($CI_{95\%}$=3-22%) of them. All patients with increased theta wave power had also an increased N3 latency. However, no technical information of EEG recording and analysis was given. Moreover, the use of N3 latency to evaluate VEP is questionable and the prevalence of cirrhotic patients with increased theta wave relative power was lower than that reported in an unselected cirrhotic population without overt hepatic encephalopathy by Van der Rijt et al. (11) and also by us (15, 16): 38% ($CI_{95\%}$=22-56%) and 31% ($CI_{95\%}$=16-50%), respectively. We found a prevalence closer to that by neuropsychological tools (17, 18).

Weissenborn et al. (19), studying cirrhotic patients with and without mild encephalopathy, compared the prevalence of positive results obtained by visual EEG reading, automatic spectral analysis, inverse pattern VEP, P300 elicited by the auditory oddball paradigm, simple reaction times and neuropsychological examination. Two main messages came from this study: 1) spectral EEG analysis did not seem to be better than visual EEG reading, 2) VEP and P300 had a greater sensitivity to detect mild encephalopathy. However, also this study did not describe how spectral EEG analysis was performed. Only a few patients were enrolled for the comparison with spectral EEG. The prevalence of positive results was low (18% $CI_{95\%}$=4-46%), the comparison with visual EEG reading was not blind, and criteria to define encephalopathy were unusual. Moreover, in the past quantitative EEG analysis was found more sensitive than visual reading to evaluate dietetic manipulation in cirrhotic patients (20).

Davies et al. (21) compared EEG spectral analysis with P300 and flash evoked VEP in 32 cirrhotics with or without mild hepatic encephalopathy. However, they used neither the dipoles of the original Van der Rijt's method, nor the same epochs, nor the same grading criteria. Therefore, no conclusion is possible, because changing technical features of spectral analysis may have sensitive effects: table 4 shows the unsatisfactory diagnostic agreement (K=0.47) of EEG spectral analysis performed with the same equipment in 2 different brain areas in 48 cirrhotic patients using Van der Rijt's classification (unpublished data).

Table 4: Diagnostic agreement applying the same criteria between spectral analysis performed in 2 different brain areas (temporo-occipital: mean values of T3-O1 and T4-O2 vs. frontal: mean values of F3-F7 and F4-F8). Analysis performed on the same recordings in 48 cirrhotic patients. Sampling rate 128 Hz, conversion resolution 400 μV/8 bit, frequency range 1-25.5 Hz, analysis of a period of 50 epochs of 2 sec. each. Equipment: Brain Quick, Micromed, Italy

		Temporo occipital recording (T3-O1,T4-O2)		
Frontal	**Grade**	**0**	**I**	**II**
recording	**0**	20	8	1
(F3-F7,	**I**	0	10	2
F4-F8)	**II**	3	1	3

Such low agreement was not due to an intrinsic low repeatability of spectral analysis, because the comparison of the original Van der Rijt' method with another one working on the same brain areas showed enough agreement (K=0.86, Tab 5).

An indirect comparison between various neurophysiological and psychometric tools is given by the research of Higuchi et al. (22) concerning the effect of branched chain amino acid infusion on CNS: the variation of spectral analysis was higher than that of VEP and P300. Such an experiment, though performed in a small group of patients, suggests that spectral analysis may be at least as useful as evoked potentials in therapeutic trials to monitor mild encephalopathy.

Table 5: Diagnostic agreement applying between spectral analysis performed on the same brain areas (temporo-occipital: mean values of T3-O1 and T4-O2) with 2 methods: A) frequency range 1-25.5 Hz, sampling rate 56 Hz, conversion resolution 5mV/11 bits, period of 100 sec. subdivided in 10 epochs of 10 sec. each; B) frequency range 1-25.5 Hz, sampling rate 128 Hz, conversion resolution 400 μV/8 bit, period of 100 sec. subdivided in 50 epochs of 2 sec. each. Analysis performed on the same recordings in 48 cirrhotic. Equipment: Brain Quick, Micromed, Italy

		Method A		
Method	**Grade**	**0**	**I**	**II**
B	**0**	23	0	0
	I	1	16	2
	II	0	1	5

Considering all this, a direct comparison of accurately described neurophysiological tools is needed in hepatic encephalopathy (23).

Recently, neuropsychological evaluation based on reaction times and accuracy measured by computerised psychometric tests was found to be linked to MDF and theta wave relative power measured by EEG spectral analysis (16).

In conclusion, quantitative EEG evaluation by spectral analysis seems to be an useful tool for quantifying central nervous system dysfunction in liver cirrhosis and monitoring dietetic and pharmacological effects, however accurate description of the applied techniques is mandatory to achieve comparable and repeatable data.

Acknowledgment: We thank Prof. S.W. Schalm (Internal Medicine II University of Rotterdam) for the cooperation in spectral analysis research and for the comments on this paper.

REFERENCES

1) Foley, J.M., Watson, C.W., Adams, R.D. (1950) Significance of the electroencephalographic changes in hepatic coma, Tr. Am. Neurol. Ass. 75, 161-165

2) Bickford, R.G., Butt, H.R. (1955) Hepatic coma: the electroencephalographic pattern, J. Clin. Invest. 34, 790-99.

3) Fisch, B.J., Klass, D.W (1988) The diagnostic specificity of triphasic wave patterns, Electroencephal. Clin. Neuroph. 70, 1-8.

4) Tyner F.S., Knott J.R., Brem Mayer W Jr.(1989): Fundamentals of EEG technology, Raven Press, New York, vol II pp. 183-197.

5) Parsons-Smith, B.G., Summerskill, W.H.J., Dawson, A.M., Sherlock, S. (1957) The electroencephalograph in liver disease, Lancet 2, 867-871.

6) Laidlaw, J., Read, A.E. (1961) The electroencephalographic diagnosis of manifest and latent "delirium" with particular reference to that complicating hepatic cirrhosis, J. Neurol. Neurosurg. Psychiat. 24: 58-70.

7) Cohn, R., Castell, D.O. (1966) The effect of acute hyperammoniemia on the electroencephalogram, J. Lab. Clin. Med. 68: 195-205.

8) Hawkes, C.H., Brunt, P.W., Prescott R.J., Horn, D.B. (1973) EEG-provocative tests in the diagnosis of hepatic encephalopathy, Electroenceph. clin. Neurophysiol. 34: 163-169.

9) Conn, H.O., Leevy, C.M., Vlahcevic, Z.R., Rodgers, J.B., Maddrey, W.C., Seeff, L., Levy, L.L. (1977) Comparison of lactulose and neomicin in the treatment of chronic portal-systemic encephalopathy, Gastroenterology, 72: 573-583.

10) Cooley, J.W., Tukey, J.W. (1965) An algorithm for the machine calculation of complex Fourire series, Math. Comput. 19: 297-301.

11) Van der Rijt, C.D.C., Schalm, S.W., De Groot, G.H., De Vlieger, M. (1984) Objective measurement of hepatic encephalopathy by means of automated EEG analysis, Electroenceph. Clin. Neuroph. 57, 423-426.

12) Van der Rijt, C.D.C., Schalm, S.W. (1991): Spectral analysis in hepatic encephalopathy. In A. Bengtsson, B. Jeppsson, TH. Almdal, H. Vilstrup (eds), Progress in hepatic encephalopathy and metabolic nitrogen exchange, CRC Press, Boca Raton (USA), 1991. pp: 59-66.

13) Van der Rijt, C.D.C., Schalm, S.W. (1985) Quantitative EEG analysis and survival in liver disease, Electroenceph. Clin. Neuroph. 61, 502-504.

14) Levy, L.J., Bolton, R.P., Losowsky, M.S. (1987) The use of the visual evoked potential (VEP) in delineating a state of subclinical encephalopathy. A comparison with the number connection test (NCT). J. Hepatol. 5: 211-217.

15) Del Piccolo, F., Quero, J.Q., Amodio, P., Gatta, A., Schalm, S.W. (1995) Comparison between computerized psychometric tests (CPTs) and EEG spectral analysis (s-EEG) in subclinical hepatic encephalopathy, J. Hepatol. 23, suppl. 1, 122.

16) Amodio, P., Quero, J.Q, Del Piccolo, F., Gatta, A., Schalm, S.W. (1996) Diagnostic tools for the detection of subclinical hepatic encephalopathy: comparison of standard and computerized psychometric tests with spectral-EEG. Metab. Brain Dis. (In press)

17) Amodio, P., Del Piccolo, F., Marchetti, P., Merkel, C., Caregaro, L., Sacerdoti, D., Angli, P., Gatta, A (1995) Comparison of computer-based psychometric tests and number connection test in the detection of subclinical hepatic encephalopathy, in L. Capocaccia, M. Merli, O. Riggio (eds), Advances in Hepatic Encephalopathy and Metabolic Nitrogen Exchange, CRC Press, Boca Raton (USA), 1995. pp: 390-94.

18) Amodio, P., Marchetti, P., Del Piccolo, F., Sartori, G., Prior, M., Merkel, C., Gatta, A. (1995) Visual attention orienting in liver cirrhosis without overt hepatic encephalopathy. Metab. Brain Dis. 10: 335-343.

19) Weissenborn, K., Scholz, M., Hinrichs, H., Wiltfang, J., Schmidt, F.W., Künkel, H. (1990) Neurophysiological assessment of early hepatic encephalopathy, Electroenceph. Clin. Neuroph. 75: 289-295.

20) De Bruijn, K. M., Blendis, L.M., Zilm, D.H., Carlen, P.L., Anderson, G.H. (1983) Effect of dietary protein manipulations in subclinical portal-systemic encephalopathy, Gut 24:53-60.

21) Davies, M.G., Rowan, M.J, MacMathuna, P., Keeling, N.P.W., Weir, D.G., Feely, J. (1990) The auditory P300 event-related potential: an objective marker of the encephalopathy of chronic liver disease, Hepatology; 12: 688-694.

22) Higuchi, K., Shimizu, Y., Nambu, S, Miyabayashi, C., Takahara, T., Saito, S., Hioki, O., Kuwabara, Y., Watanabe, A. (1994) Effects of an infused of branched-chain amino acids on

neurophysiological and psychometric testing in cirrhotic patients with mild hepatic encephalopathy, J. Gastroenterol. Hepatol. 9: 366-375.

23) Van der Rijt C.C.D., Schalm S.W. (1992) Quantitative analysis and evoked potentials to measure (latent) hepatic encephalopathy, J. Hepatol. 14: 141-142.

CHAPTER 33

INTERACTION BETWEEN NON STEROIDAL ANTIINFLAMMATORY DRUGS AND INTERFERON-α SYSTEM: MECHANISMS AND BASIS FOR THE CLINICAL USE IN THE TREATMENT OF CHRONIC VIRAL HEPATITIS.

P. ANDREONE, A. GRAMENZI, C. CURSARO, F. FELLINE, G. GASBARRINI[1], M. BERNARDI.

Patologia Medica I, Università di Bologna; [1]Clinica Medica, Università Cattolica del Sacro Cuore, Roma; Italy.

SUMMARY

The mechanisms by which IFNs induce the activation of related genes are not completely understood. Increasing evidence indicates that metabolites of arachidonic acid may act as IFN second messengers. Several studies have hypothesized a defective antiviral and immune response in patients with acute or chronic viral hepatitis. Recently, *in vitro* and *in vivo* studies showed that inhibitors of cyclooxygenase pathway of arachidonic acid (non steroidal antiinflammatory drugs) are able to amplify both the antiviral and immune response induced by IFN-α. These findings may represent the basis to evaluate the efficacy of combined therapy, IFN-α plus non steroidal antiinflammatory drugs, in chronic viral hepatitis.

Interferons (IFNs) are proteins produced and secreted by cells in response to viruses, bacteria, foreign cells, foreign macromolecules, and other compounds. There are three known types of interferon (α, β and γ), that once produced, induce antiviral, antimicrobial, antitumor, and immunomodulatory actions. The cellular response to IFNs depends on the reaction with specific receptors on cell surfaces to activate cytoplasmic signals that enter the nucleus to stimulate cellular genes

P. Gentilini and M. U. Dianzani. New Trends in Hepatology, 306-314

encoding a number of proteins which carry out a defensive action. IFNs may also enhance immune responses by increasing expression of lymphocyte surface antigens and by increasing the cytotoxic activity of natural killer cells (1). The important role played by IFN as a natural defense against viruses is documented by a number of experimental and clinical observations (1). The role of IFNs during different virus infections varies. Much depends on the effectiveness of the virus in stimulating IFN production and on the susceptibility of the virus to the antiviral action of IFN. The high biological activity of IFNs has represented a new therapeutic approach for the treatment of viral infections. To be therapeutically effective in viral infections, IFN has to be given at concentrations exceeding those endogenously produced. For this reason, chronic viral infections, when little or no endogenous IFN is produced (1), are better targets.

IFN-α was the first IFN to be utilized in the treatment of chronic viral hepatitis in 1976 (2). Today, IFN-α is the only agent of proven efficacy in the treatment of both chronic hepatitis B (HBV) and C (HCV). However, even with a prolonged course, IFN-α therapy is not straightforward: a durable response occurs in only 20-40% and 15% of HBV and HCV-infected patients respectively, and it appears that eradication of the infection is unusual in most patients (3, 4). The cause of the resistance to exogenous IFN-α is unknown, but it might be the result of defects in the IFN-α response at several levels along the pathway. At least for HBV infection, patients seem to have lower levels of IFN-α, 2',5'-oligoadenylate synthetase (an IFN-induced antiviral enzyme) and IFN-γ (5-7), suggesting a reduced antiviral response or the possible release of inhibitory factors. Among the immunosuppressive factors, prostaglandin E_2 (PGE_2), an arachidonic acid metabolite through the cyclooxygenase pathway, seems to play an important role due to its ability to reduce lymphokine function (8), decrease antigen- and mitogen-induced lymphocyte proliferation (9) and class Ia and class II MHC expression *in vitro* (10, 11). Thus, it may constitute a negative feedback mechanism for regulating the extent and duration of cellular immune reactions.

Evidence of immunosuppressive activity of PGs has also been demonstrated in viral liver diseases. In a previous study, we demonstrated an increase of plasma levels of bicyclo-PGE_2 (a stable metabolite of PGE_2) concentration during the acute phase of type A, B and non-A, non-B viral hepatitis (12). Interestingly, after the acute phase, serum levels dropped to normal values only in patients with viral hepatitis A, while they remained high in patients with hepatitis B or non-A, non-B. This finding suggested a putative role of this PG in the mechanism of chronicity.

Further evidence of immunosuppressive activity of PGs came from the study of Sinclair et al (13). They *in vivo* documented that the intravenous infusion of PGE_1 dramatically improves the survival of acute fulminant viral hepatitis, a disease characterized by an exaggerated host immune response to the virus.

IFNs and IFN inducers have been shown to be able to stimulate PG production (14, 15), and a uniform relationship between IFN induction and cellular PG synthesis in virus-infected cell cultures was observed (16). Fuji et al. reported an increased IFN-γ release by peripheral blood mononuclear cells (PBMCs) cultured with indomethacin in patients with chronic hepatitis (7). Furthermore, we found an increased PGE_2 synthesis by PBMCs of patients with acute hepatitis B during the first 2 weeks of the disease (17). In the same study IFN-γ production was not enhanced, suggesting that PGE_2 might play an inhibitory role on IFN-γ synthesis.

In spite of great progress in IFN research, the molecular mechanism underlying the mainfold actions of IFN-α remain poorly understood. The detailed mechanisms whereby signal transduction in IFN-treated cells leads to the transcriptional induction of specific genes have yet to be resolved. The signal transduction pathway is undoubtedly complex, and it is likely that a number of overlapping pathways are involved. In 1991, Hannigan and Williams demonstrated that exposure of cultured fibroblasts to IFN-α results in hydrolysis of phosphatidylcholine by phospholipase A_2 to release arachidonic acid (18). It is well known that arachidonic acid is metabolized by cyclooxygenase to PGs or by lipoxygenase to leukotrienes that might act as second messengers. Hannigan and Williams found that metabolites of arachidonic acid by enzymes other than cyclooxygenase or lipoxygenase are the specific IFN-associated eicosanoid second messengers. One possible path is arachidonic acid metabolism by way of the epoxygenase enzyme family. Interestingly, they demonstrated an enhanced production of 2',5'-oligoadenylate synthetase (2-5OAS) by cultured fibroblasts incubated with inhibitors of the cyclooxygenase (indomethacin) or the lipoxygenase (nordihydroguaiaretic acid) pathways (18). Previous observations demonstrated that indomethacin was also able to *in vitro* enhance the immune response increasing IFN-γ production (19). To confirm these observations obtained in cultured fibroblasts, we evaluated PGE_2 production by cultured liver specimens of patients with chronic viral hepatitis (20, 21). We found that PGE_2 synthesis was significantly increased in the presence of IFN-α but not in the presence of IFN-α plus indomethacin. Furthermore, we showed that indomethacin resulted more efficacious than IFN-α in increasing 2-5OAS production by liver tissue of patients with active HCV infection. Interestingly, incubation of liver tissue in the presence of IFN-α plus indomethacin determined a significant increase of the enzyme suggesting a synergistic effect of the two drugs. These data were also confirmed *in vivo* in patients with viral chronic hepatitis after the acute administration of IFN-α, indomethacin and IFN-α plus indomethacin (22). Compared to pretreatment values, we found that indomethacin alone was able to triple endogenous 2-5OAS production, IFN-α alone led to only a 1.5-fold increase, whereas the association of the two drugs led to a 4-fold increase. In cultured fibroblasts, Hannigan and Williams demonstrated that IFN-α plus indomethacin produced three times as much 2-5OAS to that obtained with IFN-α alone, while indomethacin alone was half as efficacious as IFN-α alone in stimulating 2-5OAS (18). The apparent discrepancy with our results could be ascribed to the antiviral status of our patients conditioning a basal activity of IFN-α system. This hypothesis had been previously suggested by the finding that, compared to HCV-positive patients, 2-5OAS in cultured liver biopsies of uninfected subjects was not enhanced by indomethacin (21).

To further investigate the relation between IFN-α and PGs, we are evaluating the effect of cyclooxygenase pathway inhibition on 2-5OAS and IL-2 synthesis by PBMCs of patients with chronic viral hepatitis (Andreone P, et al; unpublished data). Our preliminary results confirm the ability of indomethacin alone or, even more, associated with IFN-α to enhance the antiviral response indirectly assessed by 2-5OAS synthesis. Concerning the immune response, the production of IL-2 seems to be greatly increased when PBMCs are incubated with IFN-α plus indomethacin.

In addition to its ability to expand activated T lymphocytes and directly activate killer activities (23, 24), IL-2 also modulates and augments natural killer cell activity (25), enhances antibody-dependent cellular cytotoxicity (26) and induces IFN-γ (27). Therefore, IL-2 synthesis could be particularly relevant in HBV infections in which an impaired immune response has been described (7). Any effective therapeutic approach for HBV chronic liver disease should also be able to modulate the immune response. In fact, the use of drugs exhibiting only an antiviral action (3) has demonstrated no efficacy in inducing HBV clearance. Concerning HCV infection, although the pathogenetic mechanism of liver damage is still unclear, it could be hypothesized that enhancing T-cell response might be critical in keeping the infection under control by the immune system.

All these data strongly suggest a complex interaction between arachidonic acid metabolites and the IFN system and seem to indicate that non steroidal antiinflammatory drugs may act as amplifiers of IFN-α antiviral and immune response (Figure 1), supporting the possibility of a combined therapy in chronic viral hepatitis. Previous experiences showed that PG inhibitors appear to enhance antitumor efficacy of immunotherapy with IFN-α or IL-2 in murine models of pulmonary metastases (28, 29). Clinically, the superiority of combined therapy IFN-α plus NSAIDs compared to IFN-α alone has been demonstrated in patients with metastatic melanoma (30) and advanced renal cancer (31).

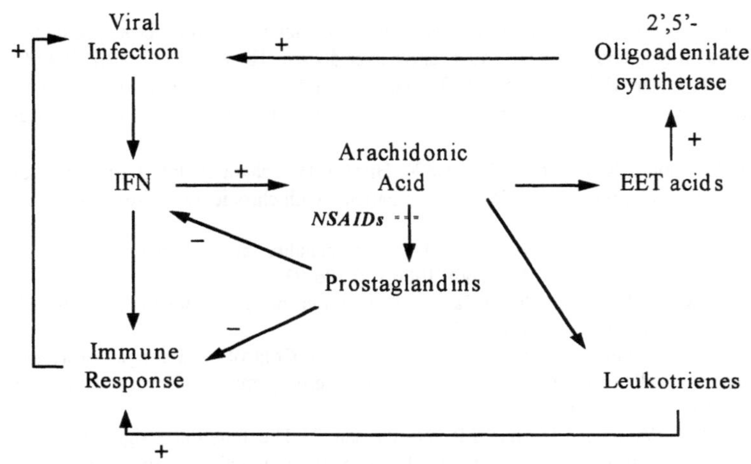

Figure 1: Possible interactions between IFN and Arachidonic Acid metabolites in viral infections

In conclusion, based on this strong evidence, we believe that the efficacy of a combined therapy of IFN-α plus NSAIDs should be evaluated for the treatment of chronic viral hepatitis, at least for patients not responding to conventional treatment, as previously suggested (20, 32, 33). However, the tolerability of such adjuvant therapy in the treatment of patients with liver diseases should be carefully evaluated, since hepatic, gastrointestinal and renal toxic effects of these drugs are possible.

References

1. Dianzani F, Antonelli G., Capobianchi MR. The biological basis for clinical use of interferon. J Hepatol. 1990;11:S5-S10.
2. Greenberg HB, Pollard RB, Lutwick LI, Gregory PB, Robinson WS, Merigan TC. Effect of human leukocyte interferon in hepatitis B virus infection in patients with chronic active hepatitis. New Engl J Med. 1976;295:517-22.
3. Lok ASF. Treatment of chronic hepatitis B. J Vir Hepatitis. 1994;1:105-24.
4. Fried MW, Hoofnagle JH. Therapy of Hepatitis C. Seminars in liver disease. 1995;15:82-91.
5. Kato Y, Nakagawa H, Kobayashi K, Hatori N, Hatano K. Interferon production by peripheral lymphocytes in HBsAg-positive liver disease. Hepatology. 1982;2:789-90.
6. Ikeda T, Lever AML, Thomas HC. Evidence for a deficiency of interferon production in patients with chronic hepatitis B virus infection acquired in adult life. Hepatology. 1986;6:962-5.
7. Fuji A, Shinichi K, Ohtani Y, Murase K, Hirofuji H, Tahara H. Interferon-γ production by peripheral blood mononuclear cells of patients with chronic liver disease. Hepatology. 1987;7:577-81.
8. Kunkel SL, Chensue SW, Phan SH. Prostaglandins as endogenous mediators of interleukin 1 production. J Immunol. 1986;136:186-92.
9. Leung KH, Mihich E. Prostaglandin modulation of development of cell-mediated immunity in culture. Nature. 1980;288:597-600.
10. Papiernik M, Dombrei H, Stefanos S, Wietzerbin J. Control of Ia antigen expression on phagocytic cells of the thymic reticulum by interferon gamma and prostaglandins. Eur J Immunol. 1986;16:296-300.
11. Tripp CS, Wyche A, Unanue ER, Needleman P. The functional significance of the regluation of macrophage Ia expression by endogenous arachidonate metabolites in vitro. J Immunol. 1986;137:3915-20.
12. Andreone P, Baraldini M, Verucchi G, Gelati G, Chiodo F, Gasbarrini G. Prostaglandin E_2 metabolite rise in acute viral hepatitis. Dig Dis Sci. 1986;10:90.
13. Sinclair SB, Greig PD, Blendis LM, Abecassis M, Roberts EA, Phillips MJ, Cameron R, Levy GA. Biochemical and clinical response of fulminant viral hepatitis to administration of prostaglandin E. J Clin Invest. 1989;84:1063-9.
14. Yaron M, Yaron I, Gurari-Rotman D, Revel M, Lindner HR, Zor U. Stimulation of prostaglandin E production in cultured human fibroblasts by poly(I)-poly(C) and human interferon. Nature. 1977;267:457-9.

15. Fuse A, Mahmud I, Kuwata T. Mechanism of stimulation by human interferon of prostaglandin synthesis in human cell lines. Cancer Res. 1982;42:3209-14.
16. Fitzpatrick FA, Stringfellow DA. Virus and interferon effects on cellular prostaglandin biosynthesis. J Immunol. 1980;124:431-7.
17. Baraldini M, Andreone P, Cursaro C, Pasini P, Verucchi G, Mazzetti M, Stefanini GF, Gasbarrini G. Role of prostaglandin E_2 on defective interferon-γ production during type B acute viral hepatitis. Res Clin Lab. 1991;21:111-7.
18. Hannigan GE, Williams BRG. Signal transduction by Interferon-α through arachidonic acid metabolism. Science. 1991;251:204-7.
19. Vervliet G, Deckmyn H, Carton H, Billeau A. Influence of prostaglandin E2 and indomethacin on interferon gamma production by peripheral blood leukocytes of multiple sclerosis patients and health donors. J Clin Immunol. 1985;5:102-8.
20. Andreone P, Cursaro C, Gasbarrini G. Interferon-α increases prostaglandin E2 production by cultured liver biopsy in patients with chronic viral hepatitis: can non-steroidal anti-inflammatory drugs improve the therapeutic response to interferon?. J Hepatol. 1993;19:228-31.
21. Andreone P, Cursaro C, Gramenzi A, Buzzi A, Miniero R, Bernardi M, Gasbarrini G. Indomethacin increases 2',5'-oligoadenylate synthetase release by cultured liver tissue of patients with HCV chronic active hepatitis. Int Hepatol Comm. 1994;2:289-94.
22. Andreone P, Cursaro C, Gramenzi A, Buzzi A, Miniero R, Sprovieri G, Gasbarrini G. Indomethacin enhances 2'5'-oligoadenylate synthetase in patients with hepatitis B and C virus chronic active hepatitis. J Hepatol. 1994;21:984-8.
23. Morgan DA, Ruscetti FM, Gallo RC. Selective in vitro growth of T lymphocytes from human bone marrows. Science.1976;193:1007-8.
24. Lotze MT, Grimm EA, Mazumder A, Strausser JL, Rosenberg SA. In vitro growth of cytotoxic human lymphocytes: IV lysis of fresh and autologous tumor of lymphocytes cultured in T-cell growth factor. Cancer Res. 1981;41:4420-5.
25. Rosenberg SA, Speiss PJ, Scwartz S. In vivo administration of interleukin-2 enhances specific alloimmune responses. Trasplantation. 1983;35:631-4.
26. Smith KA. Interleukin-2: inception, impact and implications. Science. 1988;240:1169-76.
27. Reem GH, Yeh NH. Interleukin 2 regulates expression of its receptor and synthesis of gamma interferon by human T lymphocytes. Science. 1984;255:429-30.
28. Lala P, Parhar R. Cure of B16F10 melanoma lung metastasis in mice by chronic indomethacin therapy combined with repeated rounds of interleukin-2: characteristics of killer cells generated in situ. Cancer Res. 1988;48:1072-9.
29. Kim B, Warnaka P. Indomethacin-enhanced immunotherapy of pulmonary metastases using IL-2 and IFN-α. Surgery. 1989;106:248-56.
30. McKnight J, Clark J, Miller R. Randomized trial of recombinant interferon alpha with OP without indomethacin in patients with metastatic malignant melanoma (Abstract). Proc Annu Meet Am Soc Clin Oncol. 1987;6:PA983.
31. Creagan ET, Buckner JC, Hahn RG, Richardson RR, Schaid DJ, Kovach JS. An evaluation of recombinant leukocyte α interferon with aspirin in patients with metastatic renal cell cancer. Cancer. 1988;61:1787-91.
32. Baskin G. Interferon signalling through arachidonic acid dependent pathway: a clue to adjuvant therapy for chronic viral hepatitis?. Hepatology. 1991;14:392-4.

33. Andreone P, Cursaro C, Gasbarrini G. Interferon-α therapy combined with nonsteroiantiinflammatory drugs for treatment of chronic viral hepatitis?. Hepatology. 1992;16:505.

CHAPTER 34

PHARMACOLOGICAL TREATMENT OF PRIMARY BILIARY CIRRHOSIS

ENRICO RODA, ALESSANDRO PEZZOLI, PIETRO FUSAROLI, CARLO FABBRI, ESTERITA ACCOGLI, ANNA MARIA CIRIACI, ANTONIO CIPOLLA AND GIUSEPPE MAZZELLA.

Dipartimento di Medicina Interna e Gastroenterologia - Cattedra di Gastroenterologia-Ospedale S. Orsola - Bologna - Italy

Summary

Primary biliary cirrhosis (PBC) is a rare hepatic disorder, but its incidence is increasing. It is chronic and progressive, eventually leading to the development of cirrhosis. During the course of the disease, symptoms such as pruritus and asthenia may appear. At present, the only successful treatment for PBC is liver transplantation. While no pharmaceutical treatment is truly effective, some newer drugs, or new combinations of these drugs, have given some promising results. In this chapter, the efficacy of the more important pharmacological agents in use, as well as some currently under study, are examined in terms of laboratory parameters, symptoms, end points, histological presentation and natural history of the disease.

INTRODUCTION

Primary biliary cirrhosis is a chronic non-suppurative inflammation of the intrahepatic bile ducts (cholangitis) that usually leads to the development of liver cirrhosis and, eventually, its complications (1). The etiology of the disease is unknown, but there is considerable evidence that immune mechanisms play a major role, with the primary pathological mechanism supposedly being an attack on components of the bile duct epithelium that are perceived as antigens by cytotoxic T-lymphocytes (2, 3).

The disease occurs much more frequently in females (male/female ratio 1/9), and peak incidence is observed in middle age. Diagnosis is hampered by the fact that early stages of the disease are asymptomatic. Fatigue and pruritus are

P. Gentilini and M. U. Dianzani. New Trends in Hepatology, 315-325

the usual presenting symptoms, whereas jaundice and portal hypertension develop later. Liver function tests (LFT) typically demonstrate a cholestatic pattern, i.e. elevation of alkaline phosphatase and gamma-glutamyl transpeptidase; but for diagnosis, circulating antimitochondrial antibodies and a high titre of IgM antibody are required.

During the past 15 years numerous drugs have been evaluated for use in the treatment of PBC. Anti-inflammatory, immunosuppressive and anti-cholestatic agents alone, or in combination, have been tested in controlled trials, but none has been proven effective in terms of improvement in liver histology, delay or prevention of portal hypertension, survival or time to transplantation. For assessing their efficacy, the following parameters have been proposed as criteria for treatment-induced remission (4): amelioration of pruritus and fatigue, with return to normal life-style; serum alkaline phosphatase level ≤ 1.5 times the upper normal limit; and normalization of ALT, bilirubin, and circulating IgM. Serum ALT concentration is an indicator of hepatic inflammation, IgM levels, of immunological activity, whereas serum bilirubin is the most important prognostic factor. Histological remission is characterised by the clearance of inflammatory cells from the portal tract and by a cessation of bile duct destruction. Some histological features, however, such as destruction of the biliary tree, are not reversible despite remission of the inflammatory process; this fact is reflected in the persistence of moderately elevated alkaline phosphatase levels even when other humoral factors may have normalized.

Considering the chronic nature of PBC, any medical treatment taken into consideration must be suitable for long-term use. Drugs with a high incidence of side-effects or that may impair vital organs, thus precluding future liver transplantation, cannot be utilized.

CLINICAL EFFICACY OF DRUG THERAPY

Immunosuppressive drugs

Corticosteroids

Corticosteroids were proposed for the treatment of PBC after good results were seen in autoimmune hepatitis. The most important studies were carried out by Mitchison et al: in a controlled trial reported by these authors in 1989 (5), 19 patients were treated with 30 mg q.d. of prednisolone for two months, followed by a dose of 10 mg q.d. for 10 months; treatment resulted in improvement of symptoms, liver function tests and IgG levels, and in some cases there was histological improvement with reduction in procollagen III, an indicator of fibrosis. Treatment with prednisolone, however, was also associated with increased bone loss equal to approximately twice the rate observed in the control group, even though all patients received calcium and vitamin D supplements. Bone loss appeared to be greater in the first two months of treatment,when the higher dosage was used. Three years later Mitchison published the results of two further years of follow-up (6) in these same patients: improvement in laboratory findings and symptoms continued throughout the follow-up period, and circulating levels of antimitochondrial antibodies were reduced. Statistical analysis of histological changes at biopsy was not done because of the small number performed; nonetheless, a definite trend towards delayed progression of the disease was observed. Although bone mineral density studies revealed greater bone loss in treated subjects, the differences between treated and untreated PBC subjects or patients having other diseases requiring treatment with corticosteroids were not significant (7, 8). The addition of calcium and vitamin D to the diet and, as has been more recently suggested by Reid et al (9), administration of biphosphonates, may be useful in the prevention of steroid-induced bone loss.

Azathioprine

Azathioprine is an immunosuppressive agent frequently used to prevent allograft rejection. Heathcote (10) was the first to report the use of azathioprine in PBC: 22 patients received this drug, and 23 controls did not; among those treated there was a reduction of pruritus, but no significant differences were observed in liver function test results. While serial liver biopsies showed that 50% of the patients in the control group and 62% in the treated group progressed to cirrhosis in two years, survival analysis after 3 years of follow-up demonstrated a slight trend toward improved survival in the azathioprine-treated group. In another study published in 1985 (11) on 248 patients of whom 127 received azathioprine and 121 placebo, preliminary results suggested that the drug had no effect on symptoms, immunological abnormalities or hepatic histology. However, after taking into consideration an imbalance of disease severity between the groups, the authors (12) found that azathioprine reduced the risk of death to 59% of that observed with placebo treatment. Few side effects have been reported with the use of this drug.

Cyclosporin

The use of cyclosporin in PBC has been reported in a few studies. This agent, known to influence T-lymphocyte-mediated immune response, appears to improve symptoms and biochemical abnormalities. One study reported no histologically evident effect (13), whereas the other (14) indicated that cyclosporin might delay histological progression. Recently, Lombard et al (15), by multi-variate analysis, showed improvement of survival rates in patients treated with cyclosporin, and also postulated that immunosuppressive agents are likely to be of most benefit when the disease is treated in its early stages.

Long-term use of this drug may cause structural and potentially irreversible changes in renal morphology (16); while nephrotoxicity is the most frequent and dangerous side-effect (17), in this last-mentioned study, significant renal impairment occurred in less than 10% of the patients.

Chlorambucil

Chlorambucil is an alkylating agent that has been shown to have a beneficial effect in the treatment of leukemia and some autoimmune diseases. In the only controlled trial performed in patients with PBC (18), chlorambucil improved hepatic biochemistry, but no effect was seen on the histological presentation. Survival was not analyzed and bone marrow toxicity in 4 of the 13 treated patients precluded further use of the drug.

Methotrexate

Methotrexate is a folic acid antagonist used in the treatment of some types of tumors, psoriasis, and rheumatoid arthritis. Kaplan tested this drug (19) in an uncontrolled study on 9 PBC patients, all of whom were symptomatic and in a pre-cirrhotic stage. Methotrexate was given at a dosage of 15 mg/week for 12-34 months. Symptoms lessened or disappeared, and alkaline phosphatase, bilirubin, and cholesterol decreased in all patients. In addition, the titre of antimitocondrial antibody decreased in seven patients. Alanine and aspartate aminotransferase increased in the first few months (< 6) after starting methotrexate, but eventually fell below baseline in all cases. Liver histology improved in 5 but remained stable in the other 4. Improvement consisted mainly of decreased portal inflammation and bile duct injury; while there was no significant change in the degree of fibrosis or duct destruction. No hepatotoxicity from the methotrexate was observed. When therapy was reduced or discontinued, as occurred with 2 cases because of thrombocytopenia or leukopenia, liver function test abnormalities recurred. These encouraging preliminary results must be confirmed by prospective and randomized trials, and the potential toxicity of this drug will have to be taken into account in assessing its utility in PBC.

Anti-inflammatory drugs

Colchicine

Colchicine, an anti-inflammatory and antifibrotic drug, has been evaluated for therapeutic effects in PBC in at least three trials (20, 21, 22). In one study (20) involving 30 treated patients (15 with early and 15 with histologically advanced disease) and 30 untreated controls, colchicine appeared to decrease mortality from liver disease after four years; it also improved serum levels of bilirubin, albumin, alkaline phosphatase, transaminases and cholesterol after two years, to a similar extent in both of the treated groups. No improvement in histology, symptoms, or physical findings were noted and, except for diarrhea, there were no side-effects. The two other (21, 22) trials also showed favorable effects on survival and laboratory findings. In conclusion, treatment of PBC with colchicine appears to be associated with improvement in hepatic biochemistry and a trend toward improved survival; these features and the low incidence of toxicity make this drug suitable for long-term use.

Anticholestatic drugs

Ursodeoxycholic acid

Ursodeoxycholic acid (UDCA), the 7β epimer of chenodeoxycholic acid, is a tertiary bile acid found in trace amounts in human bile; it is the most hydrophilic and least detergent bile acid among those occurring naturally (23). UDCA was initially used only for treating cholesterol gallstone disease, but Leuschner observed (24) that UDCA given for gallstones in patients with liver disease significantly improved liver function tests. Parenchymal damage in cholestatic liver disease is thought to be due, at least in part, to intrahepatic retention and accumulation of toxic bile acids (25). Several mechanisms have been proposed to explain UDCA's efficacy in chronic liver disease: 1) enrichment of the circulating bile acid pool with UDCA through decreased intestinal absorption of more toxic endogenous bile acids by competitive inhibition (26); 2) the ability of UDCA to protect membranes by modifying their fluidity and stability (27); 3) an immunomodulatory effect through reduction of aberrant expression of major histocompatibility complex antigens on hepatocytes (28), modulation of interleukin production (29), reduction of circulating T-lymphocytes or reduction of circulating IgM levels (30). Numerous studies have confirmed that UDCA improves the results of several liver function tests in PBC (31, 32); moreover, since it is non-toxic and well tolerated, it is also suitable for long-term use. However, controlled investigations have failed to demonstrate a clear beneficial effect of UDCA on the symptoms, liver histology or clinical progression of this disease. Of the nine major randomized controlled trials, a positive effect of UDCA on pruritus was reported only in three (31, 33, 34) and, of the five reporting its influence on fatigue, a favorable effect was established in only one (33). At present there is also limited documentation of a beneficial effect of UDCA on liver histology. Poupon et al (35), in a study carried out on 95 patients who had undergone two years of treatment with UDCA, reported improvement in portal inflammation, bile duct proliferation, and piecemeal necrosis; perhaps more importantly, however, they were unable to demonstrate any effect on fibrosis or fibrogenesis. Although Leuschner (36) and Turner (32) both reported improvement in liver histology, statistical significance was not achieved; in 1991, Hadziyannis (33) observed no differences in histology with this drug. In 1994, Poupon (37), Lindor (38) and Heathcote (39) published the results of their studies, each of which involved about 200 patients followed for at least two years: one reported favorable effects on histology (39), in one the authors did not observe any differences (38), and in one this aspect was not evaluated (37). In these three studies the effect of UDCA on end-points such as death, time to transplantation, histological progression of at least 2 stages, development of varices, ascites or encephalopathy and doubling of bilirubin levels were also assessed: when controls were compared with the UDCA treated patients, statistical significance was reached only for the doubling of bilirubin levels. In Poupon's study (37), mortality and the need for liver transplantation were decreased in the treated patients relative to those who had been given a placebo, and the authors concluded that these findings indicated a definite trend towards slowed progression of the disease; these findings, however, were not confirmed by the other two studies (38, 39). These results indicate that, while UDCA does positively influence some important prognostic indicators for PBC, e.g. bilirubin, for others, such as mortality and the need for transplantation, the results are contradictory. In conclusion, many trials indicate that UDCA improves biochemical parameters in nearly all patients with PBC, and that it is safe and well-tolerated, even with long-term use. There is little conclusive evidence that UDCA ameliorates symptoms or slows progression of the disease, although there may be a beneficial effect of UDCA on liver histology. Considering the overall benefit/risk ratio, UDCA is currently the most attractive therapeutic option for PBC; the need remains, however, for more effective treatment.

Other drugs

Penicillamine

Penicillamine is a cupreretic drug with known efficacy in Wilson's disease. Because PBC is associated with increased hepatic accumulation of copper, the major rationale for trying this drug was its presumed ability to reduce hepatic levels of copper in PBC as well. Despite encouraging preliminary results, final evaluation (40, 41, 42) has shown that penicillamine (250-1000 mg q.d.) has no effect on survival, histological progression of the disease, or improvement in any of the prognostically important laboratory tests; moreover, use of the drug was also found to be associated with a high incidence of serious side-effects. The reason for the lack of a beneficial effect of penicillamine in PBC may be that liver copper is not localised in the same organelles as in Wilson's disease (43).

Combination Therapy

Although a number of drugs have shown some efficacy in the treatment of PBC, major effects on the ultimate course of the disease have not been demonstrated. In an attempt to improve the effectiveness of currently available drugs, newer treatment strategies are focusing on using them in combination, in particular, UDCA with an immunosuppressor or anti-inflammatory agent.

Kaplan studied the effects of UDCA and methotrexate in combination on 14 patients with PBC (44) and found more improvement in symptoms, serum alkaline phosphatase and bilirubin than occurred with either drug alone, with no evidence of methotrexate toxicity. In another study by Buscher (45) on 8 patients, the addition of methotrexate to UDCA improved symptoms and hepatic biochemistry; transaminases increased during the first months of treatment, after which they gradually improved, but albumin and cholinesterase did not change. Contrasting results were reported in an abstract published in 1994 by Lindor (46) in a study involving 32 patients treated with UDCA and methotrexate, this author observed that biochemical changes, histological findings and symptoms were comparable to those of patients receiving UDCA alone; moreover, 7 patients were withdrawn beacuse of pulmonary toxicity or oral ulcers.

The effect of combined treatment with UDCA and prednisone was retrospectively evaluated by Wolfhagen et al (47) in 7 patients. After starting combined treatment, 5 patients became asymptomatic and in all 7 both serum alkaline phosphatase and AST decreased. These preliminary results suggest that the addition of low dose immunosuppressive treatment may enhance the effect of UDCA alone.

The combination of UDCA with colchicine has also been investigated. In 1992 Raedsch (48) performed a randomized controlled study in 22 PBC patients. All were pretreated with UDCA alone for 12 months, and then randomized to UDCA + placebo or to UDCA + colchicine (1 mg q.d.). No effect on symptoms, liver function tests or histology was observed with the addition of colchicine. However, several abstracts published in 1994 on the use of this combination in PBC reported some positive results: Poupon (37 patients with a follow up of two years) (49), Goddard (57 patients with 15 months mean follow up) (50) and the Italian PBC study group (90 patients with a follow up of three years) (51) found that, while symptoms and laboratory findings were unchanged, there appeared to be some evidence that progression of the disease was slowed. The authors concluded that this combination may have a beneficial effect in PBC and that, since it was well-tolerated by all patients, long term use is feasible.

CONCLUSIONS

Despite some favorable results, treatment of PBC with current drug regimens is unsatisfactory, especially as regards slowing the progression of the disease. Improvements have been observed mainly in liver function tests and, in general, best results are obtained when PBC is treated in its early phases. While some past studies (52) have reported normal life-expectancies in asymptomatic PBC patients, later papers (53) have demonstrated that some of these patients will eventually develop symptoms and have shortened lifespans. These findings indicate that treatment of PBC should be initiated as early as possible in order to obtain the best therapeutic response.
At present, given its efficacy and safety, UDCA is the most promising agent for the treatment of PBC. Encouraging results are also coming from studies investigating the combination of immunosuppressor or anti-inflammatory drugs with UDCA.

The authors wish to thank Miss Janice Capan for her assistance in preparing the text of this article.

References

1) Kaplan MM. Primary biliary cirrhosis. N Engl J Med 1987; 316:521-528.
2) Ballardini G, Bianchi FB, Doniach D et al. Aberrant expression of HLA-DR antigens on bile duct epitelium in primary biliary cirrhosis: relevance to pathogenesis. Lancet 1984;ii: 1009-13.
3) Sprengler U, Pape GR, Hoffmann RM et al. Differential expression of MHC class II subregion products on bile duct epithelial cells and hepatocytes in patients with primary biliary cirrhosis. Hepatology 1988; 8: 459-62.
4) Beukers R. Schalm S.W. Immunosupressive therapy for primary biliary cirrhosis J Hepatol 1992; 14: 1-6.
5) HC Mitchison, Bassendine MF, Archie JM et al. A pilot, double-blind, controlled 1-year trial of prednisolone treatment in primary biliary cirrhosis: hepatic improvement but greater bone loss. Hepatology 1989; 10;4;420-429.
6) Mitchison HC, Palmer JM, Bassendine MF·et al. A controlled trial of prendnisolone treatment in primary biliary cirrhosis. J Hepat 1992; 15: 336-344.
7) Sambrook Pn, Eisman Ja Yeates MG et al. Osteoporosis in rheumatoid arthritis: safety of low-dose corticosteroids. Ann Rheum Dis 1986;45 950-3.
8) Dykman TR, Gluck OS, Murphy WA et al. Evalution of factors associated with glucocorticoid-induced osteopenia in patients with rheumatic disease. Arthritis Rheum 1985;28:361-367.
9) Reid IR, Alexander CJ, King Ar et al. Prevention of steroid-inducet osteoporosis with (3-amino-1-hydroxypropylidene)-bisphosphonate APD). Lancet 1988; i:143-6.

10) Heathcote J, Christensen E, Smith M et al. A prospective controlled trial of azathioprine in primary biliary cirrhosis. Gastroenterology 1976; 70: 656-660.
11) Crowe J, Christensen E, Smith M et al. Azathioprine in primary biliary cirrhosis: a preliminary report of an internetional trial. Gastroenterology 1980; 78: 1005-1010.
12) Christensen E, Neuberger J, Crowe J et al. Benefical effect of azathioprine and prediction of prognosis in primary biliary cirrhosis. Gastroenterology 1985; 89: 1084-91.
13) Minuk GY, Bohme CE, Burgess E et al. Pilot study of cyclosporin A in patients with symptomatic primary biliary cirrhosis. Gastroenterology 1988; 95: 1356-63.
14) Wiesner RH, Ludwig J, Lindor KD, et al A. controlled trial of cyclosporine in the treatment of primary biliary cirrhosis. N Engl J Med 1990; 322:1419-24.
15) Lombard M, Portmann B, Neuberger J, et al. Cyclosporin A treatment in Primary Biliary Cirrhosis: Results of a long-term placebo controlled trial. Gastroenterology 1993;104:519-526.
16) Palestine AG, Austine III HA, Balow JE et al. Renal histopathologic alterations in patients treated with cyclosporine for uveitis. N Engl J Med 1986; 314:1293-8.
17) Kahan BD. Cyclosporine. N Engl J Med 1989;321:1725-38.
18) Hoofnagle JH, David GL, Scafer DF et al. Randomized trial of chlorambucil for primary biliary cirrhosis. Gastroenterology 1986; 91:1327-34.
19) Kaplan MM, Knox TA. Treatment of primary biliary cirrhosis with low-dose weekly methotrexate. Gastroenterology 1991; 101:1332-1338.
20) Kaplan MM, Alling DW, Zimmerman HJ, et al. A prospective trial of colchicine for primary biliary cirrhosis. N Engl J Med 1986; 315;1448-1454.
21) Warnes TW, Smith A, Lee F et al. A controlled trial of colchicine in primary biliary cirrhosis. Hepatology 1984; 4:1022 (abs).
22) Bodenheimer H, Schaffner F, and Pezzullo J. Evaluation of colchicine therapy in primary biliary cirrhosis. Gastroenterology 1988;95:1:124-129.
23) Matschiner JT. Naturally occurring bile acids and alcohols and their origins. In: Krichevsky D, Nair PP, eds. The bile acids. New York: Plenum Press, 1971:11-46.
24) Leuschner U, Leuschener M, Sieratzki J et al. Gallstone dissolution with ursodeoxycholic acid in patients with cronic active hepatitis and two year follow up: a pilot study. Dig Dis Sci 1985;30: 642-9.
25) King JE, Schoenfild LJ. Lithocholic acid, cholestasis and liver disease. Mayo Clin Proc 1972;47:725-30.
26) Stiel A, Raedsch R, Rudolph G. Acute effects of ursodeoxicholic and chenodeoxycholic acid on the small intestinal absorption of bile acids. Gastroenterology 1990; 98: 424-8.
27) Goldutuna S, Zimmer G, Imhof M et al. Molecular aspects of membrane stabilization by ursodeoxycholate. Gastroenterology 1993; 104:1736-44.
28) Calmus Y, Gane P, Rouger P, et al. Hepatic expression of class I and class II major histocompatibility complex molecules in primary biliary cirrhosis. Hepatology 1990; 11: 12-5
29) Yoshikawa M, Tsujii T, Matsumara K et al. Immunomodulatory effects of ursodeoxicholic acid on immune responses. Hepatology 1992:16:358-64.
30) Lacaille F, Paradis K. The immunosuppressive effect of ursodeoxicholic acid: a comparative in vitro study on human peripheral blood mononuclear cells. Hepatology 1993;18:165-72.
31) Hwang SJ, Chan CY, Lee SD, et al. Ursodeoxicholic acid in the treatment of primary biliary cirrhosis: a short-term, randomized double-blind controlled, cross-over study with long term follow up. J Gastroenterol Hepatol.1993;8:217-23

32) Turner IB Myszor M, Mitchison HC et al. A two year trial examining the effectiveness of ursodeoxycholic acid in primary biliary cirrosis. J Gastroenterol Hepatol. 1994;9:162-8.
33) Hadziyannis SJ, Hadziyannis ES, Lianidou E et al . Long-term treatment of primary biliary cirrosis with ursodeoxycolic acid: the third year of a controlled trial. In: Paumgartner G, Stiel A, Gerok W, editors. Bile acids as therapeutic a gents. Dordrecht: Kluwer; 4, 1991:287-96.
34) Lindor KD, Baldus WP, Jorghensen RA et al. Ursodeoxycholic acid is beneficial therapy for patients with primary biliary cirrhosis. Hepatology 1992;16:91A(abs).
35) Poupon RE, Balkau B, Eshwège E et al. A multicenter, controlled trial of ursodiol for the treatment of primary biliary cirrhosis. N Engl J Med. 1991; 324:1548-54.
36) Leuschner U, Fischer H, Kurtz W et al. Ursodeoxicolic acid in primary biliary cirrhosis: results of a controlled double-blind trial. Gastroenterology. 1989;97:1268-74.
37) RE Poupon, R Poupon, B Balkau, et al. Ursodiol for the long-term treatment of primary biliary cirrhosis. N Engl J Med 1994; 330:1342-1347.
38) Lindor KD, Dickson ER, Baldus WP, et al. Ursodeoxycholic acid in the treatment of primary biliary cirrhosis. Gastroenterology 1994; 106: 1284-1290.
39) Heathcote EJ, Cauch-Duder K, Walke V, et al. The Canadian multicenter double-blind randomized controlled trial of ursodeoxicholic acid in primary biliary cirrhosis. Hepatology 1994;19:1149-1156.
40) Dickson ER, Fleming TR, Wiesner RH et al. Trial of penicillamine in advanced primary biliary cirrhosis. N Engl J Med 1983; 308:1-7.
41) James OFW. D-penicillamine for primary biliary cirrhosis. Gut 1985; 26: 109-13.
42) Neuberger J, Christensen E, Portmann B et al. Double blind controlled trial of d-penicellamine in patients with primary biliary cirrhosis. Gut 1985;26 :109-13
43) Epstein O, Arborgh B, Sagiv M, et al. Is copper hepatotoxic in primary biliary cirrhosis? J Clin Pathol 1981: 34:1071-5.
44) Kaplan MM. The therapeutic effects of ursodiol and methotrexate are additive and well tolerated in primary biliary cirrhosis. Hepatology (Abs).
45) Buscher H.P., Zietzschmann Y and Gerok W. Positive responses to methotrexate and ursodeoxycholic acid in patients with primary biliary cirrhosis responding insufficiently to ursodeoxicholic acid alone. J Hepatol 1993; 18; 9-14
46) Lindor KD, Jorgensen RA, Anderson ML et al. The combination of ursodeoxicholic acid (UDCA) and methotrexate (MTX) for patients with primary biliary cirrhosis (PBC): the results of a pilot study. Hepatology 1994;20:4 421 (abs).
47) Wolfhagen FHJ, Van Buuren HR, Schalm SW. Combined treatment with ursodeoxycholic acid and prednisone in primary biliary cirrhosis. Neth J Med. 1994;44:84-90.
48) Raedsch R, Stiel A, Rudi J et al. Combined urso plus colchicine treatment in primary biliary cirrhosis: efficacy, pharmacology and urso-colchicine interactions. Proceedings of the XII internetional Falk bile acid meeting, Basel 1992:48-9.
49) Poupon RE, Niard AM, Huet JP et al. A randomized trial comparing the combination ursodeoxycholic acid (UDCA) and colchicine to UDCA alone in primary biliary cirrhosis. Hepatology 1994;20:4 217(abs).
50) Goddard CJR, Hunt A, Smith A et al. A trial of ursodeoxycholic acid (UDCA) and colchicine in primary biliary cirrhosis (PBC). Hepatology 1994;20:4:218 (abs).
51) Almasio P, Provenzano G, Battezzati PM et al. The italian multi-centre randomized controlled trial of ursodeoxycholic acid vs ursodeoxycholic acid plus colchicine in symptomatic primary biliary cirrhosis. Hepatology 1994;20:4:683 (abs).

52) Beswick DR, Klatskin G and Boyer JL. Asymptomatic primary biliary cirrhosis: a progress report on long term follow-up and natural history. Gastroenterology 1985;89:267-71.
53) Balasubramaniam K, Grambsch PM, Wiesner RH et al. Diminished survival in asymptomatic primary biliary cirrhosis. Gastroenterology 1990;98: 1567-1571.

INDEX

P. Gentilini and M. U. Dianzani. New Trends in Hepatology, 327-336

MIX
Papier aus verantwortungsvollen Quellen
Paper from responsible sources
FSC® C105338

If you have any concerns about our products,
you can contact us on
ProductSafety@springernature.com

In case Publisher is established outside the EU,
the EU authorized representative is:
Springer Nature Customer Service Center GmbH
Europaplatz 3, 69115 Heidelberg, Germany

Printed by Libri Plureos GmbH
in Hamburg, Germany